Received On:

SEP 16 2019

Ballard Branch

NO LONGER PROPERTY OF
SEATTLE PUBLIC LIBRARY

D0044547

THE

STRENUOUS
LIFE

ALSO BY RYAN SWANSON

When Baseball Went White: Reconstruction,
Reconciliation, and Dreams of a National Pastime

THE

STRENUOUS
LIFE

Theodore Roosevelt and the
Making of the American Athlete

RYAN SWANSON

DIVERSION
BOOKS

To Carter, Tyler, and Kate who—yes—at times make life seem a little bit too strenuous, but are the source of more joy, pride, and insight than they will ever realize.

To Jackson, since he actually watched me (tennis ball at the ready) write most of this book.

And to Rachael, of course. There's nothing without you.

Copyright © 2019 by Ryan Swanson

All rights reserved, including the right to reproduce this book or portions thereof in any form whatsoever.

For more information, email info@diversionbooks.com

Diversion Books
A division of Diversion Publishing Corp.
443 Park Avenue South, suite 1004
New York, NY 10016
www.diversionbooks.com

Book design by Aubrey Khan, Neuwirth & Associates

First Diversion Books edition August 2019
Hardcover ISBN: 978-1-63576-612-7
eBook ISBN: 978-1-63576-611-0

Printed in The United States of America

1 3 5 7 9 10 8 6 4 2

Library of Congress cataloging-in-publication data is available on file.

CONTENTS

INTRODUCTION

"This is the White House. The president would like to have you to play tennis this afternoon at 4, if you are free."

Years later, Lawrence Murray still remembered the thrill of receiving this call. Of course he was free; Murray had recently been appointed assistant secretary of the Department of Commerce and Labor. He was new in town, or at least newly back in town. He also happened to be a decent tennis player. So, suspecting nothing other than some important face time with the president of the United States, Murray showed up at the appointed time and place. But first, he shopped for the occasion. Thus Murray, "a round young man with a pleasant laugh and a calm manner," looked downright resplendent when he arrived, sporting a brand new, white, "spick and span" tennis getup.

President Theodore Roosevelt, in contrast, wore a brown "army shirt," thick, well-worn khaki knickers, and black boots. This was the official uniform of "the Strenuous Life," the athletic crusade for which Roosevelt had become so well known. Roosevelt greeted Murray warmly. Rounding out the playing group were Director of Forestry Gifford Pinchot and Secretary of the Interior James Garfield.

Right away, things went poorly for Murray. Feeling a bit overwhelmed, he prayed silently that he would not be paired with the commander in chief. Too much pressure there. He did not want to bear responsibility for a presidential loss—even if it was only on the tennis court. But when the four men tossed their rackets in the air to select teams, Murray's and Roosevelt's landed facing the same direction. Partners.

"I did not know the president at all then, and to find myself his partner in tennis, when I had not had a racket in my hand for months, while he was in good practice, and so were the others," Murray remembered, "was a little upsetting to say the least."

The reality here is a timeless one: the nervous, subordinate employee paired with the overly competitive, gung ho, and somewhat-skilled boss. The sport could well have been golf or ping-pong (all the rage during the first decade of the twentieth century) or badminton. Workplace anxiety was Murray's primary opponent for the day.

Play commenced. Despite his nerves, Murray managed to bat a few balls in the right direction. Things were going OK. At least he avoided pulling an Archie Butt—an invited bureaucrat who actually hit the president with a tennis ball. So that was good.

Murray had his hands full on the court. Garfield and Pinchot both played splendidly. Roosevelt, on the other hand, played with...well...great enthusiasm. "Somehow his racquet seemed too short, and the little, tantalizing ball too small," reported the *Washington Post* of the president's game on a rare occasion the press was allowed to observe a White House match. Roosevelt had the bad habit of drifting into no man's land as his partner served. "The President stands too close to the net for so stationary a player as he is. Ball after ball goes by him." Thus the partner—Murray in this case—raced around trying to pick up the slack. "The other fellow in the back court, chasing from side to side, does all the work," the *Post* explained, summing up the Team Roosevelt tennis experience.

The whole group was sweating profusely. President Roosevelt had outfitted his White House tennis court (installed in 1903, replacing several of William McKinley's greenhouses) with a twenty-foot-high canvas fence. The canvas worked perfectly in terms of privacy, but it also created an airless womb of athletic activity. Only a few games in, Murray had serious doubts about his ability to survive due to the stifling environment. "This barrier of canvas," Murray lamented, "kept out every breath of air, so on a hot afternoon when the mercury stood around ninety in the shade, and with a seven set tennis match ahead of us, it required much of the vigor of life not to wilt completely." Roosevelt, for his part, considered the heat to be a benefit in his long-standing quest to keep his weight under control.

Fortunately for Murray, a summer thunderstorm intervened before too long. The group ducked into the president's office as the skies opened up. The White House tennis court was attached directly to the Executive Mansion. The play-to-politics proximity had actually been one of the first things that Murray noticed upon entering the White House grounds. The president could, basically, step "from his office door on to the court."

So close was the court to the office, in fact, that a White House bay window could be opened at midcourt, allowing the president's secretary, William Loeb, to interrupt at any time. When an important telegram buzzed in, Loeb would lean out, practically over the net, and alert the president. The president then would attend to political matters—trust-busting, empire building, Progressive reforms, or whatever—while his partners waited. Decisions rendered, play resumed.

Certain benefits came to those who played with the president, these members of what would become known as TR's "Tennis Cabinet." To take up a racquet at the White House meant access to information and opportunity. A quick entry into James Garfield's personal diary communicated how this blend of the casual and significant sometimes happened. December 1, 1906: "Tennis with the President...Afterwards which the President showed us a telegram he just received notifying him that the Norwegian Parliament had awarded him the great Noble Peace Prize."

Murray rejoiced at a reprieve by rain. He had been saved. However, visions of handshakes and drinks were summarily dashed. With rain pummeling the District, the president pivoted quickly. He had a new, adventurous plan. "To my utter amazement Roosevelt said: 'Just the day and time for a long walk and run. We will go!'"

Murray panicked. He was dressed in tennis whites. As the president tossed his racket in a corner and headed for the door, Murray observed that Garfield and Pinchot, who also "wore the lightest tennis shoes, sleeveless shirts and white flannel trousers" seemed strangely resigned to the turn of events.

They headed out. For Murray, they might as well have been stomping into the Amazon rainforest. He was aghast at the thought of leaving the landscaped White House grounds. "Within a few roads of the White House was then a marsh, or rather an almost impenetrable jungle of weeds, marsh grasses, cane brakes covering a soft black muck," Murray recalled. Into the slop they went. Roosevelt, not completely inconsiderate of his newcomer's plight, offered a quick bit of advice: "Tie your shoes on extra tight, or the muck will pull them off."

The foursome sloshed its way through thick underbrush and across a small creek. Roosevelt could not get enough, comparing the relatively tame mud and mild conditions of Washington, DC to the brutal conditions he had confronted on a recent hunting trip to Louisiana. While the president beamed and bounded, Murray pouted. "I could not get much amusement out of such a mess." Murray also fell back quickly, "losing time here and there as the black sticky muck pulled off first one shoe and then the other."

The group crossed into the Old Dominion and plowed ahead. Just when poor Lawrence thought he couldn't take any more, Roosevelt announced that it was time to pick up the pace. The group, Roosevelt estimated, had to cover about four miles to return to the White House. "We will now run every step of the way back!" announced the middle-aged, stocky leader of the group.

At this point, Murray needed no further convincing: Roosevelt was crazy. "If at first I had my doubts of his sanity, I was now firmly, finally, and totally convinced. I was already tired out getting through the jungle, we were all completely covered in mud, the rain was still falling in torrents and four miles yet to go and on the run."

Roosevelt, Pinchot, and Garfield trotted away at a steady pace, ambling back toward the White House, keeping up a lively conversation along the way. Murray was left for dead. "After about a mile I was in agony...I was entirely out of condition, having had no exercise like that for years. After another mile between walking and running, I stopped, but the others never looked back, so

I saw them disappear while I was utterly unable, if my life depended on it, to barely move."

Lawrence Murray did not perish in the wilds of northern Virginia. Upon reaching the White House and realizing just then (or so they said) that Murray had failed to keep up, Pinchot and Garfield reversed course to recover their fallen comrade. They found him a mile back. "One took one arm, the other another, and hustled me along to the hotel." Murray, disheveled and dirty beyond what any politician could have rightfully expected from a tennis date at the White House, insisted on sneaking back into his hotel through the basement. He would hide his shame. Once in the safety of his room, Murray stripped off his clothes. In defeat, he threw away his muddy, torn tennis attire.

Murray later found out that Garfield and Pinchot indeed knew what was coming. The two men had been on Roosevelt's impromptu jaunts before—across all manner of terrain, in violent weather, and always with their boss, the president, annoyingly declaring how wonderful it was to be out in nature. "Bully!" this and "Deeelightful!" that. More than being mentally prepared, Garfield and Pinchot actually trained to keep up with the president. They advised Murray to "get into good physical condition as quickly as possible." They even recommended an athletic trainer for the task, one whom Murray had hired within twenty-four hours of his muddy embarrassment.

After all, Murray—like all Americans—had to keep up with his president.

* * *

This is a book that began because of a question, one asked in both scholarly settings and on the sidelines of youth sporting events: How did we get this way? In terms of sports and athletics, that is. This first question then, as initial questions often do, splintered in all sorts of directions. Why does the United States, unlike most civilized countries, comingle education and athletics? What's the deal with the Army–Navy football game? Has the United States always dominated the Olympic Games medal count? Is baseball (or football or basketball—it's obviously not soccer or hockey) really America's "national pastime?"

Mostly we don't ask. Most Americans *just do* sports—from Little League to Super Bowl parties—simply because it's the red-blooded American way.

The search for answers to the above questions led, eventually, to the first decade of the twentieth century. And the search zeroed in on one US presidential administration. During the time Theodore Roosevelt occupied the White House, modern sports emerged in America. In essence, the period was a super-collider. Sports banged around in a pressurized drum at speeds and volumes previously deemed impossible. Out of the pressurized period came a labyrinth of infrastructure, tradition, and sporting norms. An American athletic paradigm emerged. It is the same athletic paradigm, to a significant extent, that still reigns today.

Thus muddy and shoeless Lawrence Murray was a casualty of a revolution he did not even know was happening. During the administration of Theodore Roosevelt, or the Strenuous Era as we might as well call it, the landscape of American sports changed dramatically—at the White House and beyond. This book will tell the tale of that change. From 1901 to 1909, the sports precedents piled one upon another. Here are just a few:

In baseball, the American and National Leagues worked out a monopolistic merger. Begrudgingly (and somewhat surprisingly), the rival circuits agreed to stop poaching players from each other. Out of this agreement came the first World Series in 1903.

On university campuses, football's popularity boomed. The game, however, was exceedingly violent. So much so, that the number of football casualties sparked outrage. With abolition efforts swirling, including one at a school close to Roosevelt's own heart, the National Collegiate Athletic Association (NCAA) emerged in 1906 as a means of regulating intercollegiate sports.

In 1904, as Roosevelt faced a presidential election, the United States hosted its first Olympic Games. To make matters more interesting (and shed some insight on baseball's Cardinals-Cubs rivalry), St. Louis stole the Games from Chicago at the last minute. St. Louis then turned the Games into a months-long celebration of American conquest.

Also during this Strenuous Era, Jack Johnson worked his way toward becoming America's first African American heavyweight boxing champion.

Johnson defeated all comers in the ring but could not get a title fight for years. Finally, during Roosevelt's last days in the White House, Johnson got his shot. The possibility of a black heavyweight champion of the world called into question many of the racist norms of the athletic paradigm in place.

Perhaps most fundamentally, leaders of the New York City public schools system created the first organized athletic league for American elementary, middle, and high school students—the Public Schools Athletic League (PSAL). The PSAL courted TR, and it considered how to serve both boys and girls. Thus a juxtaposition that we take for granted today—that of the "student athlete"—had its start here. From its epicenter in NYC during the Strenuous Era, interscholastic sports boomed across the country.

Roosevelt deserves a lion's share of the credit, or blame (depending on one's opinion of sports in America), for the rise of modern sports. Sure, Progressive reforms, Social Darwinist fears, and an international muscular Christianity movement, among other factors, fueled this sports revolution. Changes had been decades in the making. And strangely, Roosevelt did not even like baseball. But Roosevelt occupied the presidency of the United States during this critical era. As president, Roosevelt participated in, commented on, and theorized about athletics more than any other US president, before or after. What's more, Roosevelt's articulation of "The Strenuous Life" translated for many Americans these broad societal changes into personal marching orders.

Making his role even more significant, Roosevelt was on his own fascinating athletic odyssey at the same time—one that reporters chronicled in a fanatical fashion. The athletic quest had begun when TR took up, as a child, his father's challenge to defeat a life-threatening medical condition. "Theodore, you have the mind, but you do not have the body," father challenged son. "Without the help of the body the mind cannot go as far as it should. You must *make* your body." Roosevelt boxed at Harvard and built a wrestling room in the New York governor's mansion. He micromanaged his children's sports pursuits, always concerned that they develop where he had struggled. He received fighting lessons in the White House. The final stop on Roosevelt's athletic journey was a two-week visit to Jack Cooper's Health Farm in 1917. There Roosevelt jogged and jiggled, strained and stretched. He pushed himself to a point of joyful exhaustion. Even at fifty-eight years old, Roosevelt was still in training for something. Perhaps it's this image of Roosevelt-the-aging-jogger that resonates closest to home for modern Americans.

Roosevelt's America was a place ripe for athletic development. Industrialization and urbanization, now unleashed for three decades, had changed the way that Americans lived and worked. Cities were dirty, crowded places. Corporations in some communities seemed more powerful than the state. Factory work, while dangerous, was boring, and it stole from men and women the physical and emotional benefits that agricultural work had given most Americans half a century before. Doctors began seeing more cases of neurasthenia, a rather amorphous condition that often included: "headaches, backaches, worry, hypochondria, melancholia, digestive irregularities, nervous exhaustion, and 'irritable weakness.'" Basically, Americans seemed to have every sign of economic progress and technological development in their midst, but instead of flourishing they were falling apart.

The Progressive reformers of this era worked to fix all manner of problems. The general belief was that society no longer worked; the nation's (and states' and cities') institutions needed to be rebuilt given the "increasingly urban, industrial, and ethnically diverse society" of the United States at the turn of the century. The Progressives were nothing if not ambitious. They targeted political corruption, overcrowding, unfair monetary policy, drunkenness, illiteracy, corporate greed, and a basic lack of hygiene, just to name a few.

The solutions for Progressives varied as much as their causes. They chased political, social, and spiritual answers. But the Progressives often ended up settling for new regulations, increased training, rigid hierarchies, and deliberate organization. In this reform context, sports emerged as one avenue for development and betterment in a rapidly changing world. Or as one scholar explained it, sports became "a strategy for regeneration and renewal."

If America faced uncertainty domestically, the international scene offered its own anxieties. "New immigrants," mostly from southern and eastern Europe, migrated to the United States by the millions—between 1890 and 1920 about eighteen million arrived. This caused no small amount of unrest, both for those arriving and those already in America. The pecking order of nations in Europe was in flux, leaving the United States scrambling for allies. As a result, the theories of Charles Darwin (and more specifically Herbert Spencer) seemed particularly relevant. It was a "Survival of the Fittest" world. In what place would the United States settle as a new century dawned? Sports—with their physicality and competitive framework—applied because they could be lumped into efforts to create a stronger, healthier citizenry. When it came to athletics in this context, most Americans did not actually assume that the Olympic Games, for example, would somehow directly secure their nation's place in the world, but it certainly could not hurt to be the nation with the most gold medals.

To be clear, this book is *both* an athletic biography of Theodore Roosevelt *and* an accounting of a period of significant change in American society. These two storylines overlap, compliment, and occasionally just stand, like two people in a line waiting for coffee, adjacent to each other. Roosevelt's boxing in the White House, for example, is butted up against the rise of the NCAA. The fact that these two happenings share a similar chronological anchor point does not necessarily mean that there is a causal relationship between the two phenomena. But there might be. We'll see. The hope is that the weaving together of these two narrative threads (Roosevelt's athletic biography and America's sport revolution) will yield a rich understanding of how sports in America came to develop as they did.

The Strenuous Life focuses primarily on Roosevelt's time in the White House. The connection between Roosevelt's personal athletic experience and the nation's broader development, however, is grounded in more than just chronology. Roosevelt used his "bully pulpit" to translate his own ideas about the significance of athletics into broader initiatives and reforms. And perhaps most fundamentally, Roosevelt told stories of athletic engagement—especially his own. When Roosevelt played tennis or boxed or tramped through Rock Creek Park the American public usually learned about it in rather short order. After time with "a real trainer of men," one New York newspaper observed,

"[Roosevelt] comes back refreshed and tells people about it with a smile." Roosevelt made himself an example and a case study and a warning to his fellow citizens.

Alice Roosevelt once famously said of her father: "[He] always wanted to be the corpse at every funeral, the bride at every wedding and the baby at every christening." Yes, Roosevelt knew how to be the center of attention. He had a near endless supply of energy and ideas. There was no topic on which he demurred. And his opinions—they never ran out. In fact, it was as if a pair of opinion-producing rabbits lived deep within Roosevelt's core, always reproducing. So, of course Roosevelt had something to say about athletics in America. He had something to say about everything! But there's more to it than that. As his daughter might have said had she considered the matter further, Theodore Roosevelt most certainly wished that he could have been the fighter at every championship bout. He would have relished being the quarterback at every big game. But it never happened. As Roosevelt admitted, "I have always felt that I might serve as an object lesson as to the benefit of good hard bodily exercise to the ordinary man. *I never was a champion at anything.*" Still, he kept striving right to the end. That was the Strenuous Life. And through the struggle, Roosevelt ended up shaping the very athletic world that he could never quite conquer himself.

ONE

HIT THE LINE HARD

In life, as in a football game, the principle to follow is:
Hit the line hard: don't foul and don't shirk, but hit the line hard.
—THEODORE ROOSEVELT

Forget pageantry or decorum, the real question was this: Was it even safe for the president of the United States to attend the Army–Navy football game? Sure, some Philadelphians worried about making their city look good when Theodore Roosevelt arrived. Others argued over where Roosevelt would sit ("It required a conference of the Cabinet yesterday to decide the matter."). Still others, including Mayor Sam Ashbridge, jockeyed to get some face time with Roosevelt. But given the state of the nation in 1901, the logistics of getting the president in and out of Franklin Field safely had to trump everything else.

The task of coordinating the security detail fell to Philadelphia Police Superintendent Harry M. Quirk. It was an unenviable position. Already Quirk was hanging by a thread; speculation regarding his removal from command of the police department had been splashed across the pages of the city's *Inquirer* and *Times* in the weeks leading up to the big game. To add to the chaos, a smallpox outbreak forced Quirk to quarantine one of his Philadelphia police stations. There were also reports that game tickets sent to dignitaries had been stolen from the mail and were "being sold promiscuously" by scalpers. Now the commander in chief, accompanied by the "heavy guns" of the cabinet, was rolling into town. And strangely, the White House had neglected to inform Quirk of exactly when and where the president of the United States would arrive in his city. "Guards were kept guessing," the *Philadelphia Inquirer* reported.*

Quirk became a battlefront general, deploying his men based on some combination of intel and intuition. He supposed that Roosevelt would arrive in his city for the November 30 Army–Navy football game at the South Street Station, this despite rumors suggesting that the presidential party would disembark at the city's towering Broad Street Station. But that was all Quirk had—a guess. Reporters watched the uncertainty manifest itself: "Consultation after consultation was held between the police, Secret Service men and railroad officials." Given the anarchy that had erupted during the previous months in the United States, most significantly the assassination of President William McKinley a mere seventy-eight days earlier, this lack of specificity and security protocol seemed like a critical mistake.

Kickoff was scheduled for 2:00 p.m. Presumably, the president would arrive sometime before then. Of course, if TR and his entourage lagged a bit behind schedule, if the president decided to, say, stop in Wilmington, Delaware, to survey the country's busiest shipbuilding yard (Roosevelt was "a die-hard navalist" after all), then the kickoff would be pushed back. Hedging his bets, Superintendent Quirk set up command at the South Street Station at noon. He also sent men to secure the station at Thirty-Seventh Street, and another squad sprinted off to the Spruce Street terminal—just in case. The US Secret Service, which still lacked official congressional approval to guard the president, provided scattered support. The whole city of Philadelphia waited in a

---

* It seems that Roosevelt's personal secretary, George Cortelyou, had in fact sent word to Col. George W. Swett of the Hotel Walton (the headquarters for the Army team) of the White House party's plan to arrive at Broad Street Station and move "as quietly as possible" to Franklin Field. See *Philadelphia Inquirer,* November 30, 1901. Swett apparently did not communicate these plans to Quirk or the police force, which was probably just as well because the train did not actually stop at Broad Street anyhow. Protocol for presidential travel was evolving by the day at this point.

state of high alert, anxious to receive the president somewhere and sometime. "Never in modern times," the *Philadelphia Inquirer* reported diplomatically, "did a President travel to an official event more unostentatiously."

Fortunately, Quirk guessed right. President Roosevelt, not yet three months into his stint in the White House, arrived—aboard the personal Pullman car of the president of the Pennsylvania Railroad—at 1:02 p.m. The conductor held the three-car train just short of Philadelphia's South Street Station as Quirk's men canvassed the area one last time. Then the train, which "bore no outward distinctive marks," pulled in. Family and friends filled TR's car. Most importantly, wife Edith, daughter Ethel, and son Kermit had also made the trip. So too had Roosevelt's sister and brother-in-law. For a voracious socializer like Roosevelt, such confined closeness during the three-hour trip was invigorating.

The train stopped. Porters served a quick lunch. Eating done, Roosevelt flipped "two shining half eagles" to the conductor and engineer, tipping them for providing safe passage. Out of the train spilled one important person after another: Secretary of War Elihu Root, Secretary of the Navy John Long, Postmaster General Charles Smith, and Attorney General Philander Knox. Most were accompanied by their wives. Roosevelt got off last. Then the race to the field commenced.

The Middies and the Cadets were going to war (at least the gridiron sort of war), and Roosevelt could hardly wait. Just a week prior, Roosevelt's avalanche of work kept him from traveling north to witness his alma mater, Harvard University, win a "smashing triumph" over Yale. Roosevelt was a football parent, a football evangelist, and a football fan all at the same time; he did not plan to miss any of this Army–Navy contest.

Pushing off so suddenly that he caused an "audible gasp" from his onlookers, Roosevelt bolted from the car stoop and set out for the stadium.

This was typical Roosevelt. While Roosevelt preached many, many doctrines over the course of his political career, he returned to a simple but transformative focus time and time again: action. To an undoubtedly overwhelmed advisee Roosevelt had once offered, "Get action, do things; be sane, don't fritter away your time; create, act, take a place wherever you are and be somebody:

get action." Roosevelt had, well, a sense of urgency about him. "We will walk," Roosevelt said, already jog-walking. He dismissed the nearby carriages; such conveniences were for the women and children. Dressed in a gray overcoat, striped trousers, a low collar shirt, a "black four-in-hand necktie," and a dark silk hat, TR strode forward at a disruptive clip. How could the president be protected if he refused to wait for his security detail? Fortunately, there wasn't far to go; the South Street Station nearly butted up against the party's destination, Franklin Field. The venue sat on the outskirts of the University of Pennsylvania's campus.

Security was everywhere. Precautions mandated closures and barricades in all directions. Trains were stopped miles down the tracks. Philadelphia police cut off traffic to the station, roped off a nearby pedestrian bridge, and formed "two solid lines of Quaker blue coats" to provide the presidential entourage unimpeded access to the stadium.

Luckily, the weather had cooperated for the president's visit. The city had received its first snowfall of the year the day before, but the precipitation had dried up. It was the type of day that makes football fans feel emboldened and vigorous, even as they do nothing but sit and watch. It's exercising by osmosis, and this Saturday was a perfect day for it. The sun shone brightly. "There was just enough frost in the air to keep the blood tingling," the *Philadelphia Times* reported. Blankets and wraps were deployed. Flags and streamers rolled and flapped in the breeze. A perfect day for football.

Probably the only one sad about the whole situation was young Kermit, TR's second-oldest son. The twelve-year-old made the trip to Philadelphia, but then for vague security reasons had been left to wait out the game aboard the train.

There was a pervasive skittishness hanging over the country. What tragedy might happen next? Anarchists had assassinated Empress Elisabeth of Austria in 1898 and King Umberto of Italy in 1900. An election dispute led to the murder of Kentucky Governor William Goebel on January 30, 1900. Then on September 6, 1901, Leon Czolgosz, a terrorist bent on defending "the good working people" of America, had shot William McKinley twice at point-blank range as the president glad-handed his way through a receiving line at the

Pan-American Exposition in Buffalo, New York. After a ghastly week-long struggle, President McKinley died from infection on September 14, 1901. Thus the United States, for the third time in fifty years (the third time in some Americans' lives!), lost a president to assassination. Within weeks, Congress was debating fourteen separate bills meant to secure protection for the president.

As McKinley's vice president, Roosevelt took over the presidency. "Oh God. Now that damned cowboy is President of the United States," New York Senator Thomas Platt (like Roosevelt, a member of the Republican Party) famously unloaded upon hearing of McKinley's death and Roosevelt's promotion.

The Philadelphia that Roosevelt visited for the first time as president was a city being jabbed and poked by grimy, lucrative industrial growth. The nation's third-largest city, Philadelphia neither had the high commerce of New York, the self-important philosophical bent of Boston, nor the political power of Washington, DC. But Philadelphia was just what it was: a sprawling nexus point for coal and steel, and a city dominated by its railroad junctions and streetcar networks. Philadelphia's workers put in far more than eight hours a day and then made their homes in racially clustered neighborhoods. At the turn of the century, Irish immigrants made up about a third of the city's 1.3 million residents. African Americans, just beginning to move to northern cities in large numbers as a part of the Great Migration, were increasingly taking up residence in the City of Brotherly Love as well.

The nation's newspapers, from coast to coast, blared the news of the president of the United States attending a football game across their front pages. "For the first time in the history of American athletics," the *Baltimore Sun* reported, "the White House was deserted because of a football game." McKinley had never made such a vigorous outing. He preferred to spend his leisure time sitting in a rocker, smoking cigars, playing cards.

Philadelphia's two leading papers, the *Times* and *Inquirer,* devoted more than a dozen pages, all of it aggressively optimistic, to the presidential visit. "The foremost spectator of the fray was the Commander in Chief of the army and the navy, President Theodore Roosevelt, and with him were the most distinguished men of the nation." Then the waxing began. "In the background was massed the beauty, the fashion and the wealth of the great Eastern cities. Under the rays of the November sun the flash of color was dazzling."

Franklin Field sported four very large but simple sections of bleachers. Wood, not cement, carried the day here. The seating along the sidelines went up twenty-five rows. The end zone bleachers were slightly shorter. No press boxes, no seatbacks, not even any handrails softened the venue; it was a sit-and-be-glad-you're-not-standing situation. Two H-style goal posts book-ended the field of play. High fences guarded the facility, partitioning off the athletic space from the streets and urbanity that surrounded it. And the Philadelphia vista in the background was one of smoke, chemicals, and steel. The fan sitting in an upper row seat could gaze upon at least a dozen smokestacks spewing forth exhaust. Machinery, chutes, factories, refuse piles—these were Franklin Field's neighbors.

Dozens of people, most concerned with security, scrambled to be a part of the presidential cluster as it careened toward the stadium. Philadelphia detectives Murray, McKenty, Gallagher, and Sell, disguised (half-heartedly) with ushers' badges, formed a ring around the president. The military academy leaders—Colonel Albert Leopold Mills of West Point and Commander Richard Wainwright of the Naval Academy—took up the James and John positions at the immediate right and left of TR. Both had served heroically during the Spanish-American War. The secretaries of the Army, Navy, and Interior and the postmaster general jogged to keep up. University of Pennsylvania Provost Charles Harrison, a prodigious fundraiser who was remaking Penn into an academic powerhouse, tagged along at the rear of the pack, barely keeping contact.

Roosevelt skipped up a few stairs and traversed a muddy embankment. Then, with lines of policemen holding back the swelling crowds, Roosevelt, trotting now, headed through Franklin Field's southeast gate.

Roosevelt's energy was palpable. Here was the man who would set a Guinness Record for shaking hands with 8,150 people in one day. Roosevelt regularly drank a gallon of coffee a day, using a coffee cup that was, according to his son Ted, "more in the nature of a bathtub." Certainly on this crisp Pennsylvania day, TR radiated positivity and action. He bounded, and pontificated, and gestured wildly—all at once, it seemed. His countrymen, having recently lost a president, pushed forward for a peek. Even the policemen, "stalwart fellows" as they were, resplendent in their "new brass buttons and white gloves" had a difficult time staying focused. They could not pull off anything close to a Buckingham Palace reserve. And what did Roosevelt leave in his wake? Smiles. "Philadelphia's finest, selected for the task, stood stately and silent" as long as they could. But once Roosevelt had passed, their decorum cracked. "As the President passed them each face broke into a smile, and remarks, such as: 'He's the real thing, is Teddy,' ran up and down the line."

The military bands knew their role, but they missed their cue because of the pace of the presidential party. One can hardly hoist a tuba without at least a few seconds of warning. The now rolling Roosevelt was well inside the gate, nearly on the field, before the military bands could strike up "Hail to the Chief." The instrumentalists scrambled to catch up. Roosevelt emerged onto the field. He strode a few yards forward and then paused at the east end goal post. Recognizing the significance of the moment, most of the security detail peeled off. And there Roosevelt stood alone for a few seconds—the former asthmatic invalid and barely competitive athlete—emerging onto an epic athletic scene.

The contemplation lasted just a couple of moments. Refocused, Roosevelt pushed off across the gridiron and then, at midfield, made an abrupt turn toward the Navy sidelines. The 25,000 fans roared. No one could hear anything but adulation. The "deafening cheer" voided the last strains of "Hail to the Chief."

Roosevelt reached the stands, ascended a few rows, and took his position in a reserved seating box. The police and Secret Service positioned themselves around the president in all directions. Roosevelt had his own impenetrable offensive line.

With Roosevelt and his accompanying dignitaries properly appreciated and seated, and with the temperature nearly at its high for the day, forty-four degrees, the game kicked off.

TR cheered both sides, favoring the rough tackle and hard hit above all else. Roosevelt was a boxer, after all. Physical contact satiated the president. Roosevelt unleashed a steady torrent of analysis and appreciation to those within earshot. He used all the football jargon of the day, plus some of his own making.

"Go it man!"

"It's a daisy tackle."

"Wasn't that tackle a sockdolager?"

Roosevelt, ever intent on being helpful and in charge, yelled instructions and chastised mistakes. He declared one player a "buster" and the next a "smasher."

The sheer enthusiasm of the president's display titillated the press within earshot. What kind of president was this? One *Philadelphia Times* reporter, who basically watched Roosevelt watching the game, simply declared Roosevelt "The Man." "More electric than [Daniel] Webster's singing and [John] Adams' digging was the honest enthusiasm of our young President. It was the emotional impulse of the lover of true sport," the paper said. Mrs. Roosevelt, Edith, looked on at her husband with bemusement. She knew this man. The two were approaching their fifteenth wedding anniversary and had been friends since childhood. She tried a few times to get her husband, the president of the United States after all, to keep it down. But she didn't try too hard; there was no quieting TR in such a space as this.

*   *   *

Early twentieth-century football was trench warfare, favoring defensive strategy and field position above all else. The game fit perfectly with an increasingly militarizing nation. Scoring was rare. The field was bigger, the ball rounder, and punting game much more important than in today's football. Banish any thoughts of a high arching Tom Brady spiral settling into Rob Gronkowski's tightly gloved hands forty yards down the field—that's twenty-first-century football. The early twentieth-century game featured barely moving masses of tangled humanity with a ball rattling around somewhere in the mix. The sport was melded to America's universities; no significant professional football teams emerged in the United States until the 1940s. The opening sequences of the 1901 Army–Navy game demonstrate this very different version of football.

After losing the coin toss, and watching as Navy elected to start on defense, Army fielded the kickoff to start the contest. Army then immediately *chose* to punt the ball back to Navy on first down. So Navy received the ball back and ran a few plays, advancing to their own forty-two-yard line. Then Navy punted. Army star Charles Daly received the ball at his own thirty and was immediately tackled. Offensive futility followed. The West Point men failed to get anything moving; they punted the ball back to Navy. Here, Navy actually made up some ground. Army's feeble punt had traveled only to midfield. Maybe there was a chance to break the stalemate?

Not really. Navy subsequently moved the ball only five yards. Then a holding penalty cost the Midshipmen. Army was awarded the ball.

At this point, midway through the first quarter, Army had the ball, first down, near the center of the field. So what did they do? Placing a premium on field position, Army punted. Again, on first down. Thus, Navy received the hot potato back, this time starting on its own thirty-five-yard line. Good sense once again prevailed; the Navy team, without running a single play meant to advance the ball, punted possession back to Army. It was a punting parade at this point.

Mercifully, finally, Army began to move the ball a bit. Daly fielded a Navy punt and weaved his way back to midfield. Then, orchestrating a straight-ahead attack, Daly and Army advanced well into Navy's territory, all the way to the twenty-eight-yard line. Some action! But alas, the drive stalled, and Army turned over the ball on downs. Navy took possession back, relatively deep in its own territory, and (you guessed it) immediately punted the ball back to Army.

College football had started in the United States in 1869. On a cold day in New Jersey, Rutgers University hosted Princeton College (officially the College of New Jersey at the time, now Princeton University). Rutgers's 6–4 victory on November 6 is recognized by scholars (who are always seduced by chronological benchmarks) as America's inaugural intercollegiate football contest. Tailgating, the Rose Bowl, the College Football Playoffs, Joe Paterno, the Heisman Trophy, cheerleaders, and Nick Saban—the starting point was here. Chalk one up (or cast another vote of blame) for New Jersey. Of course, the creation story is hardly that definitive. American football had really evolved over the course of decades, primarily pulling its players and rules from soccer and rugby. Football's playing standards remained malleable well into the twentieth century.

College football historians Ron Smith and John Watterson point to two rule decisions in particular as vital to making American football its own unique, violent game—one fitting for the men of Army and Navy. First, during the 1870s, a series of rules were adopted that allowed blocking, or "interference with those attempting to tackle the runner." Such interference was, and is, distinctly forbidden in rugby and soccer. The acceptance of this interference not only created new tactical opportunities (the forward pass would ultimately result from it) but it also made football much more dangerous. Collisions now occurred all over the field. No one could hide. As a result of blocking, equipment and padding also became more important. Players needed protection from their hard-hitting opponents, who might come from any direction.

A second change during the 1870s was even more vital in making American football its own brand of sport. The creation of the line of scrimmage revolutionized the game. The manner in which football players line up, neatly and orderly, before each return to action is unique in the world of sports. The ability to retain possession of the ball "marked the great gridiron divide that led American football down the opposite slope from the British rugby." Certainly basketball and soccer, with their constantly ebbing mix of offense and defense, have nothing remotely like a line of scrimmage. Neither does hockey. Baseball has somewhat stilted rules of engagement—the pitcher holds the ball, waits for the batter to enter his designated box, makes sure that his catcher is ready and his defense correctly positioned, and then finally pitches to the batter—but with none of football's violence, save for the occasional beanball or bench-clearing brawl. The roots of football's scrimmage, like much of the game, can be traced back to rugby. In rugby, the scrum, or "scrummage," starts and restarts control of the ball. But the scrummage was still marked by movement; football's line of scrimmage was a much more regimented beginning to each play.

The question of why the leaders of early football picked the rule changes that they did is one of the side arguments that can derail a whole afternoon at a sports history conference (and yes, sports history conferences are a real thing). We won't spend much time on it here. But one interesting theory is that football became more regimented and controllable at this time because of the changes in America's business culture happening at the same time. Efficiency expert Frederick Taylor's "Scientific Management" ruled the 1890s and emphasized that through training and optimal movements businesses could maximize their profits. With football's start and stop rules in place, a football coach could employ similar strategies on the field.

As football evolved, the line of scrimmage became the game's most sacrosanct concept. More than the violence, or the field, or the ball, or the number of players, it's football's stop and start orchestration that most distinctly sets it apart. When "mass momentum" plays—like the "flying wedge" which involved players getting a running start before the snap of the ball and then crushing a predestined target across the line after the play started—resulted in rising injuries tolls, the answer was even further control of the line of scrimmage. So in the 1890s, rules were adopted which expressly limited who could be in motion before the snap of the ball and to what extent. *Stop and be still before you lunge violently at each other,* the rules basically said. Changes in rules to tackling (in 1887 below the waist tackles became legal), the forward pass, and scoring ensued throughout the late nineteenth and early twentieth centuries, so that when Roosevelt arrived at the 1901 Army–Navy football game, he was taking a seat at a highly orchestrated and complicated sport that fit just right for an increasingly industrialized and militarized nation.*

---

* The Canadian Football League (CFL) emerges as an interesting point of comparison here. While the basics of the games are the same (although the CFL allows one more player on the field and has a slightly larger field) on both sides of the border, the CFL has much more liberal pre-snap motion rules. Basically, the CFL is not quite so pharisaical about the line of scrimmage as its American counterparts. Unlike in American college football and the National Football League (NFL), any CFL non-lineman can move, in any direction, before the play begins. Thus wide receivers in the CFL can get a running start and then time the snap of the ball. In contrast, the NFL allows only one player to be in motion before the snap, and that player cannot be moving toward the line of scrimmage. The NFL player can basically move back and forth across his team's formation, but he can't build up a head of steam before the play begins.

It was the late George Carlin, the prolific comedian—not some historian—who most memorably explained the long-standing connection between American football and America's military.

In football the object is for the quarterback, also known as the field general, to be on target with his aerial assault, riddling the defense by hitting his receivers with deadly accuracy in spite of the blitz, even if he has to use the shotgun. With short bullet passes and long bombs, he marches his troops into enemy territory, balancing this aerial assault with a sustained ground attack that punches holes in the forward wall of the enemy's defensive line.

Indeed, even beyond the verbiage, the military and football go together in the United States like country music and pickup truck sales. There's a codependency at work. The available database of football-to-military metaphors, comparisons, and connections is too vast to fully mine. But for the sake of perspective, consider three of the most enduring juxtapositions. First, as Carlin points out, football is a warlike struggle for the control of territory. Protect yours; invade theirs. The militarized rhetoric of football plays—sweeps, shifts, long bombs—emphasizes this commonality. The points awarded in football generally go to the team that has dominated control of the field. Wars have a similar emphasis on geography.

Second, Americans tend to believe, even if they don't outright say so, that football prepares men for military combat, or at the very least for robust citizenship. Men weren't men at the dawn of the twentieth century, not compared to previous generations. Fewer Americans worked on farms, and more entered into white collar, middle management each year. Thus, football served to protect the nation from an increasingly effeminate and soft citizenry. This theory of football as training for life became gospel during the Roosevelt era. Indeed, Roosevelt himself pushed such narratives constantly. "In life, as in a football game," Roosevelt wrote, "Hit the line hard; don't foul and don't shirk, but hit the line hard!"

Third, football games functioned, and continue to function, as venues for patriotic, militaristic displays. Soldiers, anthems, and flags showed up nearly from the start at American football games. While the fighter jet flyovers had to wait until the technology caught up with the sentiment, the military has always been much more than a welcome guest at the gridiron.

In this context, the development of the Army–Navy football game makes perfect sense. One might wonder, in fact, why it didn't happen earlier. The Naval Academy began training America's sailors in 1845. George Bancroft became secretary of the Navy that year, and finding his men woefully undertrained and comically undisciplined, he commandeered Fort Severn in Annapolis, Maryland, for a naval school. The Navy had a lot of catching up to do. The United States Military Academy—West Point—is almost as old as the United States itself. In 1801, Thomas Jefferson—hardly a warrior, but concerned about the safety of the United States nonetheless—directed that the nation begin training members of its army. Both the Naval Academy and West Point (and the Air Force Academy later on for that matter) emphasized physical training alongside academics.

Football came to the service academies in, basically, the same manner as other universities. The men could only do so many pushups and run so many training loops. Cloistered from girls and pushed relentlessly on all fronts, the soldiers-in-training needed an outlet—"more wholesome outlets." Slowly at first, the men of Army and Navy took to the gridiron. In 1879, Navy played its first game. The 0–0 tie versus the Baltimore Athletic Club, described by Baltimore's *New-American* as a spectacle of "living, kicking, scrambling masses of humanity chasing the ball to and fro," only whetted the Middies' appetite for the game. The Naval cadets developed a rivalry with nearby Johns Hopkins. Certainly the Naval Academy posed little threat to the football powerhouses in the Ivy League, but the game grew steadily in the military academy world.

Army lagged behind on the football front. During the 1870s and '80s, the football games at West Point remained mostly unorganized affairs. Only when football became a mechanism by which Army men could compare themselves to their Navy counterparts did the game really take off at West Point. Accord-

ing to Army historian Gene Schoor, Army cadet Dennis Mahan Michie basically goaded his institution into taking up competitive football. Michie had
learned the game as a child growing up in West Point. In 1890, frustrated that
his classmates did not take the game seriously, Michie arranged for an acquaintance at Annapolis to send a challenge to West Point: The two schools should
have a game. Michie seized on the planted message and took the matter from
there. The son of an influential Army professor, Michie pushed the challenge
up the ranks at West Point. Certainly the men of Army could not let this Navy
probe go unchecked, could they? The catch, though, was that the Army, while
certainly familiar with football, had never actually fielded an organized squad.
Michie assured the higher ups that this was not a problem. Nothing to worry
about; he would coach and captain the team himself. What could go wrong?
Thus, on November 29, 1890, on the Plains of West Point, the first Army–
Navy football contest took place. Navy romped to a 24–0 victory.

"It was a battle royal," the *New York Times* reported. "The onlookers stood
around the ropes of the West Point ball field Saturday, and, when the game
grew hot, openly demanded that the players should inflict all kinds of punishment on their adversaries."

A tradition had been established. The first game had been "an exhibition of
pluck and grit that promises well for the future," the *Times* concluded.

*　*　*

Probably very few of the players and spectators at the 1901 game were aware
of the history of the Army–Navy matchup, including the fact that the contest
had been shut down by military leadership for a few years in the mid-1890s.
Most cared only about the game at hand. Navy entered the 1901 matchup with
a record of six wins, three losses, and one tie; Army stood at 4–1–2. Could
Army avenge its close loss (11–7) of the prior year?

The first half dragged along in a back and forth, stunted manner. The teams
traded halted drives and punts. The Navy punter, Charles Belknap, enjoyed a
steady breeze at his back, which helped him drive Army deep toward its own
goal line time and time again. Finally, though, Army broke through. Captain

Adam Casad took a handoff, picked his way carefully through the left side of the offensive line, and then burst through the other side. A fifty-yard scamper followed, ended only by a diving tackle ("flinging himself on the heels of the runner") by Navy's F.B. Freyer. But then the stalemate resumed. Blocked from the end zone on three successive plays, Army elected to try a dropkick from the twenty-yard line. Charles Daly, who had already played four years of intercollegiate football at Harvard before enrolling at West Point, "put the ball beautifully over the goal posts" giving the West Point men a 5–0 lead.

Yes, 5–0. In 1901, football's rules awarded teams five points for drop-kicking the ball through the goal posts. The same five points resulted for scoring a touchdown. An additional point was awarded for successfully kicking the ball through the uprights following a touchdown. Further stupefying to today's football's viewers would be the fact that Army received the ball back after scoring its five-point goal. It was make it, take it.

The Navy defense, perhaps chastened by Army's score, held fast and got the ball back for its offense. The gridlock finally eased at this point for the Midshipmen too; Navy returned Daly's fifty-yard punt...well...fifty yards, placing the ball right back where it started, at the twenty-five-yard line.

At this point Roosevelt couldn't hold back any longer. Ignoring the phalanx of security personnel surrounding his position in the stands, and for that matter the pressures of his office and the pallor of McKinley's assassination, the president of the United States jumped up from his seat. Down the steps and toward the field went the man tasked with guiding the United States into the twentieth century. Roosevelt pommel-horsed a barrier separating the crowd from the players and let out a yell. Roosevelt then attacked the unsuspecting Navy football players on their own sideline with enthusiastic claps on the back. In his excitement, Roosevelt hugged one Navy scrub and gave another "a poke in the ribs that he probably remembered after supper, but for which he was none the less proud and happy." The president had closed in on the action.

With Roosevelt on the sidelines, Navy sent a series of plunges through the line, pushing their cause deeper into Army's territory. Finally, the ball rested a mere two feet from the end zone. The stadium pulsated with expectation. Navyman Newton Nichols took the snap, hesitated for a moment, and then "galloped over the center for a touchdown." The Navy stands went berserk. Roosevelt, for his part, whirled around toward the Navy fans, lifted his hands in triumph, and "grinned with such hearty approval that every tooth in his mouth was exposed." It was the full, signature Roosevelt smile.

Navy missed the point after. The teams ended the first half tied 5–5.

What a strange scene. Making sense of Roosevelt the sideline hugger, and the reaction of the crowd to their new president, deserves some pause. On the one hand, these were just fans doing things that fans typically do at football games. And Roosevelt was simply acting with characteristic enthusiasm and gusto. But the coming together of young and virile Roosevelt, with the football squads made up of future sailors and soldiers, and the citizens of a nation still considering what it meant to lose another president to an assassination, made for a unique moment. The *St. Louis Post-Dispatch* started its extensive coverage (nearly five pages worth) of the Army–Navy game with Roosevelt's run onto the field. Here hope and excitement seemed to override the tensions the nation had been experiencing. This was the first scene that readers needed to see in their minds' eye.

> **Special to the *Post-Dispatch*. PHILADELPHIA, Pa., Nov. 30 —**
> Theodore Roosevelt, the President of the United States leaped a fence today while 25,000 persons cheered until they could not see straight. It was not much of a fence, a boy could have cleared it, but it was the motive back of the act that made the hit with the crowd.

The reporter grasped that someone not present at the scene would protest this act being the lead story. "It was not much of a fence," but then again it was. Roosevelt broke the rule that all sports fans know as a fundamental one: Stay off the field!

The army and navy were battling for supremacy on the football field of old Penn...when the strenuous young man who is the chief of both of these great arms of the government found a fence an obstruction to his better view of the contest, he leaped it...It was too much for 'Teddy' Roosevelt. He was no longer the dignified guider of a great nation's fortunes. He was a robust exuberant boy again and with a yell that was distinguishable above the pandemonium there he sprang from his seat, leaped the fence in front of him and was on the sidelines...'Teddy' was a boy again and he was happy. It was a great day for the President.

A great day for the president? It was a great day to be an American!

* * *

Theodore Roosevelt had connections to both the US Army and Navy, and to the Army–Navy game itself. As assistant secretary of the Navy, Roosevelt helped reinstitute the contest. The rivalry game had been canceled from 1894 to 1898. The reason for the cancelation, basically, was that the game became too raucous. It compromised the very institutions it meant to benefit. At the 1893 contest, there was nearly a duel when a scuffle between a Navy rear admiral and an Army brigadier general got out of hand. Following the '93 contest (won by Navy 6–4), President Grover Cleveland shut down the still relatively new tradition.

Roosevelt, however, believed that the virtues of the game outweighed its flaws. And what was a little dueling among military leaders anyhow? So on August 17, 1897, Roosevelt penned a letter to the secretary of war, Russell A. Alger, urging for the resumption of the Army–Navy football game. At the time, Roosevelt had been assistant secretary for less than four months.

My Dear General Alger: For what I am about to write you I think I should have the backing of my fellow-Harvard man, your son. I should like very much to revive the football games between Annapolis and West Point. I think the Superintendent of Annapolis, and I dare say Colonel Ernst, the Superintendent of West Point, will feel a little shaky because undoubtedly formerly the academic routine was cast to the winds when it came to these matches, and a good deal of disorganization followed. But it seems to me that if we would let Colonel Ernst and Captain Cooper come to an agreement that the match should be played just as either eleven plays outside teams, that no cadet should be permitted to enter or join the training table if he was unsatisfactory in any study or conduct and should be removed if during the season he becomes unsatisfactory, if they were marked without regard to their places on the team, if no drills, exercises or recitations were omitted to give opportunities for football practice, and if the authorities of both institutions agreed to take measure to prevent any excesses such as betting and the like, and to prevent any manifestations of an improper character—if as I say all this were done—and it certainly could be done without difficulty—then I don't see why it would not be a good thing to have a game this year. If you think favorably of the idea, will you be willing to write Colonel Ernst about it?

Here Roosevelt's optimism shone through glaringly. The game resumed in 1899. How much credit Roosevelt deserves for this resumption is debatable. Though he was never one to shy away from claiming an accomplishment, Roosevelt failed to mention the triumph himself in his voluminous writings.

Roosevelt's military service shaped his view of football, and nearly everything else. Before his White House turn, TR had a short but distinguished military stint. This story is well churned over—but still important in terms of understanding Roosevelt's militaristic take on athletics. When the USS *Battleship Maine* exploded on February 15, 1898 in Havana, Cuba's, harbor, Roosevelt immediately declared the blow a direct and purposeful attack on the well-being of the United States. "A number of peace-at-any-price men," Roosevelt said, "of course promptly assumed the position that she had blown herself up; but investigation showed that the explosion was from the outside." The road to war between the United States and Spain, in Cuba, had been paved.

Approaching the official onset of middle age (his fortieth birthday), Roosevelt refused to sit out the conflict in Cuba. He received a commission as second-in-command (serving under his close friend Leonard Wood) in the First US Voluntary Cavalry. He became the public face of the unit. "Teddy's Terrors," "Teddy's Cowboy Contingent," "Teddy's Riotous Rounders." The nicknames were tried out as newspapers quickly focused in on Roosevelt as one of the more interesting subplots in the escalating conflict. One nickname in particular stuck: The Rough Riders. More than 23,000 applications poured in from around the country, submitted by men, many of them bloodthirsty for any sort of fight, anxious to serve in TR's unit. Roosevelt combed through the applications and selected a thousand individuals. There were two basic proto-types Roosevelt favored in choosing his fighting force. First, he wanted men— "tall, and sinewy, with resolute, weather-beaten faces"—from America's southwest territories. And second, Roosevelt wanted college athletes. "Proba-bly no regiment contained so many men well known in the athletic world as the First Volunteer US Cavalry," noted one journalist, who headlined his arti-cle directly: MEN OF MUSCLE ARE MEN OF COURAGE. The Rough Riders included Bob Wrenn, four-time winner of the tennis US Championship, and Dudley Dean, Harvard's All-American quarterback. The unit also had cham-pion rowers, half-milers, high jumpers, polo players, sprinters, and too many football players to list.

Roosevelt and his men arrived in Cuba on June 21, 1898. There the Rough Riders picked their way through the thick underbrush, trying to locate and support regiments already in place. Spanish snipers killed seven Rough Riders on the unit's first day on the island. Hamilton Fish, previously the captain of Columbia University crew team, was the first Rough Rider to die. Roosevelt barely noticed. "Roosevelt, literally jumping up and down with excitement... made no effort to run for cover; somehow the bullets missed him."

When General Wood was transferred to take over the second Brigade, the Rough Riders became Roosevelt's responsibility. "To my intense delight," Roo-sevelt recalled, "I got my regiment." On the morning of July first, Roosevelt and the Rough Riders advanced toward Santiago. The temperature soared above one hundred degrees. The distance wasn't far—only a mile and half— but the geography made coordinated movements a ridiculous prospect. A dense forest separated the US troops from the San Juan Hills. A single, ten-foot-wide road cut through the trees. Unfortunately, the road had become a muddy quagmire due to a series of thunderstorms. The Americans' plan called for moving 16,000 troops through the narrow passageway, toward Spain's entrenched guns. Not surprisingly, the relationship between volume and space did its deadly work. As the Rough Riders reached the end of the road, they confronted a gruesome pileup, a "Bloody Ford," created by the wholescale emergence of men, away from the protection of the forest, into the face of the enemy's weaponry.

With nowhere else to go, TR pushed his men forward, over bodies and through the chaos, to the base of the hills as quickly as possible. There Roosevelt and his men laid prostrate for several hours as Spanish sharpshooters used the Americans for target practice. Finally, word came that Roosevelt could advance to support the ongoing, badly flagging assault on San Juan Hill. Charge! Roosevelt's men surged forward, intermixing with other units already at work. For Roosevelt, the rush of battle took over. His "crowded hour" had arrived. Colonel Roosevelt pushed his men forward until they met a confused captain who was stuck midway up the hill. No one had given the final order for an all-out assault, this captain equivocated. "Then I am the ranking officer here," Roosevelt roared. "And I give the order to charge." Still nothing. Refusing to stall another second, Roosevelt simply ordered his Rough Riders to go around and through the more timid unit.

Bullets whizzed by, artillery fire rang out, and Roosevelt's glasses fogged up. Roosevelt kept pushing forward, upward. Then they were there. Roosevelt, "resplendent in a uniform custom-made by the Brooks Brothers," and the Rough Riders stood atop Kettle Hill. The men caught their breath. Then Roosevelt ordered another charge, this time up San Juan Hill, the height most immediately protecting Santiago. By nightfall, the Americans controlled the elevation. Santiago was within the grasp of American army. A siege began. The war was effectively won.

Roosevelt came home a hero. As the regiment decamped on Long Island to wait for official mustering out, the spoils of war spilled forth. Roosevelt's name appeared daily on the front pages of American newspapers throughout the summer of 1898. The rank and file got something out of it too: LONG ISLAND WOMEN WORSHIP ROOSEVELT'S REGIMENT, reported one daily. While tactlessly referred to as "A Splendid Little War," as if blood had not been shed and bones had not been shattered, eighty-nine Rough Riders, every bit a gallant as their colonel, died in the July 1–3 assault on Santiago. Hundreds of Americans, up to 1,071 according to one source, perished in the battle for San Juan Hill. Among the fallen was a twenty-eight-year-old West Point graduate, a former football player: Dennis Michie. Michie, "the Father of Army Football," died at the Bloody Ford. West Point named its football stadium in his honor.

*   *   *

"Football coaches love to equate themselves with military leaders and talk about battles in the trenches and going to war," sportswriter John Feinstein wrote in his book about the football struggle between Annapolis and West Point. "At Army and Navy, the players understand the difference between football and war."

As recently as 2004, the Army–Navy game remained a dead heat. After Navy trounced Army 42–13 in the 2004 contest, the series stood tied at forty-seven wins each, plus seven ties. Navy, flourishing under the leadership of option experts Paul Johnson and Ken Niumatalolo, won the next eleven contests, often trouncing Army. The vast majority of these games had taken place in Philadelphia. Franklin Field hosted the football men of Annapolis and West Point through 1935. Philadelphia's Municipal Stadium hosted from 1936–1979; the city's Veterans Stadium (a utilitarian dump that "smelled like rotten meat") took over from 1980–2001. Then naming rights got involved. The Army–Navy game at Lincoln Financial Field commenced in 2002.

The Army–Navy game continues to matter. CBS televises the contest; the network owns the broadcast rights through 2028. For this privilege, CBS pays the two service academies (and thus the federal government, basically) nearly $10 million annually. Interestingly, the Army–Navy game has also conquered a Saturday at the tail end of the football season. No other Division I football games are played on Army–Navy Saturday, usually the second weekend in December. It's a football-military holiday of sorts.

In 2018, a 3–9 Navy team lost to Army (9–2) in front of 67,000 fans in Philadelphia. More than eight million viewers tuned in on television. President Donald Trump attended the contest with his secretary of defense, secretary of state, secretary of the Interior, and attorney general. Asked about the game, Trump said, "I just love the armed forces. Love the folks. The spirit is so incredible. I mean, I don't know if it's necessarily the best football. But boy, do they have spirit."

*   *   *

At halftime (back to the 1901 game), Roosevelt cut directly across Franklin Field. The temperature was dipping now, plunging into the thirties. No fewer than twenty-five men—basically the same group of security, military, and university leaders—accompanied the president as he switched sides. Roosevelt walked quickly, doffing his hat occasionally in response to the cheering crowd. TR then took a seat in Army stands. As commander in chief, he had to espouse neutrality. And since he had been both a Navy (assistant secretary) and Army (colonel of the Rough Riders) man within the past four years, the mixture of support was genuine for Roosevelt. "You know I am occupying a position of rigid impartiality," he explained to Secretary of State Elihu Root. "I am quite diplomatic because I shall divide myself between the Army and the Navy." Both sides were his. For their part, the cadets of West Point were glad to have the president. Seeing Roosevelt heading over, the Army band blared "Hail to the Chief" and the corps "wildly welcomed" TR to their side—the winning side, as it would turn out.

At 3:30 p.m., Navy kicked the ball off to Army, starting the second half. Charles Daly, "this Napoleon of football," fielded the ball cleanly at the ten-yard line and then "ran straight down the middle of the field." The sea parted. The Army blockers made Daly's task a simple one: just run—fast. "He took a straight course, without any deviation, and by the time he reached the center line both teams were behind him." They wouldn't catch the five-foot-seven, 150lb speedster. Daly raced across the goal line, having carried the ball 105 yards to score a touchdown. The stadium rocked. This time, the kick after touchdown was converted. Army seized an 11–5 lead. Only ten seconds had elapsed in the second half, only ten seconds with the president on their side, and the men of Army had scored a decisive blow for victory.

The second half was dragged out by injuries. The toll of eleven men pounding back and forth, urged on by 25,000 spectators, wore the college players down. "Time was being continually taken off for injuries to players of both teams." This came as no surprise; injuries were a fundamental part of the football experience. On the day after the 1901 Army–Navy game, the *Chicago Tribune* published its list of "THE DEAD" and "THE INJURED," a football casualty list if you will, for the 1901 season. "Football kills 8, Injures 75, during the season that has just ended," the *Tribune* reported. Fortunately, the men of Army and Navy avoided the worst of these maladies on the day that the president looked on.

As the game clock wound down, the substitutes on the Army sideline silently urged the referee to blow his whistle and call time. Then he did; it was over. The Army men rushed from the stands to celebrate. "The President was our mascot," Secretary of War Elihu Root rejoiced. "With the score tied, his coming over to the army side so encouraged the cadets that they went in to do or die." The Philadelphia police encircled Roosevelt and moved him toward the southeast exit of the field. The "boys in gray" had their celebration as the president headed back to his waiting train. The band played "I want to be a military man." The Army players and fans paraded around the field once, and then again carrying aloft a few of the victorious players.

"The President's stay in the city was short—four hours, perhaps—but during that period Theodore Roosevelt probably had a better time and was more like the 'impetuous Teddy' of younger days than at any period since he scrambled up San Juan Hill," boasted one Philadelphia writer. It was a nice thought. But the affairs of the nation were too unsettled to allow for such a reprieve. During Roosevelt's seventy-eight days in the White House, controversy and tumult had been constant. Inviting Booker T. Washington to dinner on October 16 caused a political firestorm. It was a meal that "shocked a nation."

Shrouding everything else, though, was the case of McKinley's assassin Leon Czolgosz. In a legal blitzkrieg, Czolgosz had been found guilty of first-degree murder on September 24—ten days from the criminal act to a conviction in a US court of law. Two days later, the presiding judge, who had rejected Czolgosz's desire to plead guilty, sentenced Czolgosz to death. On October 29, 1901, the punishment was carried out: three charges, 1800 volts each, were passed through Czolgosz's body. Thus, the nation dealt swiftly and harshly with its latest assassin.

But what came next? Was Roosevelt—a young, energetic, football crazed man—the president to stabilize the nation? And even if he was the right leader, did the United States possess the right type of citizenry to protect itself from the craziness of the twentieth century? It would come out in the following days that a would-be assassin had been stalking Roosevelt even as he attended the Army–Navy game. The "Philadelphian who wanted Mr. Roosevelt assassinated" was arrested shortly after Roosevelt left the city.

There were no easy answers to the question of how America should face a new century. Certainly a fall football game, on the very cold last day of November involving two teams of soldiers, did not guarantee anything. But the game was a start. Football was a start. Sports were a start. Right?

TWO

THE STRENUOUS (LIKE, REALLY STRENUOUS) LIFE

He has developed all his muscles by rigorous training and has expanded his chest till his capacious lungs are qualified to feed his blood with oxygen; and his vigorous heart sends that rich, vitalized fluid through his big neck into his active brain. And the result is what has come to be known as strenuosity.

—*The Many-Sided Roosevelt: An Anecdotal Biography*

In 1902, Theodore Roosevelt's first full year in the White House, US newspapers—from the *New York Times* to the *Winona* (Mississippi) *Democrat*—described the forty-four-year-old president of the United States as "strenuous" more than ten thousand times. Strenuous this, strenuous that; strenuous here, strenuous there. It was as if the journalists covering the new president received a commission—maybe quarters were dropped into Mason jars on their desks—each time they could jam the word "strenuous" into one of their stories.

Roosevelt, the nation would come to learn in 1902, was a man of "strenuous horsemanship and sportishness." He had a "strenuous speaking face." Roosevelt ate with a strenuous appetite, which was fitting for such a "great exponent of strenuosity." He wanted strenuous policies enacted and had a "strenuous attitude against trusts." Roosevelt forced his children, especially his "strenuous boys," to take on strenuous tasks. In July 1902, the Roosevelt family took a "strenuous holiday." The First Family was so strenuous, in fact, that the White House staff begged them to slow down. Finally, it got to the point where the *Houston Post* on September 2, 1902, cried uncle: "The public is sick of stories regarding Mr. Roosevelt's strenuous bravery." *Enough already*!

The root of the strenuous chatter is not all that difficult to find. It was a speech that Roosevelt made in Chicago in 1899—entitled, not surprisingly, "The Strenuous Life." The speech became the basis for Roosevelt's thirteenth book, *The Strenuous Life*, in 1900.* In 1902, with Roosevelt having ascended to the White House, the book was reissued to wide acclaim. Queen Alexandra of England bought a copy and urged her countrymen to read the work. Scott Joplin, one of America's most famous composers, penned a musical score (fittingly called "The Strenuous Life") to accompany the volume. *La Vie Intense*, the French translation of the work, also appeared in 1902, touting Roosevelt as "the virile champion of a nation which has become powerful in deciding the destinies of the world."

The three words, "the Strenuous Life" gave a name and a pleasantly malleable tagline to the athletic revolution underway in the United States. The phrase was perfect; it had just the right balance of ambiguity, transferability, and panache. It was suitably militaristic. It suggested a choice between a promising but difficult path and one of relative ease. One might compare it to Nike's trademarked "Just Do It." And as became the case with Phil Knight's sneaker slogan, Roosevelt's words ceased to be his own once he shared them. Original intentions morphed with a multitude of other causes, some of which were downright parasitic. Above all other claimants, however, the advocates for a more robust sports and athletic paradigm in the United States won control of "the Strenuous Life."

---

* Yes, thirteenth. His previous published works were: *The Naval War of 1812* (1882); *Hunting Trips of a Ranchman* (1885); *Thomas Hart Benton* (1887); *Gouverneur Morris* (1888); *Ranch Life and the Hunting Trail* (1888); *The Winning of the West* (1889–1896); *History of New York City* (1891); *The Wilderness Hunter* (1893); *Hero Tales from American History* (with Henry Cabot Lodge, 1895); *American Ideals and Other Essays* (1897); *The Rough Riders* (1899); *Life of Oliver Cromwell* (1900).

Roosevelt had first unveiled the phrase at Chicago's Hamilton Club. More than six hundred guests crowded the venue to hear Roosevelt give the "The Strenuous Life" speech on an unseasonably cold April 10, 1899. The speech marked Roosevelt's arrival as a player on the national political scene. "Seldom, if ever, in Chicago has a more enthusiastic body of men met around the banquet table than the one which met tonight under the auspices of the Hamilton Club," reported the Associated Press. When Roosevelt took the lectern, the room exploded in applause. "The hall was a mass of waving handkerchiefs and napkins, and the cheers that greeted him as he rose prevented the speaker for many minutes from beginning his speech." The din continued even as Roosevelt motioned for quiet.

The crowd, finally done with its long, noisy thank-you to their Rough Riding hero, settled in. Roosevelt took over. He spoke, in his distinctively nasally tenor, always gesturing and pointing and jabbing the air for emphasis, for thirty minutes.

"I WISH TO PREACH, NOT THE DOCTRINE OF IGNOBLE EASE, BUT THE DOCTRINE OF THE STRENUOUS LIFE, THE LIFE OF TOIL AND EFFORT AND STRIFE..." ROOSEVELT BEGAN.

The speech centered on foreign policy and on the future of the Monroe Doctrine. It tested out the tenets of the Roosevelt Corollary, which would be unveiled several years later. Would the United States police the Western Hemisphere? Would the turn-of-the-century generation meet its challenges? "If we are really a great people, we must strive in good faith to play a great part in the world." Roosevelt urged the United States to build up its military. The Army and Navy needed to be expanded and modernized. "Our army has never been built up as it should be built up. I shall not discuss with an audience like this the puerile suggestion that a nation of seventy million of freemen is in danger of losing its liberties from an existence of 100,000 men," Roosevelt said.

"IT IS HARD TO FAIL, BUT IT IS WORSE NEVER TO HAVE TRIED TO SUCCEED. IN THIS LIFE WE GET NOTHING SAVE BY EFFORT."

The speech drew sharp and unfair distinctions. Some Americans, Roosevelt reasoned, would live bold, aggressive lives. Others would "shrink from danger." The speech contained parenting advice. "You will teach your sons that though they may have leisure, it is not to be spent in idleness..." Roosevelt conceived of the nation as an entity that drew its strength and ultimate direction from its smallest cogs—the individual citizens. "A healthy state can exist only when the men and women who make it up lead clean, vigorous, healthy lives, when the children are so trained that they shall endeavor, not to shirk difficulties, but to overcome them..."

Roosevelt's idea of the Strenuous Life advocated for strict, patriarchal gender barriers. While men fought, whether in boxing rings or on the battlefield, women remained anchored to the home. "The woman must be the house-wife," Roosevelt concluded simply, "the helpmate of the homemaker, the wise and fearless mother of many healthy children." Still, women could fail and disappoint the nation just as readily as men. They could fail to have and raise athletic, physically strong children. "When men fear work or fear righteous war, when women fear motherhood...they are fit subjects for the scorn of all men and women who are themselves strong and brave and high-minded."

Part of the speech's appeal, and part of the success of Roosevelt's emerging persona, came from the clarity. Winners and losers; the strong and the weak; the diligent and the shirkers. The sides were easy to identify, and few missed the message on which path *should* be selected.

Roosevelt's storehouse of varied knowledge shone through the longer he spoke. Civil War tales juxtaposed references to French philosopher Alphonse Daudet. Roosevelt tramped unabashedly between disciplines: history, politics, literature, philosophy, science, educational theory—he owned them all. The core of the speech, even though "the Strenuous Life" would become mostly widely applied to Roosevelt's athletic ideas, was a specific call to military action in the Philippines. The military victories of the past two years, including Roosevelt's own in Cuba, demanded US follow-through. "The army and the navy are the sword and the shield which this nation must carry if she is to do her duty among the nations of the earth..." The former Spanish colonies needed order and guidance, whether they wanted it or not. Roosevelt embraced a new order, a new version of imperialism. "Until order and stable liberty are secured, we must remain in the island to insure them," Roosevelt challenged, referencing Cuba particularly.

Roosevelt shamed his audience toward taking action to solve problems ("If we are too weak, too selfish, or too foolish to solve them, some bolder and abler people must undertake the solution"); he also tried his most inspirational material. Wrapping up the speech, Roosevelt dug once more into his crisis-or-conquest toolbox. "The twentieth century looms before us big with the fate of many nations. If we stand idly by, if we seek merely swollen, slothful ease and ignoble peace, if we shrink from the hard contests, then the bolder and stronger peoples will pass us by."

But Roosevelt did not see that happening.

"ABOVE ALL, LET US SHRINK FROM NO STRIFE, MORAL OR PHYSICAL, WITHIN OR WITHOUT THE NATION... FOR IT IS ONLY THROUGH STRIFE, THROUGH HARD AND DANGEROUS ENDEAVOR, THAT WE SHALL ULTIMATELY WIN THE GOAL OF TRUE NATIONAL GREATNESS."

This was a military speech, which created a phrase that summarized an athletic revolution—all of which seems strange only if you actually stop to think about the exact ways that ideas gestate.

* * *

The speech was personal. As a child, Theodore Roosevelt might have been a decent, strenuous athlete himself except for the fact that he couldn't see and he couldn't breathe—at least not very well. As a result, this boy who would go on to be so good at so many things—author of at least thirty-five books, victor of nearly every election he entered, graduate of Harvard, winner of the hands of two delightful brides (although not at the same time), father of six children—struggled to attain even B-team status, athletically speaking, during his childhood. Roosevelt was always behind. He was always fragile. He couldn't hit a ball; he dared not step onto a football field. He certainly did not have the stamina to run around Brooklyn's Union Grounds or hurdle anything that a boy his age might deem worthy of hurdling. According to one description, Roosevelt was "a pale scrawny boy with thin legs, a sunken chest, knobby knees, scant sandy hair, protruding teeth, and a speech defect." So there was room for improvement. It was from this humble position that Theodore Roosevelt began his lifelong validation-quest for "the Strenuous Life."

Most significantly, Roosevelt suffered from asthma. It's difficult for those who've never had asthma, who rarely think about their own breathing patterns, to understand its crippling nature. "Breathing through a straw," "choking," "drowning," "suffocating." These are a few of the descriptors used by asthmatic children to explain the ravages of their condition. Asthma produces cycles of fear and frustration. The condition rules as a dictator, denying its victims the key to life: the reliable delivery of oxygen to one's lungs. Jackie Joyner-Kersee, a six-time Olympic medalist in the heptathlon and long jump, summed it up as a matter of control. "It's frustrating. I can control so much of what I do and I can't control this asthma."

This chronic respiratory disease kept young Roosevelt from attending school and making friends. Theodore, or "Teedie" as his family called him, was first felled by a coughing and wheezing attack in November 1861. After that, "nothing seemed to relieve him from [asthma's] strangling grip." Nothing could be normal. The family tried sending Teedie to John McMullen's school for boys when he was eight but had to quickly withdraw the overwhelmed, scared child. Teedie's mother Martha (Mittie) and father Theodore Sr. (Thee) did everything they could to bring relief to their child.

The resources at the family's disposal were significant. Unlike his political hero Abraham Lincoln, Roosevelt could make no up-by-the-bootstraps claims. The Roosevelts were New York City rich. Roosevelt's paternal grandfather, Cornelius Van Schaack Roosevelt, had built the family's fortune through real estate in Manhattan. The family controlled pivotal piers on the city's waterfront and nearly cornered the glass plate importation business for a time. They also had a majority interest in New York's Chemical Bank and stock in the New York Central Railroad. Cornelius's son, Thee (Teedie's father), had secured the family's philanthropic reputation through an aggressive charity portfolio. Thee founded the New York Museum of Natural History and built a Young Men's Christian Association (YMCA) facility in Manhattan. He visited the city's poorhouses and orphanages on a weekly basis. Thus, the family had the financial resources and connections to go after the newest remedies and most expensive treatments. Unfortunately, though, the best medicine one could buy in the mid-nineteenth century was not very good at all.

Theodore Roosevelt Jr. was born on October 27, 1858, at the sensible but ready-to-go time of 7:45 a.m. The birth took place at the family's home, a stately brownstone with glass enclosed sitting rooms at the street side of each floor. The home featured all the high-end finishes of the day—hardwoods, chandeliers, floral wallpapers, and enough rigid and formal furniture to ensure straight spines for generations of Roosevelts. The delivery of baby Theodore went smoothly, requiring neither chloroform nor "instruments."

Teedie joined a burgeoning New York City family. Sister Anna had arrived three years earlier; Elliott (1860) and Corinne (1861) followed close on TR's heels. The family resided on East Twentieth Street, between Broadway and Park Avenues, in New York City's affluent Manhattan district. Glancing at the front page of the *New York Times* on the day of Teedie's birth, the times seemed stable and affluent. Upcoming elections dominated the news. The Tammany Hall political machine pushed its candidates aggressively throughout the state's wards. The Civil War, which would commence in two years, was buried far beyond the front page.

From age three until twelve, Teedie and his family lived with the permeating fear that the next "shattering, numbing" asthma attack was just around the corner. The condition terrorized and embarrassed Roosevelt. Part of the shame came from the fact that during the nineteenth century, asthma was understood as a nervous, neurotic affliction. Henry Hyde Salter, a London researcher and asthmatic himself, published the definitive *On Asthma: Its Pathology and Treatment* in 1864, arguing that many asthmatic children used asthma as an excuse—to stay home from church or school, to avoid uncomfortable social encounters, and to earn attention. "When the asthmatic was a little boy," Salter explained, using what he deemed to be a typical case, "he found in his disease a convenient immunity from correction; 'Don't scold me,' he would say, if he had incurred his father's displeasure, 'or I shall have the asthma'; and so he would; his fears were as correct as they were convenient." Thus, the asthmatic child was often viewed as having something wrong with his mind or even character, rather than his lungs.

Explaining his weakness over and over, in letters and in person alike, grew tiresome for Theodore. He hated it. When the family was in Europe in 1869, Roosevelt wrote to Edith Carow, explaining the predicament his condition created for the entire Roosevelt family. "A little while ago, I was threatened with an attack of asthma. A Doctor was sent for who sent me to the coast where I got the original disease." This treatment plan didn't make sense to the struggling child. "Father explained this and [the doctor] said that my disease had changed its character and so off we went." The shame in this situation stayed with Roosevelt. Here was a ten-year-old boy, writing to the girl who would one day become his wife, describing how his "disease"—which might just be a conjured-up malady at that—had once again derailed the family's plans.

Parenting such a suffering child was heartbreaking. Thee and Mittie tried everything. They had their son eat a variety of herbs, experiment with mustard plaster, ingest ipecac, and smoke cigars in efforts to calm the inflammation in his airways. The family's doctors tried controlled blood-letting. Midnight jaunts in the icy winter air became regular occurrences. One physician gave young Theodore electric shocks through his feet and head. Roosevelt endured it all. In his diary, Roosevelt noted with almost clinical detachment that a particularly vigorous rubdown, a tactic thought to loosen the lungs, resulted in bleeding. October 15, 1869: "I was rubbed so hard on the chest this morning that the blood came out." Still, no predictable treatment stood ready when an attack came. Roosevelt viewed coffee as his "trump card," but caffeine stimulation could only do so much. Albuterol inhalers, the most common treatment method currently, did not emerge until the 1950s.*

As an adult, Roosevelt remembered his younger self—Teedie—with a disgusted air. "His eyes flamed as he recalled his determination to overcome his infirmities," was how one reporter described TR discussing his past. "I was a sickly, delicate boy, suffered much from asthma, and frequently had to be taken away on trips to find a place where I could breathe." Roosevelt would relay this weak image of himself so frequently during his adulthood that newspapermen and biographers repeated it as simple fact. "A mere wisp of a boy, pale and puny, without health or strength," was how the *Ladies' Home Journal* in 1901 described Roosevelt as a child. The only reliable comfort for Roosevelt during this terrorized period of his life was his parents. "One of my memories is of my father walking up and down the room with me in his arms at night when I was a very small person, and of sitting up in bed gasping with my father and mother trying to help me."

---

* According to the CDC, the United States remains, as of 2019, in the midst of a prolonged asthma spike. Since 1980, the percentage of Americans struggling with asthma has grown steadily. Roughly 1 in 12 Americans, nearly twenty-five million individuals, struggle with the effects of the disease. Thousands die every year from asthma attacks. In 1999, the CDC launched a "National Asthma Control Program" meant to coordinate efforts to mitigate the condition, particularly in children. In essence, even with increased treatment options—the availability of quick-relief inhalers particularly—Roosevelt would still be in good company today. He would sit on the sidelines in PE class, a casualty of his breathing troubles. See Center for Disease National Asthma Control Program, *An Investment in American Health* (CDC: 2013); *New York Times*, July 22, 2008; *Guardian*, December 14, 2014; Allison S. Larr and Matthew Neidell, "Pollution and Climate Change," *The Future of Children*, Vol. 26, No. 1 (Spring 2016), 93–113.

Even as Teedie approached adolescence, there seemed to be no light at the end of the tunnel. Discouraged and worn down from the chaos wrought by his son's asthma, Thee called his eldest son into his book-lined office. Thee was a "big, powerful man" with an intense stare, a long-bridged nose, and a full, perfectly manicured beard. He had a faint resemblance to Ulysses S. Grant. He was also an intensely moral individual, a man known to attend not one but two church services on Sundays. Like many sons, Teedie felt he never quite measured up to his father. He had a "hopeless sense of inferiority" when it came to Thee. Teedie called his father "Great Heart," "the Ideal Man," and "the best man I ever knew."

Things had to change. And so Thee challenged his son directly. He nearly taunted Roosevelt, in fact, to cure himself. "Theodore, you have the mind, but you do not have the body," Thee began. "Without the help of the body the mind cannot go as far as it should. You must *make* your body." It wouldn't be easy. Teedie needed a plan, his father continued. "It is hard drudgery to make one's body, but I know you will do it." At his wits' end over his son's long delayed physical development and continual bouts with asthma, TR's father put the onus on his child.

How does one respond when he is commanded to, in essence, start breathing better? What was there to say? Teedie contemplated his father's challenge for a moment, likely running a montage through his head of his countless suffocating incidents. Then he responded. "The little boy looked up, throwing back his head in a characteristic fashion," his sister remembered. "He said—'I'll do it; I'll make my body.'" And that was that. Or so Roosevelt would remember years later. "From that day this little boy...started to make his body, and he never ceased in making that body until the day of his death."

The first thing Teedie did to make his own body was have his father build him a personal gymnasium. Considering both Teedie's struggles and those of Roosevelt's older sister Anna, who suffered from a spinal disorder, most likely Pott's disease (tuberculosis of the spinal cord), Theodore Roosevelt Sr. had "a kind of open-air gymnasium" constructed on the second floor of the family dwelling. This was bourgeois fitness at its finest; the rich children loved it.

"What fun we had on that piazza!" The room was cleared out of all domestic accoutrements and retrofitted with "every imaginable swing and bar and see-saw." The space had boxing gloves and a punching bag for scrawny Roosevelt to pound.

Young Roosevelt may have been privileged and his father may have built him a gymnasium for the task, but he also began doing his part to gain strength and stamina. "[I'll make my body] was his first important promise to himself," his sister wrote. "For many years one of my most vivid recollections is seeing him between horizontal bars, widening his chest by regular, monotonous motion—drudgery indeed—but a drudgery which eventuated in his being not only the apostle but the exponent of the strenuous life."

Shortly after their father-son talk, Thee paid for his son to begin training with "Professor" John Wood—a former professional boxer. Wood's Gymnasium, located on West Twenty-Eighth Street in New York, was the most prestigious training facility in the city. Foreshadowing fitness club trends that would emerge decades later, Wood's establishment was a place to sweat *and* a place to be seen. The Vanderbilt family, for example, claiming a net worth of nearly $100 million through their shipping and railroad businesses, sent several of its sons to Wood's Gym. When the oarsmen of Columbia University needed to conduct their out-of-water training, they used the "spacious and lofty hall" at Wood's Gym. In the years before the prestigious New York Athletic Club completed its own facility, NYAC membership—$25 per month—included access to Wood's. Small and scared, Roosevelt trained alongside the best athletes New York City had to offer.

Pay a membership fee to work up a sweat—this idea seems perfectly normal to most Americans now. After all, today Americans spend more than $24 billion annually on fitness memberships. When the Roosevelts joined Wood's, though, there was a novelty to not only having the means to pay for fitness but also to even conceiving of needing exercise as a standalone activity at all. Gymnasiums were springing up in cities across the United States during the last decades of the nineteenth century. For generations, exercise had been tied to work, warfare, and outright survival. There was something new, and a bit bizarre, about a world in which it was perfectly acceptable to arrive at the end of a day's work without having broken a sweat at all.

As he trained, Roosevelt received regular reminders that he had a long way to go. During a train ride to Moosehead Lake, several years into his physical training, a couple of bullies approached Roosevelt. An awkward fight broke out. Humiliation ensued. "I discovered that either one singly could not only handle me with easy contempt, but handle me so as not to hurt me much and yet prevent my doing any damage whatever in return." Roosevelt was such a pitiful specimen that stronger boys did not even see fit to engage him in a full-fledged fight. As a result, young Roosevelt intensified his boxing training.

Roosevelt approached his athletic development as a natural scientist. He kept copious records. No event was too trivial to record. After all, this was the same boy who wrote page after page in his journals, filled with very specific scientific terms, about family vacations. "The driver told us that there are wolves (lamis occidentalis), bears (ursus americanus), and numbers of deer (bevis virginiansas)," Roosevelt wrote of one trip. Roosevelt's 1875 "Diary of Athletic Achievements" is particularly informative regarding how a young boy tried to improve his physique. First, Roosevelt, ever fastidious, began with an outline of his shorthand system for measurements. Then the scorekeeping began.

> **Saturday, August 21, 1875.** 100 yds. Footrace between West and Theodore. Theodore won in 13 seconds. Standing jumps. T[heodore] 7"2' Running [jumps]. T[heodore] 11"5' W[est] 11"1'

> **Monday, August 23, 1875.** Standing Jump. Emlen 8"6' Elliott 7"3' Running Jump. Emlen 13'4"

> **Thursday, September 16, 1875.** Standing high jump. Theodore 3"2' West 3"

> **Thursday, November 25, 1875.** Theodore vaulting against West, beat. Vault 5"7'

Monday, November 29, 1875. Vaulting. Theodore, Elliot and [illegible] T[heodore] won...Wrestling Theodore beat Elliot.

Tuesday, December 7, 1875. Boxing. Theodore beat Buckmeister (John Longs)

Saturday, December 11, 1875. Theodore, running. Quarter of a mile 1 minute, 7 seconds. 100 yards 12 seconds.

Roosevelt's co-conspirators were family members. Elliott Roosevelt was the younger brother, born two years after Theodore. Emlen and West were cousins—William Emlen Roosevelt and James West Roosevelt. The boys spent hours and hours together during their formative years.

Poor Elliott. He almost never won at anything. And, in a rite that younger siblings everywhere would categorize as downright criminal, his older brother stood ready with a pen and paper to record his brother's losses almost immediately after they occurred.

Roosevelt rarely wasted the appendix pages in his journals. He often recorded his expenses or savings in the appropriate grids. Similarly in his athletic diary, Roosevelt filled the last pages of the volume with numbers. Roosevelt—

fastidious and self-important—recorded his measurements as of November 1, 1875. At the cusp of manhood, Theodore Roosevelt stood five foot, eight inches tall. He was a rail thin 124 lbs. His chest to waist ratio, however, provided Roosevelt with a somewhat impressive build. He had come a long way; he had the data to prove it.

The final page in the diary was as telling as any in the pocket-sized book. After noting his times and victories for the year (and how Elliott lost time after time), and then his physical measurements, Roosevelt circled back to provide the baseline standard that he expected of himself. "Regulations," of TR's own making of course, determined that a certain threshold had to be met in order to report an athletic activity. Not just any athletic happening could go into the book. In light of the many contests with younger brother Elliott that Roosevelt felt compelled to record, this seems somewhat beyond the pale. But still, Roosevelt had his standards. "Of the jumps," Roosevelt sternly noted, "none under the following amounts shall be measured." Then he listed a series of relatively meager standards—eleven feet for the running long jump; seven feet for standing jumps; three feet, six inches for running high jump; and three feet even for standing high jump. Thus, the image that emerges from this strange diary is one of a committed and detail-oriented boy making small strides toward athletic vitality.

Gradually, slowly, Roosevelt won some small victories. Another former prizefighter, John Long, later took an interest in Roosevelt. "I can see his rooms now," Roosevelt remembered decades later, "with colored pictures of the fights between Tom Hyer and Yankee Sullivan, and Heenan and Sayers." Under Long's tutelage, Roosevelt made slow progress. Long frequently held intra-gymnasium contests. TR entered one particular low-stakes competition as a lightweight contestant. He got a noticeably fortuitous draw, facing "a couple of reedy striplings who were even worse than I was." This was saying something. Still, to Roosevelt's and Long's surprise, Roosevelt emerged as the champion of his division. He won! As a reward, Long handed Roosevelt a small, pewter mug. It became one of Roosevelt's most prized possessions.

I kept it, and alluded to it, and I fear bragged about it, for a number of years, and I only wish I knew where it was now. Years later I read an account of a little man who once in a fifth-rate handicap race won a worthless pewter medal and joyed in it ever after. Well, as soon as I read that story I felt that that little man and I were brothers. This was, as far as I remember, the only one of my exceedingly rare athletic triumphs which would be worth relating.

While Roosevelt kept athletic statistics in his diary, it would be too much to call him a statistician. Statisticians deploy methodologies. They train themselves to remember, among other things, that "correlation is not causation." The point of this axiom being that just because two things are juxtaposed, concurrent, or related, we should not suppose that one caused the other. This methodological discipline, even for those who devote their lives to the study of data, is easier said than done. Blanket causation is an alluring, seductive temptress. It's so easy, but it still feels smart. It's satisfying. But assigning correlation where it does not exist causes problems.*

Roosevelt made a rather spurious connection that fundamentally shaped his view on the Strenuous Life. During the first half of the 1870s, as Roosevelt boxed with professionals, stretched and grunted in the family gymnasium, and recorded his athletic improvements in his diary, a stunning development occurred: his acute asthma subsided. It did not go away completely—it never would—but the crisis-attacks decreased markedly. Asthma bouts for Roosevelt ceased to be the Shakespearean tragedies they had been during the first decade of his life. The more Roosevelt pushed himself into athletics, the fitter he became; and the smaller the gap between TR and his peers. The challenge to "make your body" seemed to have worked.

Theodore Roosevelt assumed that a very strong, nearly exact causal relationship existed between his athletic activity and his rise to mostly normal health. Wouldn't we all? The relationship seemed obviously intertwined. A little exer-

---

* Tyler Vigen's "spurious correlations" research presents a warning about correlation with a touch of Mel Brooks subtlety. Vigen, a Harvard Law graduate, created an algorithm to produce graphs taken from publicly available data sets. Vigen's graphs demonstrate that phenomena such as (a) "The number of people who drowned by falling into a pool" are almost exactly linked to (b) "Number of films Nicolas Cage appeared in." Or that the (a) "Divorce rate in Maine," ebbs and flows in relation to (b) "Per capita consumption of margarine." Look it up; it's true. "Finding causal mechanisms is the key goal in a lot of scientific research because when we find causal mechanisms, we learn that much more about the world around us," Vigen says. His point is to be careful in assigning causation. "Correlations between two variables could be merely coincidence, or they could be the result of an underlying causal link." "Every time we see a correlation, we have a marvelous opportunity to try and figure out which one it is," Vigen concludes. See, Tyler Vigen, *Spurious Correlations* (New York: Hatchette Books, 2015).

cise begot a little progress. Then as Roosevelt neared college age and increased his athletic training to a near maniacal level, the asthma, right on cue, decreased more rapidly too.

Adding to this powerful self-healing dynamic was the fact that Roosevelt was also fitted with glasses for the first time just as he was taking up his athletic training. Fuzzy shapes became vivid. Thrown balls became more easily catchable. His athleticism, although never much, increased overnight. The first glasses changed everything; they "literally opened an entirely new world to me," Theodore said. "I had no idea how beautiful the world was until I got those spectacles." The (nearly) blind could now see.

Just as the glasses get the credit for Roosevelt's improved vision, so too there is a non-TR hero to the "almost miraculous" trailing off of Roosevelt's asthma. It wasn't just the vigorous exercise. Rather, more simply, Roosevelt's asthma subsided into a quiescent state as he entered adolescence. The gym work was at least partly a coincidence. This pattern of aging out of asthma is well documented and acknowledged today; in the nineteenth century though there was no such understanding.

But Roosevelt knew, he just knew, that exercise had cured him. He'd lived it. The connection was clear. His was a story of self-reliance. "The worst lesson that can be taught to a man," Roosevelt would declare, "is to rely upon others and to whine over his sufferings." Fix your own problems. Strengthen your own weaknesses. TR had exercised his asthma off. To be clear, there was nothing fraudulent in Roosevelt's claim. But the result of Roosevelt's conviction would play out over the coming decades. For if Roosevelt could do it—empower himself through exercise and sports and the Strenuous Life—the rest of the nation could be compelled to do the same.

THREE

HARVARD AND ITS HARVARDNESS

I am very glad I am not a Yale freshman; the hazing there is pretty bad.
The fellows too seem to be a much more scruffy set than ours.
—THEODORE ROOSEVELT

E SPN's College Game Day made its first ever visit to Harvard University in November 2014. The show descended upon Cambridge for "The Game," the annual Harvard–Yale football contest. Harvard's students didn't disappoint, showing up to fill the background of the live show with anti-Yale signs such as, "For a safety school, your defensive backfield sure sucks!" and "Yale Cites Wikipedia." It made for a fun and lively setting for ESPN's popular pregame telecast. If anything though, the visit was a bit late. It came more than a century after Harvard's football glory days.

Today Harvard University, and the rest of the Ivy League, reside far on the periphery of major college athletics. ESPN rarely cares what's going on at Harvard. Ivy League institutions (Brown, Columbia, Cornell, Dartmouth, Harvard, Penn, Princeton, and Yale) don't offer athletic scholarships. Because the schools don't offer athletic scholarships, they typically can't compete for national championships, especially in men's basketball and football. While athletic success stories still arise at Harvard (see Jeremy Lin, aka "Linsanity"), most student athletes attend the Cambridge institution for the academics more so than for the athletic opportunities the school can provide.

Harvard University during Roosevelt's era, though, was *the* powerhouse in intercollegiate sports. Thus the university played a pivotal role in defining the emerging relationship between universities and sports in America, and its teams enjoyed nearly unmatched success.

Harvard was there, in fact, at the beginning of college sports. On August 3, 1852, Harvard and Yale Universities competed in the first intercollegiate athletic competition. The event only happened because a railroad magnate, James Elkins, recognized that college students competing against each other might just have economic possibilities. If only he knew. "If you will get up a regatta on the Lake between Yale and Harvard," Elkins promised Yale rower James Whiton, "I will pay all the bills." Elkins wanted to promote his new rail line to the White Mountains resort region for affluent northeasterners.

By the time Roosevelt arrived on Harvard's campus in fall 1876, the Harvard Athletic Association managed an active sports docket. Football, crew, and baseball contests dominated campus life. Positions for the various crew teams, divided by class rank and boat size, were fought for aggressively by Harvard men desperate to test their mettle on the waters of the Charles River. Track-and-field and gymnastics competitions also attracted dozens of participants.

But as is the case now (see: the College Football Playoff), football dominated the intercollegiate athletic world. Harvard and Yale faced each other on the gridiron for the first time in 1875. They did so amidst an argument over football rules. Would the game resemble soccer (or football as the rest of the world calls it), rugby, or something as ill-defined as fightum? At issue was whether the ball could be advanced by a runner carrying it. Harvard's version of the emerging game allowed for such ball control. Yale, Princeton, and Rutgers, among others, advocated for a game that consisted solely of kicking the ball.

Harvard traveled to New Haven for the inaugural Harvard–Yale contest. More than 150 Harvard men accompanied the team. The rules were loose. Fifteen players lined up on each side (Yale had advocated for eleven) with the negotiated ability to carry the ball and tackle their opponents. "Touchdowns" counted for nothing other than the ability to then try for a kick, which made, counted for one point. The game started at 2:30 p.m. at Hamilton Park in New Haven. A small stand of bleachers allowed several hundred of the nearly 2,000 spectators to sit and watch. The rest crowded around the field. Having strong-armed Yale into accepting the rules that its men had played with at least a few times, Harvard romped to victory, 4–0.

After the game ended, the Harvard and Yale players and fans celebrated together. For those assuming that things were so very different at this early juncture of football's history, they were; the Harvard and Yale men joined together for a postgame sing-along. But one can also note that five Harvard men were arrested for, basically, public drunkenness as they celebrated their team's victory.

* * *

When Theodore Roosevelt arrived on Harvard's leafy, red-bricked campus for his freshman year in September 1876, a year's tuition cost $150. Room and board, another $175. Harvard University was, to put it in modern terms, the Harvard of American higher education in the nineteenth century. But not by such a large margin. Roosevelt joined 231 men in the class of 1880. More than half came from the state of Massachusetts. Charles Eliot, who was on his way to becoming one of the most influential university presidents in American history, welcomed the new Harvard men. Mostly local, nearly entirely American, all white (although Harvard had admitted a handful of African American students in prior classes), all male—Harvard's freshmen of 1876 looked the same as the classes the university had been assembling for decades.

The college experience for Roosevelt did not involve cinderblock dorm rooms or monochromatic cafeteria food. Rather he settled into comfortable, private accommodations located at 38 Winthrop Street (a site today near Harvard's Malkin Athletic Center). The Winthrop house was a two story, traditional home. A modest front porch, two brick chimneys, and dark shutters gave the structure a conservative, dignified air. The location put Roosevelt just three blocks from the Harvard Yard. He wrote to sister Anna shortly after getting settled in September 1876 to report on his setup: "The curtains, carpet, furniture—in short everything is really beautiful; I have never seen a prettier or more tasteful wall paper."

Roosevelt joined as many Harvard clubs as he could. It was as if he intended to make up for his cloistered childhood by accepting every offer and joining every roster. The list is impressive. During his four years in Cambridge, Roosevelt managed to involve himself with the *Harvard Advocate* newspaper, the Greek, art, finance, rifle, and glee clubs, the Hasty Pudding Club, the Class Day Committee, and the Institute of 1770. He served as a steward for the Harvard Athletic Association. Most formatively, Roosevelt joined the school's Natural History Society and gained a nomination to the exclusive Porcellian Club.

For Roosevelt, Harvard served as a finishing school—physically, intellectually, and emotionally. On the first front, Roosevelt entered university life on nearly equal footing with his classmates. He had made incredible progress. Harvard tallied the measurements of Roosevelt's entering class. The average Harvard freshman in 1876 stood five-feet, seven-inches tall and weighed 145 pounds—nearly twenty pounds less than the average male freshman today. The tallest member of Roosevelt's class measured six-feet, three-inches tall. The heaviest Harvard man who graduated with Roosevelt weighed 217 pounds. Only a handful were overweight.

Roosevelt had caught up, but he still stuck out. "There was no question about his being 'different,'" remembered one of Roosevelt's Harvard classmates. Roosevelt collected things. He kept a large turtle, a gaggle (herd... pack?) of salamanders, and several snakes in his room, unnerving his visitors. Roosevelt, despite his Knickerbocker, high-society upbringing, never dressed completely with the times either. Roosevelt's exercises, including skipping rope in red stockings, came off to some as "lady-like." In short, meeting TR was an experience. "He was using a set of parallel bars between which another freshman pushed himself backward and forward more violently and rapidly than any one else," remembered one classmate. "When all out of breath, he dropped to the floor and gasped: 'My name's Roosevelt. What's yours?'"

Roosevelt tried to visit the school's Rogers Gymnasium and his boxing "tutor" five times a week. There he hit the heavy bag, worked with weights, and sparred regularly. Roosevelt's confidence as an athlete vacillated. In January 1878, he recorded in his diary that he intended to compete for the school's lightweight championship (or "cups") in both boxing and wrestling. Defeats were mostly taken in stride ("was rather beaten in a boxing match with Bob Bacon, not much though") as Roosevelt remained doggedly convinced of the idea that he could become at least competent athletically.

Roosevelt continued his athletic note-taking. The results always mattered: "Beaten by Dick Trimble, boxing," "threw" four competitors, "thrown by Davis." Roosevelt had impossibly high standards for his athletic partners. He wanted manly, almost knightly, competitors who understood the proper place of athletics, demonstrated constant personal discipline, and appreciated ideas and intellectual debate. Even at Harvard, such men were in short supply. Occasionally though, things came together. "I was especially struck by this the other night, when, after a couple of hours spent in boxing and wrestling with Arthur Hooper and Ralph Ellis, it was proposed to finish the evening by reading aloud from Tennyson, and we became so interested in *In Memoriam* that it was past one o'clock when we separated." This was Roosevelt's idea of balance—wrestling, boxing, and then hours with Alfred Tennyson.

In February 1878, during the second half of Roosevelt's sophomore year at Harvard, everything changed. Roosevelt's father died unexpectedly from a stomach tumor. In his diary, TR wrote simply: "My dear Father. Born, Sept 23rd, 1831." For once, he had no more words. Although Roosevelt knew his father had been sick, Theodore Sr.'s death at age forty-six caught Roosevelt by surprise. Unable to make it to his father's bedside during the last hours of his life, Roosevelt collapsed into a prolonged period of grief. "He was the most wise and loving father that ever lived," Roosevelt wrote of his father a week after his passing. "I owe everything to him." Suddenly the championships Roosevelt had eyed lustily a few months prior ceased to be worth going after. The wrestling championship occurred at Harvard on March 9, 1878—exactly one month after Roosevelt's father had died. Roosevelt noted the passing as an indication of his new priorities. "The lightweight wrestling occurred today," he commented. "It is funny to look back and remember how I had trained for and anticipated it. It seems as if it was years ago."

Theodore retreated from the gymnasium as he grieved. His training schedule was pared down. He instead considered his faith and his finances. Not even two weeks had passed since his father's death when Roosevelt jotted down, in passing, that his inheritance would be $8,000 a year, making him "comfortable although not rich." In reality, it made him quite rich. The yearly sum would equal about $200,000 in 2019 currency.

Roosevelt's retreat hinted at the challenge that athletics continued to pose for him. Yes, he had improved, but he went to the gymnasium always conscious of his flaws. He struggled against his faulty physical genes and his childhood weaknesses. TR did not have a reservoir of confidence to draw upon in this area. As he would confess later, when asked about the role of boxing in his formative years, "I intended to be a middling decent fellow, and I did not intend that any one should laugh at me with impunity because I was decent." Roosevelt struggled to make sense of his new fatherless reality. "Lord I believe," he quoted from Mark 9:24 in his diary, "help thou mine unbelief."

When Roosevelt returned home to New York for the summer between his sophomore and junior years, solitary exercise gradually reemerged as a healing, strengthening antidote to his mourning. Self-medicating meant sweating. Roosevelt rowed miles and miles in the Long Island sound, strengthening his arms, bronzing his chest, and at least somewhat soothing his cracked heart. Thus even in death, Thee continued to push Theodore toward strenuous physical improvement.

Theodore Roosevelt, twenty years old, would make his father proud, especially now that he was gone. He would grow stronger and more competitive. "I often feel badly that such a wonderful man as father should have had a son of so little worth as I am," Theodore lamented during his grieving summer. Looking to jumpstart his progress once again, Roosevelt laid out a new plan of athletic improvement. Always a plan. "Ran a mile through the woods at speed; shall probably repeat this every day." While the physiological effects of the plan might be dubious, the reality of Roosevelt sprinting as hard as possible through the tulip trees and white pines of Long Island in order to improve himself seemed to fit.

The Harvard athletic class of 1880, not helped much by Theodore Roosevelt, went a long way toward cementing their university as the dominant intercollegiate athletic program in the United States. The crew team won thirty-seven events. The Harvard baseball team by this time had claimed 160 "base-balls" for victories over other collegiate teams. This was the tradition of nineteenth-century baseball; the losing team turned over a ball to the winning one.

As for Roosevelt, his contribution was mostly metaphysical. He homed in on what it was that motivated the Harvard athlete. It was simple. Roosevelt argued that the optimal manner by which to push Harvard athletes toward excellence was to give them a singular opportunity: the opportunity to defeat their Yale counterparts. "Now what induces men to train so well and faithfully for the Football Team, Crew, or Base Ball Nine?" Roosevelt asked in a letter to the *Harvard Advocate* in 1879. "Simply the desire to beat Yale. Would they not train equally well for our athletic sports if they were to try against Yale there too? It seems probable that the mere desire to win from Yale is all that is now needed to make our athletic meetings a success."

The intense sadness and mourning that dominated Roosevelt's sophomore year gave way to success and contentment as a junior, and then buoyant jubilation as a senior. During his junior year (1878–1879), Roosevelt became increasingly involved with Harvard's Porcellian Club. The finishing club's motto, "While we live, Let us live," certainly appealed to Roosevelt. That such an elite, utterly aristocratic group of Boston Brahmans would accept Roosevelt, with all his eccentricities, gave Roosevelt a new confidence during the second half of his Harvard tenure. On the night of his Porcellian initiation, Roosevelt became drunker than at any time in his college years. Roosevelt was not above wanting to fit in; in this instance it led to a compromise of TR's usual abstention from alcohol and tobacco. Only months earlier, he had declared, piously, in his diary: "I get rather tired of seeing such a drunken club…I shall not begin smoking til I am twenty-one; as it is, I drink very little." Still, on November 2,

1878, Roosevelt drank with his new Porcellian Club brothers. He woke up badly hung over the next morning "owing to last night's spree." Tellingly Roosevelt analyzed just how sloshed he had been with a judging system calibrated entirely on his own. He had been intoxicated, he remembered, but even "higher with wine than I have been before—or will be again," he could function. "Still, I could wind up my watch." Head pounding and tongue thick, Roosevelt showed up as usual to teach his Sunday School class the following morning.

There was reason to celebrate membership among the Porcellians, especially for an ambitious New Yorker such as Roosevelt. The organization was Harvard's most prestigious. Members enjoyed access to Boston's most elite clubs and institutions. And practically speaking, Roosevelt joined a moneyed and privileged fraternity with the Porcellians that had seemed out of reach during Roosevelt's first awkward semesters. The Porcellians dined together frequently. The "Porcs," after all, had initially come together out of opposition to subpar dining options at Harvard. Getting its start in the 1790s, the young men simply intended to roast pigs together instead of eating the food provided by the university. Roosevelt enjoyed the multicourse meals and ready-made camaraderie. He craved fine things and formality. It would be the Porcellian Club that would summon Roosevelt back to Harvard thirty years later to make a speech on athletics in America. And more directly, the Porcellian Club helped Roosevelt court his chosen target, Alice Lee, with all the aristocratic flair necessary for such a nineteenth-century match.

On March 22, 1879, in Harvard's perpetually cold gymnasium, Theodore Roosevelt fought for his first real, first worth-telling-someone-about athletic championship. He had advanced to the semifinal bout of the Harvard Athletic Association's lightweight boxing tournament to face a senior classmate, Charles Hanks. While not on par with, say, a Harvard football game, the *New York Times* and *Boston Globe* covered the event; it was big enough. Adding even more importance to the contest, a young woman that Roosevelt had fallen madly in love with, but who showed surprisingly little inclination to return his feelings, looked on with dozens of Roosevelt's classmates. So here was a chance at athletic glory, one that had been a decade in the making.

The match took place in Harvard's small, "circular-angular" Rogers Gymnasium. The venue looked nothing like a modern athletic structure. Instead of high ceilings and wide-open spaces, the Harvard gymnasium had too much architecture. Too much character to be practical. A hexagon dome topped the building, with beams and ropes cluttering the athletic space below. Ventilation and temperature control were constant problems. The gym did not have nearly enough space for Harvard's growing student body. "One has to wait his turn at almost every piece of apparatus, and several pieces it is impossible to use at all, on account of the lack of room," complained one of Roosevelt's (rather entitled sounding) contemporaries. Built in 1859, Rogers Gymnasium, and the eventual hiring of Dr. Dudley Sargent to run it, were Harvard faculty's begrudging acquiescence to students' demands for athletic space and sports teams on their Cambridge campus.

Roosevelt's future romantic happiness also stood at least partially in the balance as he fought Hanks. Alice Hathaway Lee, a mesmerizing seventeen-year-old beauty from one of Boston's most elite families, joined a large, "densely packed" crowd for the fighting festival. She was accompanied by a small cadre of similarly well-heeled young women. Apparently teenagers have always traveled in such packs. While Roosevelt was working himself to exhaustion in order to win Alice's heart ("I loved her as soon as I saw her sweet, fair young face"), she remained cool to his charms. Alice, with her chestnut hair, petite figure, fine features, and family money had plenty of suitors. She certainly didn't need this overly aggressive young New Yorker to secure her place in Boston society. Still, she liked him just enough to be on hand as he fought for his first championship.

Roosevelt weighed 140 pounds and stood five-feet, eight-inches tall in 1879. He wore his hair closely cropped. The hair on Roosevelt's cheeks in fact, at the nadir of his sideburns, was nearly longer than that on his head. Taut, well-defined arms and calves gave evidence to TR's time in the gymnasium.

But then there were the glasses. TR wore glasses because he suffered from grossly nearsighted vision. So even though Roosevelt desperately wanted to look rough and manly, he entered the gymnasium with a "delicate appearance" and "a pair of big spectacles lashed to his head." Combining these traits with average foot speed, a less-than-stellar reach, virtually no experience in organized athletics, and only minimal experience against seasoned fighters made Roosevelt a frightening opponent to, well, almost none of his fellow collegiate boxers.

With no undue festivities, the fight began. Hanks outreached TR and "weighed more by six pounds." Trying to make up for his lack of depth perception and his shorter reach, Roosevelt pushed his way inside during the fight's first round. He let fly all manner of punches, a few of which he even managed to land. "There would have been little left of the men had all the blows aimed at each other reached their destination," the *Boston Globe* reported. Roosevelt outpointed his opponent to secure the first round for his side of the tally sheet. Hanks adjusted his strategy in the second. Working carefully to limit Roosevelt's opportunities to get inside, Hanks jabbed steadily. Performing as a tactician now, in the style that would be perfected by Heavyweight Champion Jack Johnson some thirty years later, Hanks won the second round.

Hanks was, to a certain extent, precisely the type of man Roosevelt aspired to be. Hanks competed on Harvard's baseball and track teams in addition to holding memberships in several campus clubs and societies. His athletic gifts were obvious. Not surprisingly Hanks's superior reach and his extra bulk wore Roosevelt down. Hanks pounded away in the third and final round while Roosevelt struggled to make substantial contact. Roosevelt, according to the *New York Times,* fought "very prettily" (hardly a compliment that Roosevelt could enjoy), but Hanks had brute force. Roosevelt's nearsightedness made positioning and feinting difficult. In the end, Hanks won the bout handily, "punishing Roosevelt severely." But Roosevelt had kept coming. "You should have seen that little fellow staggering about, banging the air," recalled one of Roosevelt's classmates. "Hanks couldn't put him out and Roosevelt wouldn't give up. It wasn't a fight, but, oh, he showed himself a fighter."

Roosevelt did not belabor the fight experience in his diary. He had fought, advanced, and then lost. "Sparred for the lightweight cup," Roosevelt penciled in on the evening of the bout. "Won against my first man but was beaten by

Hanks, the champion." Roosevelt then continued down the diary page detailing his academic work. "I have been studying extremely hard the past week…" Roosevelt did not get his championship, but all was not lost. By the end of the fight, Roosevelt had left his onlookers with an inspiring foreshadowing of what he might one day become. The TR legend got one of its first bullet points. Roosevelt showed himself to be violent, relentless, and gentlemanly—all at the same time. Not a bad day's work.

Ironically, the most memorable moment in Roosevelt's Harvard boxing career was not a glorious punch he landed but rather one he took to the face. Once, hearing a round-ending signal, Roosevelt dropped his tired arms and let his boxing gloves fall from their defensive position. Then, just a moment later, the gloved fist of his opponent connected squarely with Roosevelt's unprotected face. Vessels ruptured, blood spurted from Roosevelt's nose. Roosevelt wobbled as his classmates booed and let loose with "loud hoots and hisses from the gallery." Roosevelt teetered, but he did not fall. Then, as Roosevelt regained his senses, he surprised his onlookers by rushing to the protection of his careless opponent. "It's all right! It's all right!" Roosevelt declared, waving his arms to get the crowd's attention. "He didn't hear the call." Blood now pouring from his nose, Roosevelt reached out to his opponent and shook his gloved hand as a sign of goodwill. After a brief rest, Roosevelt raised his fists back to a fighting pose, protecting his now damaged nose, and the bout continued. Thus Theodore Roosevelt, a mutton-chopped and moderately skilled university boxer, made his first public stand for athletics.

It's stunning, given his lineage and the political heights to which he would ultimately ascend, that Theodore Roosevelt made what amounted to his public debut in this musty boxing gymnasium. Questioned years later, after Roosevelt became president, many of Roosevelt's Harvard classmates could not remember much at all about the future president during his time in Cambridge. But of those who did recall young Roosevelt, many remembered his exploits as a boxer. They remembered his fight with Hanks. They remembered Roosevelt taking a sucker punch. Roosevelt had bled; he had rushed to the defense of his opponent. Then he kept fighting.

"A huge roar of clapping went up from the audience," recalled Owen Wister, the future Wild West novelist and a Harvard freshman in 1879, of the illicit blow. "The bloody nose would have been a great card: but a fair game proved to be a greater one. You may imagine what ardent champions Mr. Roosevelt had during the final round." With the passage of time and Roosevelt's elevation to the presidency of the United States in 1901, his boxing career became downright heroic. Fact and myth merged. "All that was near a quarter century ago," Wister waxed, "that stormy gust of sympathy in the gymnasium, that roomful of applauding spectators set boiling by the warm contagion of generosity, is merely the prophetic symbol of the present to the American people."

Although the tales of the sucker punch and the championship fight would be embellished as years passed, simply by winning a bout and advancing in the March 1879 intraschool boxing tournament during his junior year Roosevelt had finally hoisted himself up and peered over the wall of athletic prowess that had blocked his path since childhood. He got a glimpse of the other side.

* * *

Theodore Roosevelt chased Alice Hathaway Lee his senior year, much more than he sought after academic success or even physical vigor. He pursued and Alice feinted, at least for a time. Alice was beautiful, alluring, and young—only seventeen years old at the beginning of Roosevelt's senior year. She was nearly as tall as Theodore. Photographs of Alice at the time of TR's full pursuit reveal a young aristocrat with an hourglass figure and fine features. Descriptions of her beauty offer a transcendent image. Alice was "enchanting," "exceptionally bright," "as ravishing a beauty as ever walked across a Boston lawn," "a strikingly beautiful blonde with vivid blue-gray eyes." And she played tennis. Roosevelt wanted to marry her almost from the moment he first saw her.

Roosevelt spared nothing in his pursuit. He was a five-foot-seven bespectacled peacock intent on winning his target. To her credit, Alice resisted Theodore's romantic blitzkrieg for months. She may have even rejected a presumptive proposal for marriage. In turn, Roosevelt grew exasperated and paranoid at the thought she might choose someone else. Certainly Alice had plenty of fine Boston men from which to select a mate. But Roosevelt's enthusiasm was tough to top: "I spent all day with my sweet, pretty, pure queen, my laughing little love. Oh, how bewitchingly pretty she is!" Eventually the overwhelming tonnage of Roosevelt's attention—the letters, the parental get-togethers, the frequent calls by Theodore to the Lee family home in Chestnut Hill—delivered the intended result. In January 1880, Alice accepted Roosevelt's marriage proposal, although not without some concern, historian Kathleen Dalton notes, "about losing all her freedom by marrying the intense jealous man she called 'Teddy.'" The couple would wed in the coming fall, just after Roosevelt obtained his degree from Harvard University.

*   *   *

Before Theodore Roosevelt could get married, he had to graduate from Harvard University. And before he could graduate, one last athletic hurdle had to be navigated. Roosevelt needed to complete a physical examination given by Harvard University's newly hired (and first ever) assistant professor of physical education and director of Harvard's Hemenway Gymnasium, Dudley Allen Sargent. Sargent was at the very beginning of a long career that would eventually establish him as the father of modern physical education. But in 1880, he just wanted three things: (1) A suitable space in which to train athletes; (2) The means to take his ideas for exercising equipment—and there were so many ideas—and build prototypes; and (3) Measurements. Sargent wanted the sort of athletic data that could only be obtained by measuring and testing hundreds of individuals. Thus Roosevelt and all other Harvard seniors were required to let Sargent poke and prod and measure before diplomas could be handed out.

Sargent had taken the position at Harvard in September 1879. Sargent looked the part; he was trim and energetic. He had a tremendous mustache. Sargent celebrated his thirtieth birthday shortly after arriving in Cambridge. The young professor did not get a particularly warm reception upon his arrival; many members of the faculty felt physical education had no place in Harvard's curriculum. Some even reacted with racially bigoted derision. Sargent recalled one Harvard man greeting him by remarking about this position in charge of the school's gymnasium, simply, "Ah...they had a nigger when I was there."

Sargent was born in Maine and earned his undergraduate degree at Bowdoin College. In 1878, he completed his MD at Yale University. After a year spent in New York City working as a personal fitness instructor, Sargent took charge of Harvard's newly opened Hemenway Gymnasium—a building that was all brick, glass, arches, and ornate touches. It was as if Harvard had realized that it had to create some athletic space, but it wasn't going to advertise the true purpose of its newest building. Sargent arrived and immediately announced that he did not particularly like the new space. He didn't think it much of an improvement over Rogers Gymnasium where Roosevelt had fought his best fights. Hemenway "was better from an architectural than from a gymnastic standpoint," Sargent pointed out. He quickly went to work reorganizing the new venue to fit his plans.

Dudley Sargent was driven by a fundamental concern that America was becoming too weak to compete in a challenging world. Men were sitting too much of the day. Children did not spend enough time outside. Women remained confined to domestic duties inside their homes. Softer work was making for a softer nation. "Steam, gunpowder, and electricity are now doing the work and fighting the battles of the world," Sargent wrote in his personal manifesto, *Physical Education*. "They have increased the power of man a thousandfold. So puny seem the efforts of a human when compared with these powerful agents that we have almost ceased to regard physical vigor as one of the factors in human progress." Although there is no evidence of Roosevelt and Sargent conversing about these ideas, TR would evoke similar concerns throughout his political life.

As a child, Sargent had constructed an iron horizontal bar in his uncle's barn and taught himself gymnastics. The bar became an obsession. Even in the frigid Maine winters, Sargent continued his work, despite the fact that his skin would freeze to the apparatus and rip his hands apart. He became so proficient at his routines, "monkey shines" as they were called by his neighbors, that a circus career beckoned. And so Sargent quit high school and went off with a traveling carnival. He did trapeze work for several months before coming to the conclusion that, while fun, the circus probably wasn't his life's work.

As the director of Hemenway, Sargent believed in resistance and weight training, and cardio work. He wanted his students to approach their physical development with both deliberation and enthusiasm. "Cultivate the physical perfection of the body, and the mental perfection will follow as a matter of course," Sargent concluded. But as much as anything, Sargent enjoyed tinkering with exercise-related inventions. He invented an industry's worth of machinery: The Abdominal Table, the Chest Developer, Finger Machine, Head Lifting Machine, Inomotor, Leg Rotating Machine, Sculling Machine, Spirometer, the Travelling Bar. Sargent developed tests, training plans, and games ("Battle Ball") too. He formalized best practices for an emerging field.

1) Be examined by a reputable physician and present a written opinion. 2) Understand that it is not desirable to engage in violent exercise until eighteen or twenty because the heart and lungs are not fully developed until then. 3) Avoid tight clothing which strains the heart. 4) See that the blood is circulated and warm before severe exertion. 5) Eat a light meal no sooner than three hours before a contest. 6) Do not take a cold shower after vigorous exercise. 7) Make careful preparation and training to attain condition.

On March 26, 1880, Roosevelt arrived at Sargent's office for his mandatory exit examination. The scene he confronted was an uncomfortable one, according to others who had gone through the process: "On the threshold of the door, three or four utterly naked young men were waiting until their names were called." Roosevelt took his place.

When it was Roosevelt's turn, Sargent, with the help of an assistant, used an "Anthropometric Chart" (of his own crafting) to take sixty measurements. "Next comes the tape measure," the *Boston Weekly Globe* explained in an 1881 feature on Sargent. "Height, weight, girth of head, neck, forearm, upper arm, chest, inflated and contracted; waist, hips, thighs, valves, feet, breadth of shoulders, length of arms and legs, all are taken." Only a few slots on Roosevelt's form (including "temperament") were left blank. The most critical finding came toward the end of the examination when Sargent tested the "strength of lungs" for young Roosevelt. Using a simple but effective tool called a manometer, Sargent recorded a lung score of ten for TR. The average college aged man blew a thirty.

After the measuring, Sargent dug further into his patient's health background, asking "about his father and his mother, his grandfathers and his grandmothers, what diseases they had died of, and which of them he looked like the most." Sargent wanted every scrap of information he could get. "Information about his heartbeat, the size of his liver, and his breathing rate were written down. He was asked if he caught colds easily, and if he had nosebleeds," reported one health-conscious reporter. Then finally, Roosevelt was allowed to get dressed. By the end of the examination, Sargent had serious concerns about the damage caused by Roosevelt's asthma.

Roosevelt graduated from Harvard University on June 30, 1880. Still euphoric over his romance and upcoming marriage with Alice, Roosevelt declared himself the most satisfied of college graduates. "I can not imagine any man's having a more happy and satisfactory four years than I have had," he wrote on commencement day. The proximity of the subject at hand, however, may have clouded Roosevelt's judgment of Harvard. In the decades following his time at Harvard, Roosevelt would consistently downplay the utility of his college degree. It had been a positive experience, but it was hardly applicable, or even relevant, to the work that he went on to do. "I thoroughly enjoyed Harvard," Roosevelt summarized years later, "and I am sure it did me good, but only in the general effect, for there was very little in my actual studies which helped me in afterlife."

This interpretation by Roosevelt revealed a strain of self-acknowledgment that hampered him throughout his life. Roosevelt liked the self-made-man narrative when he could swing it, even if it meant categorizing something as significant as family money or a Harvard education as a mere bystander to his success.

Roosevelt counted down the fall days until his wedding. His excitement overflowed from the pages of his diary. "I am so happy that I hardly know what to do," he wrote on September 30, 1880. "I am living in a dream of delight with my darling, my true-love," he declared a few days later. Looking toward the future, Roosevelt enrolled in Columbia University's Law School. Dreams of becoming a natural scientist had receded to a desire to provide the material comforts that both he and Alice had grown up enjoying. Finally, after an intense, ten-month engagement, Roosevelt and Alice wed on October 27, 1880. It was Roosevelt's twenty-second birthday. Elliott (he of the slower race times and short jumps) served as his brother's best man. "At 12 o'clock, on my 22nd birthday, Alice and I were married. She made an ideally beautiful bride; and it was a lovely wedding. We came on for the night to Springfield, where I had taken a suite of rooms for the night. Our intense happiness is too sacred to be written about."

The couple honeymooned twice, first for several weeks on Oyster Bay, then for five months in Europe. Alice enjoyed it all. "Teddy and I take lovely drives every morning and in the afternoon we either play tennis or walk," Alice wrote to Corinne. That the two young lovers could share physical, athletic pursuits together was an immeasurable bonus to their union. Then the couple moved in with the Roosevelt family, securing the third floor as their own in the New York City home. Roosevelt, somewhat reluctantly, entered Columbia University's Law School. Alice began an aggressive slate of social networking.

When it became clear that he had no interest in pursuing work as a lawyer, Roosevelt dropped out of Columbia. He turned to politics and in 1882 won election to the New York State Assembly. Theodore and Alice moved into a boarding house in Albany.

While the political victory was satisfying, Roosevelt loathed his time in New York's assembly. The problem from TR's perspective stemmed from the fact that he had almost no leeway in Albany under the machine leadership of Roscoe Conkling. His position amounted to rubber stamping. Only a few days into the 1882 session, just days into his political career, Roosevelt was pouting. "January 7, 1882: Work both stupid and monotonous," Roosevelt wrote in his diary. Roosevelt's ideas went nowhere: "I have introduced several bills, the most important being one to build a new aqueduct which has no chance of passing." Furthermore, Roosevelt had a particular spite for his political opponents, especially those that came from a different strata of society than his own. "There are some twenty-five Irish Democrats," Roosevelt noted in 1882, "all either immigrants or the sons of emigrants...They are a stupid, sodden vicious lot, most of them being equally deficient in brains and birth."

The couple had some concerns about fertility; Alice had a gynecological surgery earlier in the marriage. Thus news in the summer of 1883 that Alice was pregnant was celebrated with abandon. "Oh how doubly tender I feel toward you now! You have been the truest and tenderest of wives," Roosevelt wrote to Alice during the pregnancy, "and you will be the sweetest and happiest of all little mothers."

After a complication-free pregnancy, the baby (named Alice after her mother) was born on February 13, 1884. Theodore did not attend the birth. This was perfectly acceptable behavior for the time. Instead he kept his normal routine in Albany, confident that his presence was entirely unnecessary. He received a telegram with the news and order to return to New York when the birth was complete. "I love a little girl," Alice gushed in the minutes after the birth. Alice held baby Alice on her chest as the doctor went through the post-delivery checkup.

Then things began to take a turn for the worse. Alice, just twenty-two years old, was reeling from the physical trauma of child birth. "Alice has had her child in her arms and kissed it," her mother reported in an ominous tone shortly before Alice lapsed into a semiconscious state.

*   *   *

Dudley Sargent traveled with Theodore Roosevelt, residing somewhere in his psyche, after the future president of the United States left Harvard.

Roosevelt entered adulthood with a prestigious degree, a beautiful bride, and considerable family wealth. The Strenuous Life seemed there for the taking. But Roosevelt had also been issued an ultimatum—stop exercising or face near certain early death. Drawing on the best medical advice available at the time, Dudley Sargent followed up his March 1880 examination of Roosevelt with a harsh, snap diagnosis and warning. Due to the strain on his lungs over the past two decades, Roosevelt risked grievous injury—a fatal heart attack, probably—if he exerted himself too fully. Sargent did not want his patient to miss his directive. There should be, Sargent chastised Roosevelt, no exertion. No athletics. No climbing or hiking. Certainly no boxing or wrestling. Sargent even warned that ascending stairs too quickly (Roosevelt was a stair bounder if there ever was one) could well result in fatal cardiac arrest.

It was a stunning, life-altering blow. Or at least it should have been. Instead, Roosevelt found whatever it was that he had summoned up when his father told him to "make his body."

"Doctor," Roosevelt said to Sargent, "I'm going to do all the things you tell me not to do. If I've got to live the sort of life you have described, I don't care how short it is."

Tragically, there was a life cut short, but it was not Theodore's. The joy of birth in the Roosevelt home was quickly clouded by crisis. Shortly after receiving a telegram in Albany announcing the birth of his daughter, Roosevelt received another informing him that Alice had some complications. Then another arrived with the devastating news that Alice appeared to be dying.

Roosevelt arrived back in New York City to find Alice slipping away. He held his wife for her last hours. At the same time, and in the same house, his mother Mittie struggled with a high fever. The next day, Valentine's Day, both women died. In a matter of hours, young Roosevelt had become a father for the first time and a grief-stricken, motherless widower.

Again, Roosevelt descended into a deep state of grief and despair.

Always one to process through the written word, Roosevelt took a compilation of news clippings and memorial remarks and fashioned them into a tribute for his wife.

She was beautiful in face and form, and lovelier still in spirit; as a flower she grew, and as a fair young flower she died. Her life had always been sunshine; there had never come to her a single great sorrow; and none ever knew her who did not love and revere her for her bright, sunny temper and her saintly unselfishness. Fair, pure, and joyous as a maiden; loving, tender, and happy as a young wife; when she had just become a mother, when her life seemed to be but just begun, and when the years seemed so bright before her—then, by a strange and terrible fate, death came near to her. And when my heart's dearest died, the light went out from my life forever.

The last line came from Roosevelt's own diary. This public, poignant passage would be one of the last times Roosevelt spoke publicly about the wife of his youth.

FOUR

THE TENNIS CABINET

*Don't ask me who won because tennis always bored me
and I didn't pay much attention to it. My impression is that
father didn't play a great game, but played very hard.*

–ALICE ROOSEVELT

After the loss of his young bride in 1884, Theodore Roosevelt declared he would never remarry. This was in keeping with Victorian traditions. The promise came from a place of overwhelming grief. Fortunately, it didn't stick. Roosevelt found "light" and love again. Rather quickly, in fact. In November 1885, less than two years after Alice's death, Roosevelt proposed to Edith Carow. She, having loved Roosevelt since childhood, accepted.

Though understandably chastened by his romance and marriage to Alice, Edith's reserve thawed quickly when she and Theodore met up for the first time in years in 1885. The sparks flew. As Edmund Morris described the romance, "Edith was as alarmingly attractive as he had feared—even more so, perhaps, for she had matured into complex and exciting womanhood. He could not resist her. Nor could Edith resist him." The passion caught TR by surprise. Roosevelt tried to explain his predicament to his sister Anna. He wanted Edith but felt trapped by his own moralism. "I utterly disbelieve in and disapprove of second marriages," he wrote. "I have always considered that they argued weakness in a man's character...But please I do very earnestly ask you not to visit my sins upon poor little Edith."

The engagement was kept quiet; Roosevelt wanted no disrespectful ideas cast upon his previous marriage. The new couple understood the timing was quick. They avoided attention. So thorough was the cover-up campaign that Roosevelt even avoided writing much about Edith in his diary, exhibiting nearly the polar opposite reaction to love as compared to his romance with Alice. Roosevelt used the abbreviation "E" to reference Edith in his diary, and even then said little. He did not describe the couple's visits or Edith's enchanting looks (Edith was a pretty, brown-haired, slender, dignified woman as the two fell in love).

Edith's childhood in New York City had been remarkably similar to Roosevelt's, primarily because she lived in the same part of the city and her family socialized in the same circles. She too came from wealth; the Carows had made their money in the shipping industry. Edith first met Roosevelt when she was four years old. And while the two developed an easy friendship as children, it was Edith's relationship with Corinne, Roosevelt's sister, which brought the two families into a close friendship. Edith spent many of her childhood summers at Oyster Bay, running and playing with all the Roosevelt children.

While Roosevelt always, *always* felt compelled to say something about everything, Edith listened first and then spoke up when she had something to say. She loved books and was content to spend long periods alone, this despite her capacity to make close friends. She was not interested in athletics or sports. When invited to participate in Roosevelt's childhood exercise regime at the piazza gym, Edith did not see the point. She was healthy and happy, so why would she submit herself to "such artificial exercise?" This view of athletic activity as something unnecessary (although fine for those so inclined) remained with Edith throughout her life.

When Roosevelt went off to Harvard, Edith could do nothing but wait—for Roosevelt or some other suitor. These were the times. Edith continued her own education, though, through the books she read. She won a prize in the *New York World* literary competition and read and reread the works of Charles Dickens. A few letters went back and forth between Edith and Theodore. But then in the summer of 1878, the two had some sort of fight. Exactly what transpired remains unclear. As Morris concludes, "History is silent as to the nature of their lovers' quarrel." Perhaps Edith rejected a marriage proposal. Regardless, what had been a slowly simmering romance turned cold.

Amazingly, when Roosevelt married Alice, Edith was there. She threw a dinner party for the Roosevelts leading up to the nuptials. Then she "danced the soles off her shoes" at the wedding. Then when the double funeral for Alice and Mittie filled New York's Fifth Avenue Presbyterian Church in 1884, Edith was there, too, consoling the mourning Roosevelt family.

On December 2, 1886, the couple—Theodore twenty-eight years old and Edith twenty-five—married at St. George's Church in London, England. The city was engulfed in typical English fog on their wedding day, and the church was nearly empty. Thus a successful marriage and partnership launched.

The two made a perfect political pair. Roosevelt ran unsuccessfully for mayor of New York City in 1886, but then he rebounded quickly to serve as Civil Service Commissioner. This post took the family to Washington, DC for the first time, from 1889 to 1895. Next Roosevelt became the police commissioner of New York City. As he rose through the political ranks, Roosevelt cultivated friendships with all the Republicans that mattered—William McKinley, Jacob Riis, Elihu Root, Henry Cabot Lodge, and John Hay. He carefully navigated relationships with party bosses Thomas Platt and Mark Hanna. It was because of these connections that Roosevelt was named assistant secretary of the Navy shortly after William McKinley's election as president in 1896. "I owed the appointment chiefly to the efforts of Senator H.C. Lodge of Massachusetts," TR admitted, in part because it was so obviously true. But TR had done his part as well. Roosevelt's highly acclaimed book *The Naval War of 1812* had come out in 1882 and was so revered by the US Navy that a copy was placed aboard every ship in its fleet.

Roosevelt's time with the Rough Riders in 1898 took what had been a promising political career and launched it to another level. The Rough Riders summited San Juan Hill on July 1. On August 15, the Rough Riders landed at Montauk Point on Long Island in order to recuperate (they were briefly quarantined for fears of spreading Yellow Fever) and await disbandment. A month later, on September 13, Roosevelt wept as he formally dismissed his beloved regiment. "Three cheers for the next Governor of New York," one bold, predictive fellow called out. On October 4, Roosevelt accepted the Republican nomination for governor. There had been a brief pause when it became known that the Roosevelt family had changed its residence from New York to the District of Columbia for tax purposes, but the Teddy wave was too strong to be held up by such formalities. Roosevelt campaigned aggressively, highlighting his war record and previous service. When Roosevelt celebrated his fortieth birthday on October 27, the press corps presented Roosevelt with a cane and a bouquet of flowers. Finally, on November 8, merely eighty-five days after returning to American soil, Roosevelt won the governorship of New York.

Six months later, Roosevelt was shooting down rumors that he would join William McKinley's cabinet or perhaps even the 1900 reelection ticket in the vice president slot. "The Governor Not to Resign," the *New York Times* reported, during the summer of 1899. "Roosevelt Will Not Accept," the *Chicago Daily Tribune* clarified shortly thereafter, referencing an undetermined cabinet post.

By all accounts, Roosevelt did not want the vice presidency. He wanted to run for president in 1904 and worried about being "buried" in the vice presidency for four years. But Roosevelt's fans couldn't wait, and his political enemies wanted TR out of Albany. The wave of support simply overwhelmed Roosevelt. At the Republican Convention in June 1900, the issue became a fait accompli. In one case a group of pushy Kansans burst into Roosevelt's private hotel room, "Fife and drum and bugle headed the delegation with more than discordant noises," remembered sister Corinne. "Round and round the room they went, monotonously singing to the accompaniment of the above raucous instruments: 'We Want Teddy, we want Teddy, we want Teddy.'" What could be done? Roosevelt accepted the VP nomination for the 1900 Republican ticket.

Once nominated to the position he did not want, Roosevelt characteristically threw himself into the task. Roosevelt made more than six hundred speeches for the Republican Party during the summer and fall of 1900. Roosevelt traveled more than 20,000 miles by rail and visited more than half of the states in the Union. It was an exhausting schedule. Roosevelt averaged five speeches a day. Roosevelt mostly did politics as he did life—with a smile on his face. He wasn't above an occasional threat ("I'll kick you in the balls," he told one adversary in the New York legislature), but charismatic persuasion usually carried the day for TR.

Baby Alice, who had been abandoned by TR for nearly two years as he roamed the Dakota Territories assuaging his grief, was quickly removed from Anna's care following Theodore and Edith's wedding. Edith insisted she would raise Roosevelt's first daughter as her own. It would not be long before she had plenty of playmates. Edith became pregnant on the couple's honeymoon to France. The Roosevelt children arrived in quick succession: Theodore Jr. (1887); Kermit (1889); Ethel (1891); Archibald (1894); and Quentin (1897). This was the family Roosevelt brought to the White House upon taking over for McKinley.

*　*　*

The one-hundred-year-old Executive Mansion the Roosevelts moved into in 1901 existed in a state of perilous decay. Initial examinations by contractors hired for the restoration project found crumbling beams in the president's offices and an unsafe floor beneath the East Room. As heating pipes had been added over the years, the structural arches in the basement had been hacked into oblivion. The walls of nearly every room needed significant plasterwork.

As workers moved their investigations to the second floor of the mansion, they found themselves stepping lightly. The upper floors had settled to such a degree that an entirely new support beam and subfloor was required. The architects added a new roof, revamped ductwork, and completely fresh electrical wiring to the to-do list as initial examinations of the project were completed.

As if this wasn't enough, the initial report also suggested that the White House might well have gone up in flames without some improvements. "The electrical wiring was not only old, defective, and obsolete, but actually dangerous, as in many places beams and studding were found charred for a considerable distance about the wires where the insulation had completely worn off," the report read. Shockingly, inspectors also found there was no readily accessible standpipe for firemen to connect to in case of a fire. "In short," the White House reported after the renovations had been completed, "it was necessary to reconstruct the interior of the White House from basement to attic, in order to secure comfort, safety, and necessary sanitary conditions."

As a father of six children, and as a child of wealth himself, Roosevelt viewed the $600,000 appropriation from Congress for the task of revitalizing the White House as one of domestic necessity. He waved off the political risks that came with a massive taxpayer-funded remodeling project so shortly after assuming the presidency. The family needed safe and comfortable domestic space, and plenty of it. Plus, the White House would function better with a clear demarcation between domestic and political space. Over the years, offices had been haphazardly added throughout the White House, encroaching on the domestic wing to an "unreasonable and abnormal extent." Moving with telling boldness, Roosevelt acquired the necessary funds, bid out the job, and demanded that the rehabilitation project be completed in six months.

The winning firm, the McKim, Mead and White group, was told that the outer appearance of the White House was to remain "as near as possible to the original design as approved by George Washington." But the interior needed to include new functional space for hundreds more civil servants and press members than Washington had ever anticipated. Additionally, the president required that a new space for state dining functions be created. McKim, Mead and White took on the challenge with good cheer "because among no class of the people was the feeling for the historic White House stronger than among the members of the profession of architecture."

Due to time and political constraints, the architects decided on a strange compromise in order to increase office space, reserve the second floor exclusively for the use of the first family, and to improve diplomatic meeting space on the first floor of the Executive Mansion. It was determined that "temporary executive offices" should be built on the site of the greenhouses adjacent to the west side of the White House. Plans called for the new "temporary" office building to include a room for the presidential cabinet, the "President's office and retiring room," and a room for the press. From these plans the space that would eventually become the West Wing sprung up in a matter of weeks.

In the midst of all of this—the beautification and safety efforts led by world-class architects paid for by the United States Congress—the Roosevelt family decided that a tennis court should be placed directly outside the window of the new office addition.

One can almost hear the groans of the architects even today.

It did not look like much, but this tennis court at the White House became a tangible manifestation of the Strenuous Life presidency. Roosevelt set about transforming the Executive Mansion into a place of athletic activity. Through the activities on and around the tennis court, Roosevelt added athletics into America's arsenal of diplomacy and debate. It was not that Roosevelt somehow invented the idea of side-by-side, on-the-move discussions instead of more formal, face-to-face talks. But rather that Theodore Roosevelt normalized a radical comingling of physical and intellectual pursuits. So in that way, this was no ordinary tennis court.

We don't know whether Roosevelt actually directed the placement of the tennis court himself. The historical record on this matter is incomplete. Not surprisingly, advocates of the sport of tennis made it all TR. The *Complete Lawn Tennis Player* placed Roosevelt squarely in the middle of the decision. "At Washington, the seat of the Government [tennis] enjoys unusual prestige," determined one 1908 article. "Mr. Roosevelt personally supervised the construction of a hard-packed clay court in a corner of the White House grounds, not forgetting to add a dark green fence which should serve the double purpose of a playing background and a screen."

Letters between Edith and Kermit, however, suggest that the tennis court was served up as a present, to the president, from Edith. Given Edith's role in overseeing the landscaping of the grounds following the White House restoration project, this makes sense. Edith Roosevelt biographer Sylvia Morris suspects that it might have been less a present and more a nudging from the First Lady that the president needed to watch his weight. Roosevelt knew he needed to pay attention to his waistline. Life as the president "has been very conducive to me getting fat," he wrote as the court was being built.

Regardless of how it got there, the proximity of the tennis court to the workspace of the president was unprecedented. A mere four feet separated the White House tennis court from the president's office.

The court was just that, a court. This was not a presidential tennis complex. Shut off carefully from the public gaze, the court sat nestled behind a grass berm and thick hedge. The court was made of a compacted, clay surface. Described as "pretty gritty" and of "the black, coarse variety," the surface was similar to that found at nearby country clubs. Roosevelt did not worry about his guests' comfort. The court had no chairs or benches. Just a court. Just tennis.

Roosevelt had little patience for sports gear or accoutrements. He wanted a place for physical exertion. Thus the Spartan White House court suited the president just fine. In his early forties as he adjusted to the presidency, Roosevelt prioritized activity and exercise. "While in the White House I always tried to get a couple of hours of exercise in the afternoons—sometimes tennis, more often riding, or else a rough cross-country walk," Roosevelt reported matter-of-factly in his *Autobiography*.

Roosevelt played tennis often with his children, and when they were away from the White House he reported, in his almost daily letters, on the state of his tennis game. "Yesterday afternoon we played tennis, Hurbert Knox Smith and I beating Matt and Murray..." Roosevelt wrote in a typical update to Kermit. Sometimes, especially when weather made the matches more arduous, Roosevelt provided significant detail. "Played tennis...ground was rather muddy and net coated with ice. First Ted beat Mat in singles; then in doubles Mat and I beat Ted and Church two deuce sets." Did the teenage Roosevelt children—away at boarding schools and Harvard by this time—enjoy such updates? It's unclear. One would imagine a warm-hearted rolling of the eyes by the Roosevelt offspring upon receiving the scores and details of recreational tennis matches. But their father's pure joy and enthusiasm for the sport may well have won over even the adolescents.

For Ethel, who turned ten just before the Roosevelts moved to the White House, tennis offered the best opportunity to compete alongside her brothers. Football, baseball, boxing, wrestling—these were off limits to young girls. The sports paradigm emerging during the first decade of the twentieth century undoubtedly favored boys and men. But tennis was a game open to both sexes. And Ethel Roosevelt could more than hold her own. She possessed a double helping of athleticism. At school, Ethel was known as the "leader of all sports among the young girls."

To the press, Ethel seemed to be the perfect balance of athleticism and femininity—a balance that was always in the eye of the beholder. "She is a type of the life-loving American girl," wrote one Washington newspaper. She was tall and slender. "None of the Roosevelt boys can outdo Miss Ethel in the sports that boys love so well." She "has her father's spirit" and was "fond of outdoors and athletics sports," the paper concluded.

Still, the White House glare inhibited Ethel to an extent. She felt more comfortable playing tennis during the family's time at Sagamore Hill than in Washington. There she was "very frequently an opponent of her father." With older sister Alice largely off on her own adventures and Edith usually content just to sit and watch, Ethel forged her own path. She demonstrated that girls could compete in certain sports, but access always remained a challenge. "At Sagamore Hill, she never misses a day and to this study exercise is due her fresh pink skin and white complexion," noted one newspaper. "She can skate as well as she can ride, and she plays tennis with all the dash of her father and brothers."

The installation of the White House tennis court cost Roosevelt a few political points. Democrats tried to use the court as a wedge issue. As the court neared completion in April 1903, both the *Washington Post* and *New York Times* picked up on the story. The "President's Children to Have a Model Playground Adjoining his Office," the *Post* reported, missing entirely the true recipient of the court. The court measured 78 by 36 feet and required a crew of a dozen from the assistant engineer of Public Grounds and Buildings to build. The workers excavated three feet down in order to construct a completely level, compacted surface. The builders used the prevailing court-construction practices of the day. A court could consist of a closely shaven lawn or of compacted soil. The latter, however, was presumed better for the climate of Washington, DC. A trap rock screen rested overtop the compacted soil, providing a relatively hard and consistent surface (although this would not prevent a tennis ball from becoming lodged in the court over the course of the years). This surface, prior to concrete courts, was the best available, the same surface as that used at the Potomac Speedway.

Roosevelt's critics seized upon the White House renovations and the new tennis court as a sign that the president was out of touch with the average American. The *Commercial Appeal* of Memphis, Tennessee, for example, suggested that the nation could hardly afford, financially, to keep Roosevelt in the White House. "We want to see a Democrat in the White House again for a number of reasons," the *Appeal* appealed. "The White House has been enlarged at an expense of $500,000, a $2,500 tennis-court has been built for his children, and the living expenses have been about triple. We would like to see a Democrat in the White House in order that a period might be put to this carnival of graft and extravagance."

Roosevelt's steadiest literary supporter, *Outlook*, argued back in defense of the court. "Is the President Extravagant?" No. "It is true that there is a tennis-court on the White House grounds, but it cost less than four hundred dollars— which is a much smaller amount than was expended upon the greenhouses under the previous administrations." The sympathetic editors of *Outlook* articulated an early form of life-balance counseling. "We think there can be no serious objection on the part of any decent American to the President playing tennis with his children, and it is impossible for them to play tennis except on the White House grounds." Pay attention to the Tennis Court oath (Hint: the French Revolution), perhaps, but the Roosevelt White House tennis court was a nonissue. The GOP entered the *Outlook* article into the congressional record.

Puck, a devilishly satirical publication, produced a story representative of many Americans' feelings about presidential tennis. "In the Spring the President's fancy turn to thought of love, forty-love, if possible, for from that to a triumphant 'game is but a swish of the racquet.'" But, many wondered, and here was the potential danger, did such cavorting lead to compromised deals and off-the-record diplomacy? "The mutter of conspiracy is heard...Words arise, harsher words than 'deuce' and 'love' of the tennis court." So, the editorial postulated, the true "mission" of the White House tennis court might well lie not in friendly games but rather in creating political opportunities. "Who questions the happy outcome of conference or confab, the parties which have previously lobbed and smashed, volleyed and served together on a common level the smooth delightful level of the White House tennis court?" Then using Roosevelt's own words, and his appreciation for tennis: "If we must have a big stick, let it be well balanced, rounded at the upper end and strung with good quality of cat gut."

If there was a saving grace to tennis, politically speaking, it was that the game wasn't golf. Roosevelt viewed golf as political suicide. He would warn his successor, William Howard Taft to stay away from links. "I myself play tennis, but the game is a little more familiar; besides you never saw a photograph of me playing tennis. I am careful about that; photographs on horseback, yes; tennis, no. And golf is fatal."

When the White House renovations were complete, Roosevelt had a handsome workspace that faced south, toward Virginia and the Washington Monument. But most immediately, right outside his window, probably less than ten steps from his presidential desk, Roosevelt could see one thing in particular—the newly installed tennis court. This presidential view did not go unnoticed by visitors. William Bayard Hale spent a week with President Roosevelt in order to write an insider's piece on TR. Hale tried to convey, as many have since, the frenetic energy and incredible capability of Roosevelt. It was in this context that Hale noted that the president had obstructed his own view for the sake of athletics. "Imagine, then, a room thirty feet square," Hale guided his readers, "with three windows looking south over the White House grounds to the Potomac and the Virginia hills, the top half of the Monument visible over the back-screen of a tennis court..." Yes, Roosevelt could stand and survey his veritable kingdom *and* consider his serve and volley game.

* * *

In terms of the actual playing of the game, Roosevelt offended many tennis purists. To Roosevelt the game was meant for exhaustion and competition. He cared little about decorum. His partners ranged from children, to diplomats, to soldiers. The conditions of the actual match did not matter all that much to the president. Captain Archibald Butt, one of Roosevelt's closest confidants and a warm, personal friend, for example, reported to his mother, perhaps looking for a bit of maternal sympathy, that White House tennis could well mean a muddy drenching. "Yesterday afternoon Fitz Lee and I went over the White House to play tennis, the other two players being the President and Postmaster-General Meyer," Butt wrote.

> Just as we began to play it began to rain, and it did not cease during the afternoon. We thought, of course, that the President would stop as soon as it began to rain hard, but on the contrary, he played all the faster. We could not make any suggestions about stopping and the second set was played in a driving rain, with water over the entire court and the balls so wet that they would not bounce. The court being dirt, we had a great fun trying to run, for at every step one would slip and someone would go down. The third set was farcical, but he said that while people looking on might think us insane, yet we could get just as much exercise playing water tennis as water polo, and since exercise was the ultimate object of all sport there was no use stopping on account of the elements.

Here Roosevelt's philosophy shone through, even as the sun did not. Exercise was the point.

The White House tennis court served as the most visible physical reminder of a simple fact: Roosevelt preferred to surround himself with athletes. He connected politics and sports. *Sporting Life* noted this proclivity with satisfaction, seeing perhaps a model of political-athletic cooperation—at the highest levels of American society—that had not been revealed before. "Everybody knows that President Roosevelt is an all-around athlete; but it is not, perhaps, generally known that he has gathered about himself a Cabinet of men whose tastes are similar to his own."

While the working definition of "athlete" was always a moving target, a Roosevelt archetype had emerged by his second full year in office. Secretary of the Navy Victor Metcalf was a former Yale crewman, baseball, and football player. Postmaster General George Cortelyou and Attorney General William Moody were former baseball players as well. Secretary of War William H. Taft, "notwithstanding his 250 pounds," rode horses, boxed, and—above all else—golfed. Secretary of the Treasury Leslie Shaw was a horseman.

More important even than his official cabinet, which was filled with ex-athletes, was a secondary group of advisors selected by Roosevelt almost exclusively because they met his need for athletic companionship. The press labeled the group, tentatively at first and then, by 1906, as a near official title, the "Tennis Cabinet."

The group got its start when Roosevelt appointed five men—Charles Keep, Frank Hitchcock, Lawrence Murray, James Garfield, and Gifford Pinchot—to a taskforce meant to reform government operations. The Keep Commission was its official name, but the fact that each of the five were tennis players caught the attention of the press. They became first the "Tennis Board," and later the Tennis Cabinet. Their numbers swelled as the Roosevelt administration worked its way through nearly two full terms of service.

There is little doubt that Roosevelt's Tennis Cabinet fundamentally shaped the way that the president operated in the White House. These were the day-to-day advisors. These were the notably *young* men giving their opinions to the president of the United States as they batted balls or trekked through the wilds of the District of Columbia.

While the particular exercise varied depending on the weather, Roosevelt liked to spend a day or two each week on each, tennis, horseback riding, and cross-country hiking. He preferred to have company. The membership of the Tennis Cabinet ebbed and flowed over the duration of Roosevelt's two terms. Roosevelt described the group simply as "Men with whom at tennis or hunting, riding or walking, or boxing I have played, with whom I have been on the round-up or in the mountains, or in the ranch country." The ranks of the Tennis Cabinet included:

John Abernathy

Robert Bacon

Seth Bullock

Archibald Butt

Alford Cooley

James Garfield

C.E. Heffelfinger

Luther Kelly

D.J. Keefe

Jean Jules Jusserand

Francis Leupp

John McIlhenny

George Von L. Meyer

William Henry Moody

Lawrence Murray

C.P. Neil

Truman Newberry

John O'Laughlin

William Phillips

Gifford Pinchot

H.C. Pritchett

J.B. Reynold

John Rose

Herbert Satterlee

William Sewall

Herbert Knox Smith

Henry Stimson

Beekman Winthrop

George Woodruff

The group reveled in physical activity and a vague notion of strenuous courage. The men promoted and supported each other, always with an absence of decorum or formality. Joyful exuberance seemed to be the goal, if not the norm, of Tennis Cabinet interactions. The opportunity to celebrate achievements was seized. Robert Bacon, for example, earned special commendation from the Tennis Cabinet for an act of valor. Traveling on a steamship headed to Boston, Bacon, then the assistant secretary of state, dove overboard to save a drowning man. When word reached Roosevelt, a surprise banquet was organized for Bacon, at which the cabinet awarded Bacon a "silver cup" for his achievement. Bacon, suddenly emotional, could barely muster a word in response. Then the silver cup became an ongoing joke. "Now let us look for the next runaway horse, and we distinguish ourselves," several of the men kidded as they left the White House.

When one member of the Tennis Cabinet had to pass on a Roosevelt invitation for a walk, begging off due to too much work, Roosevelt dashed off a letter suggesting that "the day was not near when he would receive a silver cup like Bacon."

The Tennis Cabinet was anchored by three men: James Garfield, Gifford Pinchot, and Jean Jules Jusserand. Roosevelt likely played more sets and tramped more miles with these three men than any others between 1901 and 1909. They were an impressive trio.

James Garfield, the son of the assassinated president, built himself a life that reached beyond his martyred father. Garfield rose steadily through the ranks of the federal government and gradually earned Roosevelt's trust and affection. He was "a pleasant genial kind that meets you half way and takes you by the hand and shows you wherein you are wrong." It was Garfield that played several sets of tennis at the White House with Roosevelt as the two waited for the 1902 election returns to come in. Garfield became secretary of the Interior in 1905.

In terms of tennis, his game lacked both power and precision. After one "unmerciful" beat down at the hands of the president, Roosevelt (usually all good sportsmanship and "nice games") had even rubbed it in a bit: "Garfield, if you make as poor a commissioner of corporations as you do a tennis player, I am going to put somebody else in your place." On another occasion, Garfield launched a ball out of the court, hitting Quentin on top of the head as he played on the seemingly safe White House lawn. "You'll never know what the strenuous life really is until you are familiar with Mr. Garfield's play," Roosevelt said. But it certainly didn't hurt Garfield's career that he spent so much social time with the president.

Gifford Pinchot, a former football star at Yale University, helped President Roosevelt translate his ideas about conservation and environmental protection into legislation. Chief of the Forest Service, Pinchot could "wield the racket as well as he can chop down a tree." Pinchot rebutted the ideas of radical preservationists such as John Muir; he saw America's forests as assets to be protected *and* used. Pinchot rarely turned down a presidential invitation to the White House court.

Then there was the Frenchman. Jean Jules Jusserand did not fit, on many levels. Most obviously, Jusserand's primary allegiance, as France's ambassador, was not to the United States and certainly not to the Roosevelt administration. Jusserand did not owe anything to the president, at least not in the same explicit way that Garfield and Pinchot did. Jusserand became the ambassador of the French Republic to the United States of America in 1903. He held the post long after Roosevelt left Washington. Jusserand rivaled Roosevelt as an author. Jusserand was a Shakespearean scholar who wrote the definitive *A Literary History of the English People.* He wrote on diplomatic history (*With Americans of Past and Present Days*), the bard (*What to Expect of William Shakespeare*), and, perhaps most poignantly, of his own experiences in the United States (*What Me Befell: The Reminiscences of J.J. Jusserand*). Jusserand won the Pulitzer Prize in 1917 for *With Americans.*

Jusserand came to Washington with an extensive background in sports. He had written a history of sports and pastimes in France, which was published just months before he received transfer to the United States. A tennis player, Jusserand was also "an ardent devotee of the lost art of walking." He arrived in Washington, DC having just turned forty-seven years of age. During his first few months, Jusserand had little contact with Roosevelt, and he worried about the closeness of the German embassy to the president. And he worried that the torrent of German immigration to the United States would ultimately sway America's allegiance toward the Kaiser.

But then an opening occurred. At a White House luncheon, Jusserand's wife dropped a casual comment regarding the focus on courage so popular in French poetry. Roosevelt locked in. "Mr. Roosevelt, immediately interrupting all other conversation, asked me across the table if I had a translation of the poem [*Chanson de Roland*] with the text, and if I could lend it to him." Jusserand did; a friendship—involving scholarship, diplomacy, and strenuous recreation—was born. More than two decades after the fact, Jusserand remembered his developing kinship with Roosevelt wistfully: "I was welcomed from the first by that extraordinary man...President Roosevelt. A variety of interests in things of the past and things of the future, a disposition to give melancholy just its due, which is nothing at all, a fondness for sport brought us together and I became one of the Tennis cabinet..."

Jusserand's first year in Washington marked a difficult time to be a Frenchman serving in the United States. It was the year the United States celebrated the centennial of the Louisiana Purchase, the monumental expansion of US territory that happened as a result of Napoleon's wars in Europe. It was a celebration of one of history's most profitable purchases, one made possible by France's shortsightedness. Jusserand attended functions in Washington, DC and New Orleans in order to celebrate the Purchase. "The transfer from France to the United States of French-founded New Orleans and French-discovered Louisiana had taken place in 1803," he dutifully recalled. Jusserand traveled to the bayou capital for the anniversary of the "cession." It must not have been an easy event, although the influence of France in the Big Easy remained reassuringly evident for Jusserand.

Jusserand had the reputation as "the best player in the diplomatic list." His game was a mix of agility and skill. A short, trim man, Jusserand could track down balls all over the court. Certainly Jusserand had an advantage over Roosevelt on the court; off it, all bets were off. Once, after a tennis match, TR persuaded Jusserand to do some jogging and calisthenics on the White House lawn. Then, and this is where Jusserand really suffered, Roosevelt coaxed his French friend into a medicine ball workout.

"What would you like to do now?" Roosevelt asked—after the tennis, jogging, and medicine ball.

"If it's just the same with you Mr. President, I'd like to lie down and die."

On the court, we know Roosevelt had significant limitations. Daughter Alice recalled, many years later in the midst of a White House tennis revival during the Gerald Ford administration, "My impression is that father didn't play a great game, but played very hard." Or as another contemporary put it: "He played tennis vigorously on the White House courts, though he never became very expert, there being no danger at any time of the President's entering the National Tennis Tournament at Newport."

A *Washington Post* report provided a rare glimpse of Roosevelt's game. First things first: Roosevelt made for a noticeably husky tennis player. He was not light on his feet. Always aware of the level of exertion (and perspiration) experienced during an athletic interlude in his busy day, TR often encumbered himself further with heavy clothing. "Even when the other players disport themselves in flannels and soft shirts with rolled up sleeves the President sticks to his sweater and his heavy trousers." On another day, Roosevelt showed up to the court in "rough-and-ready flannels, neither new nor fashionable." TR wanted to sweat and, hopefully, lose a few pounds each time he took to the court.

Partnering with the president in a doubles match was often a difficult task. The pressure of disappointing the thoroughly engaged president loomed. Additionally, TR needed his partner to cover significant ground.

[His partner] dances nimbly about the court, covering about ten miles to the President's one. At the same time the President, though a rather ponderous player, seems to keep up his end of the game. He gets most of the balls that come his way, though if he were to try singles it might be a very different story.

Roosevelt also served the ball in a singular fashion. He held the ball and his racket aloft, at precisely the place where a direct, straight shot could be orchestrated. Then, "the ball itself he holds right against the racquet. For several seconds he stands absolutely motionless in that position and then, smack! He hits the ball one of these hard, short, straight blows." The serves nearly always went in with plenty of pace. Still the privileged journalist who assessed Roosevelt's game estimated that the deliberateness of the process (along with a complete lack of deception) made returning the president's serves quite simple for a competent player.

Perhaps above all, Roosevelt wanted effort. Those who postulated that the tennis matches at the White House were simply politicking in a different venue would have been surprised at the decorum of some of the participants. Roosevelt did not play "hit and giggle" sports. Archibald Butt, writing to his mother, explained the focus expected on TR's tennis court. "Yesterday I played tennis with the President again, but this time got licked by him," Butt wrote in June 1908. "The Tennis Cabinet is supposed to be that coterie which plays tennis with the President and between plays gives him points on people and things. If some of them could see how little talking there was at these alleged tennis cabinet meetings." Instead, Butt clarified, the hours spent at the tennis court with the president were strictly about tennis. "The only way for one to make himself solid with this man when doing anything is to do it hard."

The game and exercise came first, but politics were indeed never far beneath the surface. The performance of a man on the court, or during a romp through Rock Creek Park, often shaped how that individual fared with the president. Nearly eighty years after the fact, *Sports Illustrated*, which judiciously stays away from diplomatic history usually, summarized French-American relations as one determined by tennis. "It is said that France's ambassador, Jean Jules Jusserand, so wowed Roosevelt with his vigorous game that TR completely changed his attitude toward the French government," *SI* clarified, forever shaping the sports-obsessed American's view of diplomatic history.

Many had the same opportunity; but countless others, including all women and American men of color, were denied even a chance. Setting up White House tennis matches ranged from a casual request, to an official invitation. On the former front, in 1907, the Lord Bishop of London, Rev. Arthur F. Winnington Ingram, found himself taking the court shortly after arriving in Washington. He had not planned for the event. He didn't bring a tennis racket or the prerequisite attire. Winnington Ingram, an accomplished theologian and preacher, was on a crusade of sorts. He sought to save souls, not serve and volley. Winnington Ingram's "The Call of the Father" urged a return toward God and away from sins. The modern age, "with telephone, telegraph, motorcars, and what not" did not necessarily cause spiritual waywardness, according to the bishop, but it surely provided a multitude of distractions.

President and Mrs. Roosevelt welcomed the Bishop of London to the White House. After proper protocol and greetings had been taken care of, Roosevelt began goading the good preacher toward the tennis court. The two men walked the White House grounds. TR mentioned the superior abilities of American athletes. Then, as the strolling men reached the White House tennis court, the bishop mentioned that "England also had a few tennis players to boast of." That was all it took. Roosevelt, having learned prior to the visit that this particular man of God was known for his prowess on the cricket pitch and tennis court, as well as at the pulpit, declared it a perfect time for some tennis.

Roosevelt sent his boys scurrying for rackets. They returned with the equipment, as well as a sweater and shoes for the visitor, and "in less time than it usually takes Mr. Roosevelt to unlimber his muscular arms the game was in progress." As usual, the game was doubles. Two members of the Tennis Cabinet, Assistant Attorney General Alford Cooley and Secretary of the Interior James Garfield, just happened to be loitering nearby. Why yes, they quickly accented, they did have time for a quick afternoon doubles match. Bishop Ingram, given the potentially awkward task of selecting his partner first, chose wisely. He picked Cooley.

The fall day was perfect for tennis. The draining humidity of the summer had lapsed. An invigorating fall wind whipped through the tiny tennis arena. The teams, however, were far from evenly matched. Roosevelt and Garfield, a politically powerful doubles pairing, could not keep up with their younger competitors.

It took the President but a few moments to realize that, in light and airy parlance, "he was up against it." Like a good fighter he is, however, there was no let up in his determination to win, but somehow his racquet seemed too short, and the little, tantalizing ball too small, and, besides, the bishop and Mr. Cooley were at their best. Several sets were played before the players laid aside their racquets to prepare for dinner. The President accepted his defeat good-naturedly, and there is promise of more tennis at the White House before the bishop departs for his native shores.

This scene, which is jarring to today's sensibilities, was remarkably common at the Roosevelt White House. A distinguished visitor arrived, prepared for discussions and diplomacy. But the president, cognizant of his daily need for physical exertion, quickly changed the course of the visit. He wanted a co-conspirator in his hourly fight against sedentary life. So the visitor became, in the simplest terms, a Rooseveltian playmate.

The nation took note. As story after story came out about the president on the tennis court (or boxing or attending football games), the point was hard to miss. Serious men, doing serious things, could include exercise and athletics as an important part of their days.

* * *

Tennis itself changed during the Roosevelt era. The game's American roots were, like baseball and football, decidedly linked to New York and New England. The first courts in the United States opened in 1874 in Staten Island, New York, and Nahant, Massachusetts. Newport, Rhode Island, became the center of American tennis when the nascent United States Lawn Tennis Association established its headquarters at the Newport Casino Club in 1881. Fitting such locales, the game catered almost exclusively to northeast elites. Wealthy socialites and cultured businessmen dabbled in tennis, often as a means of hierarchical climbing. Critics of the game tabbed it as too feminine, too haughty, and too refined to be worthy of "real" athletes. In short, the game didn't sound very Rooseveltian at all.

Change came to tennis, as Theodore Roosevelt might well have predicted, due to a Harvard man. Dwight F. Davis established the International Lawn Tennis Challenge Cup, later to become the Davis Cup, in 1900. The competition pitted American players versus their British counterparts. The matches would eventually expand to be an international competition, the American team versus all others. This patriotic component marked an important shift for the game. International competition, especially against Britain, fueled American interest. The competition also helped shift the reputation of tennis away from the women in white dresses and frilly hats image to that of a tactical, athletic game.

Even with the changes brought by Davis and others, tennis still provided the most developed athletic structure in which women could compete during the Roosevelt era. Wimbledon had begun hosting a women's singles tournament in 1884. The US Open followed in 1887. Two American women emerged as stars on the tennis circuit at the turn of the century: May Bundy and Hazel Wightman, both from California. Both won US Open championships and emerged as two of the first female athletic stars in the United States. They did so wearing dresses that went to their ankles. But they still competed; they still won. When Bundy dared to roll up her sleeves at Wimbledon in 1905, she was derided as the "Pasadena Washer Woman"—an insult on the class front. To a certain extent, the ability of women to compete in tennis was offset by the fact that these women had to be rich. Tennis at the turn of the century took place at "the summer resort and the country club." In these cloistered environments women could compete.

Even beyond the athletic clubs, however, there was an idea of the "athletic girl" emerging more broadly. The obvious fact was that many of the same concerns about the enervating effects of industrial life applied to girls and women. So, if athletics were fit to solve such problems for boys and men, the thinking might have gone, they would benefit female Americans too. But the gender politics of the time did not allow such a simple conclusion. Opportunity came, but within strict constructs. The chance to compete in tennis, for example, and the successes of Bundy and Wightman did indeed represent some progress. However, the scales remained grossly out of balance. Progress occurred mostly in areas of the athletic world that men did not particularly care about. "The 'athletic girl' won acceptance," Susan Cahn, an expert on gender and sport, suggests, in part, "because as long as the numbers of women participating in sport remained small, the female athlete did not yet jeopardize men's actual control over the sporting world."

So in Roosevelt's world, Ethel could play, sure, but usually after Ted, Kermit, Archie, and even Quentin had their chance first. And not until the Tennis Cabinet had cleared the court. This despite the fact that by the time Ethel turned sixteen she could bring all the game to the court that any Roosevelt could handle. Perhaps she was even the best in the family. "She can beat all four of her brothers at tennis," the *Chicago Tribune* reported, matter of factly.

FIVE

CREATING THE ROOSEVELT
ATHLETIC LEAGUE

*I do not mean to say that a very bright fellow can play
football well, or that a tolerably dull fellow cannot; but
if you find a boy who is too shiftless to work at his books he
will also be too shiftless to work at sports in the long run.*

—THEODORE ROOSEVELT

The headline kept it simple and got it right: the story was in the size.

SCHOOL ATHLETICS ON A BIG SCALE

On November 29, 1903, the *New York Times* printed the announcement by General George W. Wingate, a partner in the Wingate & Cullen Law Firm and the president of the National Rifle Association. A new venture had been formed—the New York City Public Schools Athletic League (PSAL). The PSAL declared a clear, ambitious purpose, "for the boys of our public schools to get the sort of exercise that could develop their bodies and bring them into sturdy manhood." Within three years, girls too would be added to the mandate, but always with the caution that "it is not the ideas to have the girls' branch resemble the boys."

There was no time to waste. While "country boys" were tossing hay bales and digging post holes to develop rugged, muscular bodies, the residents of cities were getting weaker by the day. Urban life was depriving children of the physical rites of passage that their ancestors had taken for granted. Therein this new organization, of which Wingate announced himself as president, had its vital cause and usefully nebulous crisis.

In the days following the announcement, Wingate moved quickly to complete the incorporation process for the PSAL. The ducks had all been lined up. Wingate—a decorated Civil War veteran, an expert in railroad law, and the "father of rifle practice in America"—was a man who knew how to get things done. Seventeen preselected directors signed the articles of incorporation. They agreed upon bylaws and put out the word that a massive inaugural PSAL athletic meet would be held December 26, 1903.

The PSAL directors themselves were a show of force. Religious and educational authority? Check. Political wherewithal? Check. Support from the athletic establishment? Check. Led by Wingate, the group included:

> Victor Dowling—Senator, State of New York
> John Finley—President, Colleges of the City of New York
> Luther Gulick—Director of Physical Training, New York
>   Public Schools
> Gustave Kirby—Chairman, Intercollege Amateur Athletic
>   Association of America
> Michael Lavelle—Rector, St. Patrick's Cathedral
> William Maxwell—Superintendent, New York Public Schools
> William Rainsford—Rector, St. George's Episcopal Church
> Henry Rodgers—President, New York Board of Education
> James E. Sullivan—Secretary-Treasurer, Amateur Athletic Union

And the directors were only the start. New York society's A-listers quickly jumped on board as patrons. The effort snowballed. "Our League was organized in December [1903]," Wingate reported in a letter to Roosevelt at the beginning of the 1905 school year. "It already numbers some 800 of the most prominent men in New York...a large number of educational leaders, many prominent athletes and leading business men, among them J.P. Morgan, August Belmont, Edward M. Shepard and many others." Andrew Carnegie and John D. Rockefeller provided their endorsements and financial support to the PSAL. The ruthless financier J.P. Morgan, renowned for his solitary character, signed on too, as did the powerful Guggenheim family. S.R. Guggenheim went so far as to accept the role of chief financial officer for the PSAL. The Guggenheim family had mostly made its philanthropic mark in the art world. New York's Guggenheim Museum holds many of the world's most valuable pieces of art even today. But the mining clan added interscholastic sports to its list of causes.*

The seemingly overnight success of the PSAL resulted from the groundwork that had been laid, culturally and politically, long before its founding. Physical education classes became popular in schools beginning in the 1880s. Tournaments and competitions involving high school aged athletes proliferated during the last decade of the nineteenth century. There were opportunities in baseball, handball, basketball, swimming, track and field, tennis, and football. There were also loose attempts at creating league structures—including several in New York City—around the turn of the century. But finding the proper level of organization proved difficult. Thus in 1902, the National Education Association issued a call for a renewed focus on the organization of school-based athletics moving forward.

The foundation was laid for quick buy-in from all manner of important individuals. The trophies told the story. The Spalding Guide for the PSAL listed the season ending trophies and awards doled out by the new organization. Dozens of awards "Presented by William R. Hearst" recognized excellence in indoor track-and-field competition. The New York Athletic Club

---

* The equivalent today is difficult to fathom. For the sake of some comparison, try mentally pairing a relatively new sporting venture—say inline hockey—with one of the country's leading businessmen and philanthropists—Bill Gates. The "Bill Gates Inline Hockey League," funded and supported by the money of Silicon Valley, is roughly the equivalent of Carnegie, Guggenheim, Morgan, and Rockefeller almost immediately supporting the PSAL.

presented the Silver Cup for the Novice Championship for elementary track and field. The A.G. Spalding Company awarded the "Sliding to Second" high school Baseball Championship Trophy. The *New York Herald* gave a plaque to the high school team allowing the fewest runs during the PSAL season. The *New York Evening World* awarded the Invitation Marksmanship Trophy. The *Brooklyn Eagle* took charge of presenting the All-Around Championship Trophy to the top Brooklyn elementary school. Alfred G. Vanderbilt presented the Junior Basketball Trophy.

Roosevelt loomed as the biggest prize for the PSAL. Would the sitting president of the United States give official sanction to the PSAL? The courting began almost immediately. Jacob Riis, the New York City reformer and a personal friend of the president, took on the task of facilitating the formal "ask" for support. Riis sent off an appeal letter from Wingate, enclosed with a letter of his own. Here was a cause that the Strenuous Life president could not ignore. "I enclose the letter from General Wingate about the Public Schools Athletic League," Riis wrote. "*The whole thing is sound, right in line with your life and work, and full of promise.*"

The founding of the PSAL revealed a group of New York City elites bent on saving their city. Good intentions abounded. But "plain, stark fear" was there too, just as it was a part of many of the reform efforts during this Progressive period. "Judicious athletic sports are particularly needed by city boys," read the opening lines in the inaugural PSAL Official Handbook. "Because of the work, which in all previous years of the world's history has been available as a source of muscular education of boys, is now done very largely by machinery."

Lest it feel like I am falling into the timeless trap of focusing too much attention on NYC sports, the PSAL matters because it created a model for interscholastic athletics that caught on quickly. Cities from Boston to New Orleans to Seattle would soon set up similar organizations. One report linked seventeen other leagues directly back to PSAL standards. "There is scarcely a day upon which your President or Secretary fails to receive one or more letters asking for information in regard to the work of the League," a PSAL official reported. According to one historian of high school sports, it was the PSAL that laid the groundwork for what would become high school hoops hysteria in Indiana and *Friday Night Lights* in Texas so many years later. "[The PSAL] was the largest school league in North America and became a model for educators not only across the continent, but overseas as well."

That work and business had changed in New York City could be seen on every street corner. In 1903, the United States was nearing the tipping point of urbanization, nearly half the country's population lived in cities—up from 25 percent in 1870. New York City was exploding, growing at a rate of about one million new inhabitants per decade during the Progressive era. Businesses seemed more imposing as a merger wave had created bigger, more powerful corporations than ever before. A transportation revolution had connected states, cities, and neighborhoods in new and sometimes disconcerting ways. Wall Street had emerged as the world's most important commodities trading center. Certainly the Americans of 1903 (the nation had nearly eighty million citizens) lived, worked, and played differently than their ancestors.

This change came with side effects. And thus the second reason for the PSAL: "The opportunity for play, under normal conditions, has been largely removed by their not having space enough in the cities for athletic sports. The boys themselves are unable to secure opportunities for their own development." Working conditions had changed living conditions, which in turn changed the way that children played.

PSAL leaders acted in concert with other movements. They themselves were byproducts of a culture increasingly emphasizing physical health. "Muscular Christianity," a doctrine that emphasized saving America—especially American men and boys—from the enervating effects of city life through a "Christian commitment to health and manliness," had been blooming in the United States for more than two decades. Strains of the movement can be traced all the way back to the 1850s in Europe. Indeed the activities of YMCAs, American universities, and Roosevelt's Strenuous Life all had tie-ins to muscular Christianity. And, on some basic level, teams composed of school boys had been competing against each other for as long as there had been schools (especially boarding schools) in the United States.

But the PSAL represented something different, something more organized. Something targeted at a younger audience. At stake, as historian Robert Pruter describes it, was the "establishment of institutional control." This is when the adults took over. Never before had the public education system been so intricately involved in creating nonacademic change in American children.

The PSAL settled on an ambitious, two-pronged approach to schoolboy athletics. First, the PSAL planned to hold championships in track and field, baseball, basketball, and other sports. "These great city games constitute dramatic elements that appear in the public press and which are talked about by the boys." Second, the PSAL also, perhaps even more radically, pledged itself to do everything in its power to encourage wide, universal if possible, participation in athletics. The athletic ringers of this school or that school, the champion of Manhattan or Brooklyn, were not the point. The championships would only function to drive broader participation. "[The PSAL's] main interests and its largest activities are to get boys having average or below average attainment, into vigorous athletic sports." The child who would never hoist a trophy or see his name listed near the top of his school's record book stood at the center of the PSAL mission. The idea was to facilitate athletic excellence *and* universal competence—a vexing balance.

The "Button Test" quickly emerged as one of the marque features of interscholastic athletics. "Each boy who attains the prescribed standard," the PSAL carrot dangling began, "shall receive from the League a bronze button."

The standards:

Boys of Elementary Schools under 13 years of age:
60 Yards Run: in 8 3/5 seconds
Pull up, or chinning on bar: 4 times
Standing Broad Jump: 6 feet

For all other boys of Elementary Schools:
100 Yards Run: 14 seconds
Pull up: 6 times
Standing Broad Jump: 6 feet, 6 inches

For High Schools:
220 Yards Run: 28 Seconds
Pull Up: 9 times
Running High Jump: 4 feet, 4 inches.

Students who achieved a "higher standard" earned a silver button. There was no gold.

The plan worked. During the course of the Roosevelt presidency, the number of badges awarded increased significantly each year. In 1904–1905, one thousand one hundred sixty-two New York City students earned their PSAL Athletic Badges. From there the numbers grew rapidly.

1905–1906: 1,654 badges awarded
1906–1907: 2,563
1907–1908: 4,000
1908–1909: 7,049

The PSAL Badge Award made the Strenuous Life quantifiable. Progress could be gauged. Schools tracked their participation rates; system administrators then pressured schools with low participation rates.

* * *

If this last part—the part about the buttons—sounds familiar, and if you now find yourself inexplicably thinking about staying home sick with a mysterious fever, you're probably remembering a twentieth-century outgrowth of the PSAL: The Presidential Fitness Award Program. From 1966 until 2012 children attending public schools in the United States earned the modern equivalent of the PSAL Button. The exercises were a bit different, but the intent to measure/encourage/embarrass children into fitness was roughly similar.

The PSAL button-to-presidential-award connection is easy to track. In 1953, Hans Kraus and Ruth Hirshland, doctors at the New York University

Medical Center, published the results of a multiyear fitness study, "Muscular Fitness and Health." Kraus and Hirshland had tested 4,264 American children and 2,870 European children. The findings startled the nation: the youth of the United States "were woefully unfit" compared to European children. Fifty-seven percent of American children failed the fitness test altogether versus only 8 percent of the Europeans. As a result, a parade of bureaucratic solutions appeared. First, President Dwight D. Eisenhower founded the President's Council on Youth Fitness, although ironically Eisenhower's heart attack forestalled the council from actually meeting until 1956. Next President John F. Kennedy established the President's Council on Physical Fitness, which—while not changing much from Ike's toothless program—expanded the scope to include all Americans. Then in 1966, President Lyndon Johnson added "and Sports" to the end of JFK's council and launched the Presidential Physical Fitness Award program (PPFA). The PPFA established tests, standards, and awards that, basically, reverted right back to the PSAL button program—but on a national scale.

In 1986, Ronald Reagan ordered a few changes. "We are a nation in search of excellence," he explained. "Promoting physical fitness in education will help us achieve that goal." So Reagan's administration expanded the test age; all students 6–17 would take up the PPFA challenge. The new test battery included five measurables designed to test flexibility, endurance, strength, speed, and agility.

Here's how test day tended to play out.

First came the sit-ups. "Pair up!" would come the order. "Student lies on back with knees flexed at ninety degrees; partner holds feet," read the standards. Partners were to count aloud the number of repetitions completed in sixty seconds. "Bouncing" sit-ups did not count.

Red-faced now, students moved on to the next task: the pull-ups/flexed-arm hang. Turns were taken, unless for some tortuous reason a school had dozens of chin-up bars. "Student raises body until chin clears the bar and then lowers body to full-hang starting position. Student performs as many correct pull-ups as possible." Only the non-swinging, "smooth and not a snapping or jerky" pull-up counted. Later, perhaps learning that American children couldn't actually do pull-ups, some Washington official slipped in an amendment that allowed students to simply hang from the bar, flex-armed, ostensibly without using their chin for support, for as long as possible.

Having suitably shamed a good portion of a given class for their complete lack of upper-body strength, the test whiplashed to flexibility. Using either a straight line on the floor or a devilishly constructed sit and reach box, students sat and strained forward as far as possible. Knees had to stay locked. Again, no bouncing. The "0 point" was at the end of one's legs; points could only be accrued by those children flexible enough to reach beyond their own toes. Everyone else got negative points. "While legs are held flat on the floor by a partner, subject holds soles of feet perpendicular to the floor (feet flexed) and slowly reaches forward along the measuring line as far as possible."

If things had started harmlessly enough, the PPFA took its pound of flesh from most American children with the fourth element. The one-mile run served as the true terrorizer in the process. "At the signal 'Ready? Go' the student begins running the mile distance. Fast times are encouraged; however, walking may be interspersed with running." For many, the mile run served as a death march. The venues for this task varied as much as the ability of students to complete it. Parking lots. Wide open fields. Cinder tracks. Around the school building. Even hallways, in some colder climates, made up the course.

Lastly came the shuttle run. The end was in sight. Instructors marked out two parallel lines thirty feet apart. Two blocks (or erasers, it was always chalkboard erasers at my school) were positioned on the far line. On "Ready? Go!" the student ran and retrieved the first and placed it on the starting line, then they returned with the second block. Not much room to get in trouble here other than cheating: "Do not allow student to throw blocks across the line," the instructions warned.

Students who scored in the top 15% in each of the five tests earned a special Presidential Physical Fitness Award. "The 8" x 10" certificate is suitable for framing and includes a Presidential Signature, Presidential emblem and a brief congratulatory message."

While the PSAL chased after Roosevelt's support beginning in 1903, President Barack Obama announced the phasing out of the Presidential Fitness Award in 2012. The nation exhaled. The memories flooded back and a form of Presidential Fitness Test Trauma Lit emerged—in print and online forums and even spoken word. The stories reflected shared national experience—albeit one that left its share of scars.

"Sit and reach. I sat, I reached, I farted. Ruined 5th grade."

"I have not attempted to do a pull-up in 20 years due to the shame scrawny grade school me felt at being unable to do even one EVERY DAMN YEAR. I also think I somehow got negative numbers on the V-stretch."

"For our Presidential Fitness test we went out into the field in front of our school and ran a mile, four laps around a rough, semi-grassy terrain. Off the start, I was kicked accidentally by someone behind me and lost my shoe. When I tried to go back to get it, my gym teacher yelled at me to keep running. I had to do the entire lap with only one shoe before I was able to get the other one back and then put it back on while running. Final mile time: 12:48."

Still, there was at least one good memory:

"I felt like I was failing my country because I was bad at pull-ups. But I kicked ass at the sit-n-reach. You could use my sit-n-reach to defeat ISIS."

* * *

The revolutionary behind the PSAL, Dr. Luther Halsey Gulick, was a tall, wiry man with a shock of red hair. Gulick was all jerky movements and gestures. He "was not," acknowledged one otherwise very sympathetic biographer, "handsome nor majestic nor austere in appearance." Gulick possessed a short attention span and quick fuse temper. He suffered from migraine headaches and depression. But somehow despite these shortcomings, Gulick fundamentally changed the course of American history.

He did so with a buckshot quality. Yes, his ideas went in the same general direction, but they still sprayed all over the place. He had strong convictions on a myriad of topics. On school: "The normal life of the child is one of steady activity during waking hours. [Because of school] we are taking away for five hours a day a large part of this activity." On play: "If you want to know what a child is, study his play; if you want to affect who he shall be, direct the form of play." On the meaning of life (with a nod toward Roosevelt): "Efficiency is the ideal. To be strenuous is no end in itself. It is only when being strenuous is an aid to efficiency that it is worthwhile; and sometimes the quiet life is more effective than the strenuous one. The pursuit of health is not an end in itself. But to live a full, rich efficient life is an end."

Gulick was born in Honolulu, Hawaii, on December 4, 1865. He was the fifth child of Luther Halsey Gulick and Louisa Gulick. Luther's father and grandfather were both missionaries. The Gulicks' moral and religious convictions had the unusual effect of actually determining how the family used its time. Jesus Christ and the spreading of the Christian gospel came first. The roots of Gulick's faith plunged deep; Luther's great-grandfather had once been called, simply, the most powerful argument for Christianity that any of his fellow townsmen had ever seen.

As a missionary kid, Luther Jr. moved from one lost civilization (spiritually speaking) to another. Spain, Italy, Switzerland, Japan—these were Luther's growing-up haunts. The movement between different cultures and peoples provided ready stimulation for Luther's curious mind. Luther was "always interested in new things, experimenting and inventing," remembered his brother Sidney. When it became clear that some effort at an organized education was necessary, the family sent Luther to attend Oberlin College in Ohio in 1880.

Oberlin was as good a place as any for Luther to try to put down roots. The bucolic liberal arts college, which had been established in 1833, was a haven for missionaries and abolitionists. The campus featured "thick, chunky, aggressively solid buildings" made from Ohio sandstone. Counter-cultural messages could be found everywhere. Under the leadership of mid-nineteenth-century President Charles Grandison Finney, Oberlin joined the fight for the abolition of slavery. Oberlin, Ohio—"the town that started the Civil War," according to one historian—itself had served as a stop on the Underground Railroad. During Gulick's time at the institution, Oberlin launched the career of Moses Fleetwood Walker—the baseball player who would become one of the first African American ballplayers in Major League Baseball in 1884.

So what was the heir of missionaries to do for a career? While his path to the mission field might have seemed preordained (and Oberlin supported numerous missionaries sent out from the school), Luther contemplated carefully the options that might become his life's work. Luther had shown a flair for entrepreneurship at an early age. He started a chicken farm while at Oberlin. The venture failed (lice), but it demonstrated Luther's willingness to jump into a capitalist world that his ancestors had largely shunned.

In terms of classes, Oberlin's records from the time are sparse. Luther took Latin and Geometry to some middling level of success. He worked at mastering the piano (Oberlin had a world-class conservatory after all). He joined the baseball team. But none of it came easily. Throughout his time at Oberlin, Luther suffered from severe, blinding migraine headaches. His vision, "trouble with his eyes," made reading difficult. As a result, Luther missed classes often. Following closely in the Rooseveltian pattern, Gulick's active mind seemed betrayed by his frail body.

Out of weakness blossomed interest. Luther became fascinated by gymnastics and physical fitness. He became a disciple of Oberlin's Dr. Delphine Hanna, a gifted, infectious, and path-breaking physical education instructor. With Hanna's help, Gulick threw himself into the study of the human body. He devoured texts like *How to Get Strong and How to Stay So* by William Blaikie. He came to think about the body as a machine: "It pays for us to learn how to run our machines on the higher levels of quality-efficiency," he concluded. Gulick also began to ponder a life that mixed the physical and spiritual. "Sitting beside a rail fence," Gulick wrote, years later. "We looked forward to the future of physical training. We spoke of the relation of good bodies to good morals, we thought of the relation of bodily training to mental training." Dr. Hanna picked up on Gulick's interests and recommended that he go where she had gone: The Dudley Sargent Physical Training School in Cambridge, Massachusetts.

"Gulick came to Cambridge in the fall of 1884 after having broken down as a student at Oberlin on account of trouble with his eyes," Dudley Sargent recalled. Luther enrolled in Sargent's Normal School of Physical Training, an offshoot school that Dudley opened in 1881. Mirroring his Harvard program, Sargent developed a curriculum to train (privately) athletes and physical education instructors. Luther jumped in, voraciously reading and studying, but he then left abruptly after only six months to take a position as director of the YMCA Gymnasium in Jackson, Michigan. He had bills to pay. Sargent was miffed that Gulick had the audacity to leave before completing the entire course. How dare he? But even Sargent had to admit that Gulick had an infectious energy about him. "He has considerable enthusiasm for Physical Training," Sargent wrote in a letter of recommendation. Further, Gulick possessed a "fund of mirth and vivacity that would enable him to inspire others."

Gulick had found his calling. Never a man for partial measures, Gulick wrestled with the carrying out of a physically responsible life. Gulick's romantic life had been one of the first casualties in this struggle. While at Oberlin, Luther met a charming young girl, a fellow redhead, who stole his heart. The two fell in love. But like Gulick, this suitor suffered from "migraine headaches" and a "highly organized" nervous system. Could love trump such physical flaws? Not for Gulick. Thus the two lovestruck teenagers wrenched themselves apart, determined not to have a sterile marriage or "to be responsible for further accentuation of their undesirable traits to their offspring."

The decision made sense, sort of. But what lovers think this way? Somehow when Luther looked at his potential mate, his mind went to places that he did not even fully understand at the time—eugenics, recessive genes, reproductive health—in order to make his decision. He would not play a part in combining two faulty gene pools in an unsuspecting child. Later a more suitable, healthier wife entered the scene. Luther met Charlotte "Lottie" Vetter on a camping trip. She too had grown up in a missionary home. Fortunately she did not suffer from migraines. The two married on August 30, 1887.

Gulick's career jolted forward. After a year in Michigan, Luther enrolled in New York University's Medical College. From there Luther took his medical degree to his first professional post: The School for Christian Workers (soon to be renamed the International YMCA) in Springfield, Massachusetts.

For the Gulicks, the children came quickly—four daughters and two sons. The family became known as "Springfield's experimental family." Luther and Lottie were "frank and enthusiastic about experimentation," wrote one biographer. "All kinds of ideas and theories were tested with the Gulick children." Luther forbade his daughters from playing with dolls. Lottie refused to plan meals ahead and usually sent several of her children to the store when dinnertime rolled around. Luther for a time adopted the policy of wearing only gray flannel shirts, insisting that the same clothes each day improved his efficiency. Lottie required that each member of the family play a musical instrument. Perhaps most disruptively, the family experimented with living aboard a boat. They would drift here and there and then sleep wherever the currents had driven them when the sun went down.

When the family did have a permanent, nonfloating, address, the Gulicks invited their neighbors on camping trips, often to Gales Ferry, Connecticut. Sometimes they rounded up a group of nearly one hundred friends for a journey into the woods. With a crowd at his disposal Gulick took charge, organizing morning sing-alongs and afternoon athletic contests. All of it—the trips and parental trial and error—seemed to be necessary to occupy Gulick's "insatiable, almost uncontrollable desire to experiment."

Gulick loved questions. He started one of his books (he wrote a dozen) with a few of his musings. "What is play? How are play customs formed? How are they passed on through generations? Can the underlying forces of play be so well understood that they may be applied in other directions, in education or morals? What light does a study of play throw on the nature of the player?"

With this seemingly endless stream of questions to answer, Gulick bounced from one experiment to the next. In order to study maternal instinct, Gulick and his colleagues turned a firehose on an innocent hen sitting on her eggs. How long would a mother's protective instinct last in such a context? Later Gulick sat one of his students in a bathtub and then proceeded to add more and more boiling water, testing how high one could raise body temperature via bathing. In order to test a theory on flexibility, Gulick sliced on the tendons in his own hand.

In essence, what Gulick was doing was grafting a new athletic tree, pulling from Christian teachings, European athletic culture, medical advances, and ideas of urban management. It was Gulick's tendency to force together topics that many of his contemporaries thought had little in common and then move on to an altogether different project that left James Naismith as sole inventor of the game of basketball—at least in the eyes of most historians. Naismith, an ordained Presbyterian minister, worked alongside Gulick as a faculty member at the International YMCA in Springfield, Massachusetts. In 1891, Gulick was teaching a psychology course that tested the very foundations of games. What were the dynamics, rules, subtle cues, and power dynamics that made people love to play a game? How did it work? Gulick, typically, obsessed on the matter. Suddenly, no game being played at Springfield's Y could be just a game. They became exhibits in a schoolwide debate on the gameness of games.

In this graduate psychology class, Gulick began working on a new game. He crafted a few provisional rules and ideas. The game was to be suitable for winter participation. Hopefully it could replace the boring calisthenic routines used by the YMCA during the cold months of the year. It should be fit for girls or boys, women or men. But then, as often happened, something clicked in Gulick's brain that told him it was time to move on. Gulick's attention shifted to the next question on his ever-fluctuating mental list. The start, not much more at this point than a handful of ideas and rules, was passed onto James

Naismith. Out of this athletic incubator, basketball, a game designed intentionally for boys and girls, was born.*

In 1900, Gulick left the YMCA for the Pratt Institute, a college and high school founded by oil tycoon Charles Pratt. At Pratt, Luther continued to try out educational ideas, usually with little regard for the traditions that he trampled upon in doing so. Luther pushed for the elimination of admissions standards altogether. He allowed any young man or woman to enroll in the school, taking part in whatever classes they might deem of benefit. There was no pressure to graduate. Physical examinations, Dudley Sargent style, were required, as was participation in either athletics or physical education. Gulick emphasized "health and vigor" as the building blocks to learning.

In January 1903, the New York City Board of Education, noting his work at the YMCA and Pratt Institute, offered Luther Gulick one of the most important positions in all of American athletics: the directorship of Physical Culture and Training for the Public Schools of New York City (PSNYC). He would be the first man to hold the position—a seat that oversaw all physical training for the newly consolidated districts of Brooklyn, Manhattan, Queens, the Bronx, and Richmond. The school system was gargantuan—the United States' largest. It contained 501 schools; 13,131 teachers; 622,201 students; 46 local school board districts; and an annual budget of $27 million (roughly $770 million in 2019 dollars). The PSNYC not only oversaw elementary and secondary education, it governed one of the world's most ambitious community education efforts. No interested man, woman, or child existed outside the reach of the PSNYC system. In 1903 and 1904, for example, the board of education organized 4,665 public lectures in New York City, which were attended by more than 1.1 million people. Night schools, playgrounds, and "vacation schools" providing after-school and summer programming—these all fell under the jurisdiction of the PSNYC.

---

* Although it does not compare to baseball's creation debate, some controversy does surround the question of who deserves credit for inventing basketball. The Basketball Hall of Fame seems to have found a middle ground, stating, "Gulick oversaw Naismith's creation of the game." Thus Gulick served as boss of the creator—not a bad title. http://www.hoophall.com/hall-of-famers/luther-gulick/; see also, Dorgan, *Luther Halsey Gulick*, 34.

It was into this enormous system, this conglomerate of learning and fund-raising and politicking, that Luther Gulick ascended in 1903. His ideas and experiments had reached the ultimate laboratory.

*   *   *

The task bordered on the impossible. Regardless of the particulars laid out by the board of education, Gulick had been hired to make New York City's hundreds of thousands of school children healthier. That was all. And he was to accomplish this feat nearly from scratch. The District had only a handful of physical education instructors, hardly any gymnasium space, and no set physical education curriculum. One of the PE instructors already working for the District, Dr. Augusta Requa, sued the PSNYC, unsuccessfully in the end, in order to undo Gulick's hire.

Undaunted, Gulick moved quickly. "One of the greatest dangers to city children," Gulick wrote in his year-end report to the New York Board of Education in 1903, "is that they may not grow up with strong vitality, with great organic vigor." Gulick saw the developmental paradigm as having flipped. Unlike in previous generations, fewer American children at the turn of the twentieth century were at risk of achieving a subpar education. Instead more children risked making it to adulthood "without the power of health."

More than a century before health experts would declare that "sitting is the new smoking," Luther Gulick zeroed in on the enervating effects of prolonged sitting, especially for children. "The general aim of the work," Gulick clarified in his long, ten-page report (the director of music by comparison needed only two pages), "is to correct the postural and other results that come from long sitting at a desk." In order to combat this mandatory sedentariness, Gulick organized the world's largest physical education effort. By the end of his first full year on the job, Gulick had hired three assistant directors, twenty-eight high school PE teachers, twenty-four elementary school PE teachers, and a handful of physical trainers and curriculum experts. This team undertook a massive training operation, teaching the District's teachers, who then carried out physical education training.

With this staff in place, Gulick organized a system designed to stimulate physical growth. As always, Gulick experimented. He wanted changes at every level. To start, teachers were instructed to give their students several two-minute exercise breaks daily. These breaks consisted, basically, of breathing and stretching exercises. On their own, the breaks did little to make children noticeably healthier, but the breaks provided teachers with a constant reminder that the physical bodies of their students needed attention too. Gulick quickly pushed through the scheduling of daily physical education classes (usually for fifteen minutes) and recess for all students aged ten and under. Teachers received physical education syllabi that delineated between those physical activities best suited for schools with gymnasiums (only 44 of the district's 478 elementary schools), those with some sort of outdoor or basement square footage available for exercise, and those with only classroom space. Additionally, hygiene instructors were brought in to teach students about cleanliness, disease prevention, and "personal hygiene and home hygiene."

At times, the fear of frailty outweighed the implementable knowledge of the public health community. Issues that Gulick could have never anticipated found their way onto his desk. Case in point, in Gulick's first year as director of Physical Education, a panic of sorts broke out regarding the rise in cases of scoliosis in the city. Why were so many children suffering from curvatures of the spine? In the panic, a theory arose that blamed the public education system directly. It was the books. It had to be. Carrying books home from school, on average 4.7 books per student (at a total weight of about five pounds) an investigation found, daily might well be the culprit. Was it possible that the children of New York City were quite literally being crushed by their educational pursuits?

With no one else interested in defending the PSNYC against such a charge, Gulick investigated the theory. He dispatched sixteen observers across the city to collect data regarding who was carrying what, how far, and how often. His researchers found that children did indeed haul their books back and forth between their schools and homes. And sometimes the children were overloaded; one child was observed balancing a stack of twenty-one notebooks as she made her way down the streets of Manhattan. This poor student was eager, the investigator surmised, "so as to appear to be in a high grade." Characteristically, Gulick devised a five-step plan to address the "problem." In addition to urging teachers to regulate what students carried, Gulick looked to Europe for solutions. European students, Gulick reported to the board of education, "carry their books home in a modified form of knapsack carried upon the back." Thus began the backpack's rise to ubiquity in American schools.

* * *

Gulick wanted to go big for the PSAL's first championship event. Although the organization had not yet secured Roosevelt's formal endorsement, Gulick had national ambitions. And so, after careful consideration, he proposed a "pyrotechnic relay race" to mark the occasion. The idea harnessed a bit of magic à la PT Barnum (who had mastered showmanship during the last half of the nineteenth century). The proposal foreshadowed the Olympic torch relay conjured up by the Nazis at the 1936 Olympic Games. For the inaugural PSAL meet, Gulick envisioned a relay from the board of education building to Madison Square Garden. Runners would carry a message from the board president to Mayor-elect George McClellan Jr., who was to preside over the games. Two automobiles, shooting off fireworks, would accompany the schoolboy runners through the dark streets of Manhattan. Every two blocks the message would change hands; another young runner would pick up the quest where his predecessor left off. Finally, the message would arrive. The evening session would commence. It would be a brilliant bit of pageantry.

Unfortunately for Gulick, and future interscholastic athletes everywhere, the board of education failed to grasp his vision. When the night-relay proposal was discussed at a December 8, 1903, PSAL meeting, "the announcement of the conditions for this novel race evoked considerable laughter." Chief Fuddy-Dud/Superintendent William Maxwell derided the relay as being "opposed to the athletic spirit of the league." Gulick offered a mild defense of the idea, but he could read the room. The "pyrotechnic relay race" was scrapped.

Gulick was left to find other ways to ensure that the meet provided the PSAL with a spectacle he believed it needed to launch a broad revolution.

Fortunately the sheer size of the event grabbed New York City's attention. One thousand five hundred twenty-three students signed up to compete. The *New York Times* concluded simply that the PSAL undertaking "was the most important athletic meeting which has ever taken place in the United States." The weather, however, made things difficult. A storm rolled into the city at nearly the same time the athletics were to begin; snow began falling around noon on December 26. All day long, the temperature plunged. Fifty-mile-per-hour wind gusts blew the powdery snow. And then when the snow and wind finally subsided, a murky fog descended over much of the city.

Still the children came. And they dragged along their parents. Perhaps because of the weather, Gulick got an athletic incubator the likes of which he could have only dreamed. Groups of school children arrived by the dozens escorted by teachers and parents. Police officers directed traffic into the Garden; each school received a designated place to sit. Those not competing had nothing to do but watch and cheer. Thus they cheered, and crazily. Hastily made school banners demarcated sections of the Garden stands for this school or that one. As the wind howled outside Madison Square Garden, a cocoon of athletic activity buzzed inside.

Since the athletic movement had preceded the manufacturing of athletic-specific clothing (it was not Nike that created athletics but rather the other way around), the competitors wore whatever they perceived to be suitable for competition. The athletic "costumes" told a story of the city's diversity. There were trousers, waistcoats, and knickerbockers. Shoes ran the gamut; some children competed barefoot. Many competitors grabbed the most comfortable piece of clothing they owned as they headed for the Garden—their bathrobes. "The spirit of the public school was everywhere manifest," the *Times* reported.

The New York City school system had desegregated in 1900, thus African American schoolboys participated as well. A considerable network of schools for African American children had existed in New York City before the Civil War. An audit compiled in 1856 counted 21 of the city's 214 schools as "specially devoted to colored children." The plan to gradually absorb the colored schools in the broader system began in 1880. But the integration effort did not come without some protest from both sides of the racial spectrum. As a result, in 1884 the city suspended the closing of the two final colored schools.

In 1900, a new governor of New York—Theodore Roosevelt—signed an order "finally and happily" abolishing racially segregated schools all together. Did the PSAL promote racial equality? Sort of. The PSAL provided the opportunity for racially integrated competition from the start. That was not nothing. The *Times,* however, followed fairly standard practice by portraying the "Negro Lads" as willing but not fully capable competitors. "Quite a few of the contestants were young negroes, whose white school mates whispered final instructions before the start," readers learned from the racially biased reporting.

The December 26 athletic extravaganza began with basketball. The elementary school tournament featured twenty-four teams. Next, nine high school teams competed for the senior title. The games took place in the center of the Garden infield with the running track encircling the action. Two games were played at a time. The situation was crowded and chaotic. Several times officials stopped a basketball game due to "anxious athletes who ran across the floor from side to side of the building in order to watch their fellows in the track events." No matter; the games went on.

The basketball contests featured fifteen-minute, running-clock halves. Very few participants actually knew how to shoot a basketball. Soccer scores abounded. Public School 30 defeated PS 123, 4 to 0. PS 8 beat PS 47, 3 to 0. These scores were typical. Although most squads managed to score at least one basket, the action was decidedly below the rim. Only one school—PS 122 (Brooklyn)—scored with any consistency. This team advanced easily to the championship match. There, the Brooklyn schoolboys defeated PS 166 from Manhattan, 40 to 2. The rout immediately aroused suspicion that PS 122 had ineligible (read: too old and too good) players. An official protest was filed.

"It is a wonderful showing," Luther Gulick told a reporter as the event buzzed on around him. "But the games, successful as they have been, are only a beginning." With the basketball competition winding down, the track portion of the competition took center stage. First came the fifty-yard dash, a race so pleasantly brief and exhilarating that every child it seemed wanted a chance at it. Thirty-eight heats of the dash ensued, one after another. The winners of those heats advanced to semifinal races. The winners of the semifinals advanced to the final. There, a lightning bug of a boy, Walter Bardell of Brooklyn, seized the prize.

After the young ones sprinted, the high schoolers lined up for their fifty-yard dashes. Next the boys from the City College of New York had their try. The events proceeded one after another. The 880-yard run. The One Mile Race. The 440-yard run. The 220-yard run. Shot Put. Running High Jump. Every boy had his turn. Fans cheered each finish. It was as much a celebration of movement and organized athletic activity as it was an athletic competition—although the leaders of the PSAL quickly took the results of the day and entered the top times in the first organization handbook under the auspicious "Indoor Records" heading. To win a race on December 26, 1903, meant setting a PSAL record. The night concluded with a series of relay races.

For Gulick, his PSAL represented something so entirely new, so stupendously exciting, and so daringly gigantic that he had to look across oceans and back millennia in order to offer some perspective. "It may surprise you when I tell you," Gulick said to a *New York Times* reporter standing beside him in the arena, "that they are the greatest games held in any country in modern times... not since the days when gladiators entered Roman arenas in thousands have so many contestants decided the question of superiority within the same time limit that we have to-night." And unlike the gladiators, some of these New York children did so in their pajamas.

*   *   *

The PSAL leadership was all white and all male. The competitors in the day-after-Christmas athletic spectacle were all boys. In the announcement of the PSAL endeavor, Wingate made the pecking order clear. "While the beginning of our work in the league will be with boys, the girls will not be neglected. It is certainly just as essential that they be strong and robust, too, but our efforts on their behalf will come later on." It was as if the nation's leaders sensed that all children needed a different, more physically vigorous, upbringing, but they could not conceive of treating boys and girls equally. The boys were the real crisis.

The PSAL echoed the priorities that President Roosevelt clarified time and again on the political stump. As Roosevelt had remarked to a group of school children on April 5, 1903, in Sioux Falls, South Dakota: "What will count in the future is the way the children turn out; how they are trained; the stuff that is in them." And then the pivot: "I like girls and boys; especially the boys; of course I am fond of the girls but the boys I like better."

Fortunately, there were a group of New York City women with the will and wherewithal to push the cause of girls' athletics to the forefront. Grace Dodge, a wealthy reformer and social activist, took charge at a meeting held on November 28, 1905. Vague hopes for girls' opportunities became a working program: "The Girls' Branch of the Public Schools Athletic League." The initial focus for girls was folk dancing (a favorite of Gulick's) and noncompetitive athletics. "It will really be athlete play," clarified one report. Certainly the demand from girls existed. "In the schools where athletics are in full swing, there is always a crowd of enthusiastic girls waiting for admittance at 3 o'clock," a New York City newspaper reported as the program was being rolled out.

Organizing financial support for girls' athletics proved difficult. Simply starting a program did not mean the New York City public school system would provide support. And so fundraising was a constant from the start. Always cautious about somehow steering girls into unrestrained competition, the PSAL Girls Division did not have the badge program but instead awarded "all-around athlete pins" to girls who participated in twenty athletic events.

At no point during the Roosevelt era did athletics for girls escape a suspicion that such physical activities might cause serious problems. Luther Gulick remained at once supportive and suspicious. "There is now sweeping over the country a wave of athleticism, especially of athletics for women, and it carries a good deal that is undesirable," Gulick said in 1905. Gulick supported basketball in particular as a girl's game but only in private. "Women should not compete in public," he said. Dodge, a talented socialite, knew enough to sell the earliest version of schoolgirls' sports as experimental and cautious. "One of the purposes of this organization," she had said at the founding meeting, "should be to discover how girls' athletic sports should differ from those of boys."

Despite all these obstacles, by 1910, more than 20,000 girls were participating, working with nine hundred teachers, in PSAL activities.

As the PSAL evolved, Roosevelt remained in the organization's crosshairs. "I feel that the work of the League is directly in line with what you have so frequently and powerful advocated that we are justified in asking you to help us," Wingate wrote to Roosevelt in 1905. Wingate wanted a letter and an official connection. "If you could honor us by accepting an office, as vice-president, honorary direct, director, patron, a life or annual member—*anything* to identify yourself with the League, it would be a tower of strength," Wingate wrote.

Roosevelt, perhaps recognizing that he had wanted such activities for his own children, agreed. He signed on and became a PSAL patron. Finally, a full-page photograph of Roosevelt adorned page two of the 1905 PSAL manual with the following caption: "Hon. Theodore Roosevelt. Honorary Vice-President, Public Schools Athletic League." Several pages later the marriage between the PSAL and the popular president became even more evident. President Roosevelt Approves of Public Schools Athletic League, blared the headline. Below appeared the nearly one-thousand-word letter from Roosevelt to Wingate in its entirety. "I most heartily believe in your league," the president wrote. Roosevelt identified "the great congestion in population" as the key challenge to overcome. New York City itself was the enemy. "It is a great disadvantage to a boy to be unable to play games; and every boy who knows how to play base ball or foot ball, to box or wrestle, has by just so much fitted himself to be a better citizen."

By 1905, the PSAL was sponsoring seven hundred events annually. When a request for funds to purchase fields for the PSAL was made in 1905, the justification rested on the numbers: "This is the big schoolboy organization that now numbers more than 100,000 competitive athletes and to which much of the present overwhelming interest in sport is due." The PSAL got its

$300,000 request from the city. The PSAL complex on Staten Island featured a large field (suitable for football or lawn tennis), a track, two baseball diamonds, and several basketball courts. Schoolboys participated in athletic events at a rate that dwarfed anything that had been done even five years earlier. "Already with its vast membership, which includes practically every boy and girl in the public schools of Greater New York," the very supportive *New York Times* gushed in December 1905, "it causes the athletic organizations of Yale, Harvard, and the triumvirate of big universities to sink into comparative insignificance."

As one final stitch in the tapestry connecting the PSAL to Roosevelt and the Strenuous Life, District No. 7 of the PSAL in 1907 officially changed its named to the "Roosevelt Athletic League." Even for a man having won a Nobel Peace Prize recently, this was an honor worth having. When Roosevelt wrote his thank-you letter to the group for attaching his name to such a worthy cause, he demonstrated a bit of progress as well. He closed his two-page letter with a simple wish: "Do let me say that I hope the girls will have their share of athletic attention just as much as the boys."

SIX

1904

The St. Louis Games were completely lacking in attraction. Personally, I had no wish to attend them...There was no beauty, no originality. I had a sort of presentiment that the Olympiad would match the mediocrity of the town.

—PIERRE DE COUBERTIN, President of the International Olympic Committee (and thus in charge of the St. Louis Olympics)

Try this for irony. For one relatively short period during his presidency, political decorum demanded that the ever-gregarious Roosevelt remain out of sight. Advisers warned him to keep his public appearances to a minimum and to avoid the big crowds that he adored. It was during that very period that the United States hosted a World's Fair (attended by twenty million people) and, for the first time, the Olympic Games.

Bizarre as it seems to us, to "act Presidential" in 1904 meant a president did not actually campaign for reelection to the office held. The dirty work of making the case for the candidate was to be done by friends and political partners. Roosevelt did not want to be accused of overt politicking. So Roosevelt knew what he had to do for the summer and fall of 1904. Stay out of trouble. Don't seem too eager. Avoid obvious vote-shilling. "My one safety at present and for the next seven months," Roosevelt wrote to Kermit in April 1904, "is to refuse to be drawn into any personal controversy or betray any irritation, under no matter what provocation." If Roosevelt could just be, well, understated, his chances for holding onto the presidency looked promising. The Republican campaign song promised as much.

All right Teddy!
You're the kind that we remember;
Don't you worry!
We are with you!
You're all right Teddy!
And we'll prove it in November Teddy!
We're going to keep you in the White House!
You're [sic] White House!

But as everyone around him knew, understated was not exactly Roosevelt's forte.

Although Roosevelt was in the process of creating the modern presidency, he remained tortured by the fact that he had not actually been elected to the office. In Roosevelt's mind, the 1904 election meant not only gaining another term as president, obviously, but also validation that the period from 1901 through the election held in November 1904 had been legitimate. He was not "His Accidency," as some newspapers, especially in the South, liked to call him. The American people had wanted him. They had understood his actions against the railroad strikers in 1902, and his support for the Panama Canal in 1903, and his use of the Reclamation and Antiquity Acts to irrigate the arid West and protect the Grand Canyon. And they understood the strength that America needed to show through (what would become known as) the Roosevelt Corollary to the Monroe Doctrine. Right?

The Mark Hanna wing of the Republican Party concerned Roosevelt the most in the early stages of the 1904 political campaign. Hanna, a senator from Ohio, reigned as the GOP's kingmaker. Hanna had emerged after the US Civil War, during which he served briefly in the Union Army, into the booming business scene in Cleveland, Ohio. The Hanna family had interests in coal, railroads, newspapers, steel, and steamships. Hanna became involved in politics to protect what he had built. Keep tariffs high and political corruption relatively low; this basically summarized Hanna's political ideology.

In the 1896 presidential election, Hanna threw his support behind William McKinley, a fellow Ohioan. Hanna took the reins; McKinley stayed at home on his front porch addressing the crowds that came to see him. The famous, and aptly named, "front porch" campaign worked brilliantly. With Hanna orchestrating a highly effective fundraising effort—he urged bankers to give a small percentage of their total wealth to defeat Democratic candidate William Jennings Bryan and his pledge to take the US off the Gold Standard—McKinley stayed at home, above the fray, and on message. McKinley was no puppet; he set the message and the overall campaign strategy. But he let Hanna serve as his major general, moving campaign troops and resources as needed. McKinley won the presidency in 1896 and then again in 1900.

Roosevelt had come on the McKinley ticket for 1900 as a result of the sudden death of Vice President Garret Hobart. Hanna had fought the Roosevelt movement at the 1900 Republican Party convention with all his political clout. For Hanna, Roosevelt's penchant for action first was a fatal flaw. The nation should not be exposed to such recklessness. When it became clear that the political tide at the 1900 Philadelphia convention would indeed turn to Roosevelt, Hanna pitched a political fit. "Do whatever you damn please!" Hanna yelled at party leadership. "I'm through! I won't have anything more to do with the convention!" It was an empty threat. Still, Hanna tried one more pleading. "What's the matter with all of you?" Hanna asked desperately. "Here's this convention going headlong for Roosevelt for Vice President. Don't any of you realize that there's only one life between that madman and the Presidency?"

Hanna's Republicans wanted a more conservative and predictable politician in the White House. Even as 1904 dawned, Roosevelt remained concerned that some sort of nomination challenge might emerge. He wrote to Ted, who begged his father for political news, "Senator Hanna and the Wall Street crowd are causing me some worry, but not of a serious kind. I doubt if they can prevent my nomination."

Roosevelt had maintained a tense working relationship with the Old Guard Republican leadership in the Senate. Hanna and his team—including Nelson W. Aldrich, William B. Allison, John C. Spooner, and Orville H. Platt—worked to rein in Roosevelt's antitrust pursuits. They sought to hold him back in the international arena as well. Coupled with longtime, crusty Speaker of the House Representative Joseph G. Cannon (described by TR as "an exceedingly solemn, elderly gentleman with chin whiskers, who certainly does not look to be of playful nature"), many of the leading GOP men in Washington, DC spent their time trying to hold Roosevelt back. And then of course there were the Democrats.

The problem for Hanna, Cannon, and the entire Democratic Party was that Roosevelt was the most popular president since Andrew Jackson. This was the dichotomy of the 1904 election. TR appealed to the American public in ways that few presidents ever have. Roosevelt had long, long coattails. Thousands of state legislators, county commissioners, and city councilors planned to claim very close allegiance to President Roosevelt as they sought to win their own political battles in 1904. Throughout the entire United States, with the notable exception of the South, which Roosevelt lost with the Booker T. Washington dinner in 1901 (among other factors), evidence of loyalty and even love for Roosevelt manifested itself everywhere.

The Democrats nominated Alton B. Parker—a conservative appeals court judge from New York. It was a terrible choice. Or as one political historian put it: "Theodore Roosevelt's landslide victory over Alton B. Parker in 1904 was a foregone conclusion from the moment of the New York judge's nomination, if not before." Judge Parker could not give a powerful speech, nor did he possess the ideological underpinnings necessary to promote any sort of aggressive agenda. He could not even deliver his own state—New York. While the Democrats felt they should not nominate William Jennings Bryan again (he had run for president in 1896 and 1900), the party missed the fire and fury of the Great Commoner.

Set against the Parker backdrop, any other candidate would have seemed personable. Roosevelt therefore was off the charts. Before the election year,

Roosevelt had built up his political balance. He toured through New England and the Midwest. Roosevelt's Rough Rider reputation still packed a powerful political punch as well. In 1903, Roosevelt had turned a soldier reunion into a long political rally. TR traveled from Washington, DC to the Grand Canyon. He invited his middle-aged (but still rough) comrades from 1898 to meet him along the way. Many were so excited at the prospect of a reunion that they celebrated a bit too much beforehand, becoming so drunk that they missed their rendezvous with the president. Still, Roosevelt traveled nearly 14,000 miles during a two-month tour of the West in April and May 1903. He made speeches (planned and impromptu) all along the way. Roosevelt even ducked his head outside the moving campaign train to shake hands with cowboys galloping alongside the railroads.

* * *

Given the political handcuffing of Roosevelt leading up to the election, it makes sense that 1904 became the busiest boxing year in the history of the White House. In terms of boxing *within* the White House that is. Roosevelt took out his frustrations in the ring. He boxed with Ted, who had left Groton to study for Harvard's entrance exams from the comfort of the White House. Roosevelt brought in a new fighter, Joseph Grant, for sparring and to teach him and his sons wrestling. Furthermore, Roosevelt invited an old friend to the White House for the first time: Mike Donovan.

Donovan was a boxing lifer. He had fought as a middleweight during the bare-knuckle era. In 1880, Donovan battled John L. Sullivan, then an unproven up-and-comer, fairly evenly. Donovan broke his hand in the Sullivan fight. A few years later, Donovan signed on to spar in nightly exhibitions with Sullivan in a vaudeville-style tour throughout the South. In 1884, Donovan, by then forty-one, fought a championship bout with Jack Dempsey (not *that* Jack Dempsey but rather Nonpareil Jack Dempsey). Donovan again held his own, fighting to a six round draw in Brooklyn's Palace Rink—"an ancient skating" facility that for this night was jammed with 2500 spectators.

As Donovan's career in the ring wound down, he transitioned nimbly into a lucrative "professor of pugilism" position, teaching society men and boys to box and telling stories about being in the ring with Sullivan. It was his boxing instructor business that had originally brought Donovan to the Executive Mansion in Albany. During Roosevelt's tenure as governor of New York, Donovan was invited for a visit under the auspices of crafting a training program for Roosevelt's sons. But as always, Roosevelt wanted in on the action. He rarely sat out—on anything. "I have a vivid recollection of my first fistie encounter with Theodore Roosevelt," Donovan recalled. "He wore a sleeveless flannel shirt, his khaki Rough-rider uniform trousers and light canvas shoes without heels."

Donovan also immediately noticed that Roosevelt lacked common sense in the ring. It was as if Roosevelt didn't know—or worse, didn't care—enough to give a former bare-knuckle champion a wide berth. "Most men, on coming to box for the first time with a champion, present or retired, show some trepidation," Donovan explained. "There was none of that here." The men fought; Roosevelt refused to be handled with extra care. He objected to soft blows by Donovan.

"Look here, Mike, that is not fair."

"What's the matter, Governor?"

"You are not hitting me. I'd like to hit you."

"All right, Governor."

Such honesty defined Roosevelt's relationship with Donovan. So when the call came to visit the White House in 1904, Donovan knew what Roosevelt needed. The presidency had not changed Roosevelt, at least not in Donovan's eyes. "I found him the same enthusiastic, simply democratic, kindly man I had boxed with four years earlier in Albany," Donovan said.

It was always difficult to find a man who would actually hit the president of the United States. Like, really hit him. Grant the wrestler, for example, constantly held back. Roosevelt protested and tried to get Grant going, but eventually there was no choice. "The day before yesterday, I bloodied Grant's nose," Roosevelt wrote to Kermit, "which made me feel ashamed as Grant was not hitting me hard, although I had besought him to do so."

Roosevelt relied on boxing more during the election year than at any time since Harvard. In one instance during the year, Roosevelt turned an interview into an afternoon of boxing and wrestling. Robert and William Mooney, brothers, came for what they hoped would be ten minutes with the president. William worked with the Post Office and was hoping for a promotion. Robert, a New York reporter, just wanted a story. But Roosevelt remembered that he had seen William knock a man out of the ring during an amateur exhibition put on for Washington dignitaries. The KO was what the president wanted to talk about. "Now," Roosevelt said upon shaking William's hand, "show me how you did it." For the next three hours, Roosevelt sparred and wrestled with the two men. It was the beginning of a boxing relationship. "When he was boxing," William Mooney recalled, "he seemed oblivious to all things else."

At the end of their time, Roosevelt confessed to the Mooney brothers that he was badly out of shape, even though he did things like turn an interview into a physical jousting match. "I am overweight," Roosevelt told the Mooneys. "Don't let anybody know if I tell you something! Promise?" The Mooneys promised; the president could trust them. "I weigh 224 pounds. I ought to tip the scales at only 198 at the most. But don't betray that to a soul."

* * *

Boxing made its debut as an Olympic sport in the 1904 games. Pugilism was not a particular highlight among the events offered, but one could make the argument that the host city St. Louis (like Roosevelt) peaked in 1904.

St. Louis's place within the hierarchy of American cities today reflects its geography—it's somewhere in the middle. It has the Gateway Arch, the Mississippi River, and the St. Louis Cardinals. The city also has its own unique pizza style, characterized by a "cracker-thin crust," Provel cheese, and square slices. But one can't expect a city to be good at everything.

In 1904, St. Louis wrested the world's attention from Boston, New York City, and (most importantly for St. Louisians) Chicago. The city that had launched Lewis and Clark pushed its way into the sun. During the course of one calendar year, St. Louis hosted the Democratic Convention, the Louisiana Purchase Exposition (called by many the St. Louis World's Fair), and America's first Olympic Games. There was a consensus that Thomas Jefferson's acquisition of 828,000 square miles for the bargain price of $15 million deserved commemoration. The Louisiana Purchase Exposition Company put it this way.

> We believe that this object be best accomplished by an exposition, international in its character, where the products of its labor, skill, genius, industry and enterprise of our country are brought into close comparison with those of all other countries where the people of the earth can have an opportunity to behold and study the mighty impress which the influence of liberty makes upon progress of man.

Representatives from St. Louis beat back a proposal from New Orleans to host the exposition.

The exposition idea was not at all original; in fact the proposed St. Louis event fit into a larger pattern of world expositions. In the second half of the nineteenth century, the Western world settled into a rhythm of gathering regularly in order to compare wares. Beginning with the Great Exhibition of 1851 held in London, England, large scale expositions occurred roughly every five years—bouncing primarily between Europe and the United States. These massive events required extraordinary efforts of planning and infrastructural development. The aim was relatively simple: bring together the world's leading technologies, ideas, and achievements in one place, at one time.

These expositions typically ran for three to six months. Visitors poured in by the millions. More than 9.2 million attendees passed through the gates of the Paris Exhibition of 1867. Barcelona's 1888 World's Fair attracted two million people. The Brussels International Exposition of 1897 drew twenty-seven participating countries and an estimated attendance of 7.8 million people. St. Louis planned to outdo them all.

A "Committee of Two Hundred" took charge of planning the event. The committee tabbed David R. Francis, a former governor of Missouri, as its leader. Split-down-the-middle graying hair, spectacles, and a full mustache gave Francis a serious, diplomatic look. Francis realized "the magnitude of the enterprise," and he got to work.

The sheer scale of the Louisiana Purchase Exposition defies easy appreciation. In some ways the escalation of its naming reflects how grandiose the event turned out to be. It started out as the Louisiana Purchase Exposition. Then it became widely referred to as the St. Louis World's Fair. By the time the event happened, many, including Francis himself, referred to the undertaking as the "Universal Exposition." From territory, to world, to universe—the expectations grew.

The planning committee wrangled use of 1,271.76 acres within St. Louis city limits for the event, mostly from Forest Park and Washington University. The Fair Planning Commission hired nine architectural firms to oversee the development of the grounds, which would include more than one thousand buildings. The budget for the event ballooned. A preliminary program for the fair detailed a $50 million cost for the preparations. Adjusting for inflation, that puts the tally around $200 million in 2019 dollars.

*　*　*

As St. Louis ramped up its planning for the Louisiana Purchase Exhibition, the International Olympic Committee—an organization founded and controlled by Pierre de Coubertin—made its own, seemingly unrelated (the two events would soon collide), plans for a 1904 event.

The IOC had resurrected the Olympics Games in 1896. The inaugural *modern* Olympic contest took place over ten days in April 1896, in Athens, Greece. The location made sense; the games built off the tradition of the ancient Olympic Games, which had served as an important religious, social, and athletic tradition for Greek city-states from the eighth century BC to the fourth century AD. The 1896 Olympic Games featured track-and-field, wrestling, fencing, gymnastics, shooting, sailing, tennis, and weightlifting competitions.

Since Pierre de Coubertin was a Frenchman, he made sure that Paris had the first crack as a non-Greek hosting city. And so Parisians welcomed nearly one thousand athletes to their city for the 1900 Olympic Games. The athletic competition was held as part of Paris's World's Fair of 1900.

This second attempt at holding a modern Olympic Games did not go nearly as well as the first. Paris's World's Fair seemed to gobble up the athletic competition. No opening ceremonies demarcated the beginning of the Games; indeed some competitors came and went not knowing that they had competed in the Olympic Games at all. Coubertin and the IOC lost control of the athletic docket as well. Events such as automobile racing, croquet, ballooning, pigeon shooting, and underwater swimming somehow made it onto the competition schedule. The athletic competition schedule stretched out over a six-month period, robbing the still embryonic Games of any sense of being its own event.

Coubertin, always a proud French nationalist, was forced to admit that the 1900 Olympic Games were a disaster.

And he'd have to acknowledge that 1904 represented a make or break year of the Olympic movement. Given the United States' booming sports culture, reflected most obviously by Theodore Roosevelt, the nation seemed to be a logical destination for the games. The question was, which city? Philadelphia, New York City, and Buffalo all submitted bids. But in the end, the IOC awarded the 1904 games to the city of Chicago. St. Louis, busy planning to celebrate the Louisiana Purchase, did not make a bid.

In 1904, there was still very significant disagreement over exactly what the Olympic Games were supposed to be. Coubertin tried desperately to control the debate. The story of the Olympics is partly the story of Coubertin, a small man sporting a wildly successful mustache with a dream to make the Olympic Games such a part of the modern world that men would unite around the purifying elements of sport without even knowing that they were performing a service to themselves, their nations, and the civilized world itself.

Pierre de Coubertin, like Roosevelt, had grown up rich. Paris rich. Coubertin was born, in 1863, into a family of French nobility. The family split its time between the French capital city and an estate in the countryside. Like Roosevelt, Coubertin lost himself in the heroism of *Tom Brown's Schooldays*. He received a Jesuit education in Paris during his teenage years. There Coubertin gained "a love of Greek antiquity," and he learned to box, fence, and row.

Coubertin believed that athletics could serve as the most powerful of teachers. "Sport leads directly to that human idea: the victory of the will," he said. "It is in this way that sport is great and philosophical, bringing us back to Stoic teaching where posterity has revealed many errors and exaggerations, but whose nobility and purity have never been challenged." The phrasing was a bit muddled, but the idea was that physical exertion opened up new learning opportunities.

Coubertin and Theodore Roosevelt first met in 1889 while the Frenchman was traveling throughout the United States gathering information for his study of educational techniques and athletic training. He found much to admire in the United States. The gymnasiums, swimming pools, and athletic fields, among other facilities, stood out as very practical and necessary investments in sport. In New York City, where the meeting took place, Coubertin complimented TR on his promotion of boxing clubs for poorer areas of the city.

Coubertin cashed in on that meeting a decade later. He waited just barely long enough after McKinley's assassination to send his first letter to Roosevelt, president of the United States. On November 15, 1901, Coubertin wrote to Roosevelt and got right to the point. "Mr. President, The International Olympic Committee having decided, in the month of May last, to accept the proposal of the City of Chicago in view of celebration of the Olympic Games of 1904 in that city..." Then the flattery began. "We know too well your Excellency's personal tastes and the reputation that it has acquired in the practice of all the sports to doubt its sympathy on this occasion." Translation: *We're assuming you, Mr. New President, will be supporting the Olympic endeavor.* Coubertin asked that Roosevelt accept the position as Honorary President of the Chicago Olympic Games.

Roosevelt, somewhat surprisingly, passed: "It is a matter of real regret that I do not feel at liberty to accept your very kind suggestion that I become Honorary President at the Chicago Olympian Games." Roosevelt may have been hesitant to put the backing of his office behind such a new event. Or, given his tendency to looks at sports through a nationalist lens, Roosevelt might have been suspicious of this European looking to trade on Roosevelt's name and office.

Undeterred, Coubertin fired back: "May I be permitted to point out that at the games of 1896, in Athens, there presided over by the King of the Hellenes, while President Loubet held the honorary leadership of the Paris games of 1900."

Roosevelt did not budge.

A turn in the relationship between Coubertin and Roosevelt occurred a few weeks later, however, when Coubertin took a different tack with Roosevelt. Rather than asking for support, Coubertin inundated the president of the United States with a torrent of his ideas about education, athletics, and the building of strong citizens. In a handwritten, 1500-word letter dated June 2, 1903, Coubertin poured out his athletic philosophy. He spared no detail.

This deluge of ideas, rather than turning off a president engaged at that moment in securing the right to build the Panama Canal and preparing for the campaign of 1904, worked. *Tons of unsolicited ideas? I'm in.* Roosevelt turned his attention more fully toward Coubertin and the Olympics. For the first time, Roosevelt engaged in the Olympic movement.

"If I were writing to any other than President Roosevelt," Coubertin wrote to, well, President Roosevelt, "I would feel ashamed." Given the demands of the job, such a letter as Coubertin had begun to pen would not have been permissible. But "we all know in Europe that President Roosevelt finds time for everything and at the same time that his interest in physical culture is so great as to allow any leader who has something to say on the subject to look on the White House for advice and support."

Coubertin then shared his philosophy of sport with Roosevelt. There were, according to Coubertin, three categories of sport that needed to be emphasized for all men.

"Life-Saving"—Gymnastics, running, jumping, climbing, and swimming

"Self-Defense"—Fencing, boxing, and shooting

"Transportation"—Animal (walking, riding), Mechanical (cycling, rowing)

"The great objective to all this was that the man would feel unable to retain what the boy had acquired; it was generally admitted that unless keeping himself in consistent training a man became rapidly unfit for anything valuable." Finally, at the end of the long letter, Coubertin returned to his regular request. The Olympics. "We hope the St. Louis games will be a great success," Coubertin wrote, hinting at his desire for Roosevelt's support.

Roosevelt could not help but engage. "My Dear Baron Coubertin," Roosevelt began, "I agree with you entirely. If a growing boy, a young fellow up to the time that he attains manhood, achieves a certain degree of mastery in such exercises as those you enumerate—walking, running, riding, shooting, swimming shooting, etc.—I fully believe that he does, through what you do aptly describe as muscular memory, acquire the capacity to retain a large degree of his powers through their comparatively infrequent use." Whether Roosevelt considered himself to be an example of this theory or a casualty of the relationship it espoused is unclear. But Roosevelt quickly turned the theory toward his own sons.

"I have four boys," he wrote. "The youngest is five and there can be left out of account for our purpose."

Here was what the Roosevelt athletic stock had produced:

TED

- "The eldest, Ted, is fifteen. He is a regular bull terrier."
- "In most branches of sport he has already completely passed me by. He can outwalk and outrun me with ease, and perhaps could outswim me—although I think not yet."
- "On account of my weight I could probably still best him at boxing and wrestling, but in another year he will have passed me in these."
- "He plays football well. In a game last year he broke his collar-bone, but finished the game all right."

KERMIT

- "The next eldest, Kermit, is thirteen. He had water on the knee [knee effusion] when young and it kept him back and has prevented his ever becoming really proficient at sports."
- "He is not at all competitive."
- "I have been utterly unable to teach him to box, but he wrestles pretty well."
- "In running he is no good at all for the sprints, but has a good deal of endurance and comes in well for the long distances."
- "He skates rather poorly. At last I have got him so that he swims fairly."

ARCHIE

- "The next eldest is nine. He is a sweet tempered little fellow, not at all competitive. He runs, walks, and climbs well, and has learned to swim fairly well."

After assessing his boys, rather critically with the exception of Ted, Roosevelt turned inward.

The sensitivity and self-doubt were always there. He could not talk about athletics without judging himself. "Personally I have always felt that I might serve as an object lesson as to the benefit of good hard bodily exercise to the ordinary man." So Roosevelt connected with the decidedly non-Olympian, even as he wrote to Coubertin. *"I never was a champion at anything,"* Roosevelt declared, admitting that he was a nonathlete talking athletics. From there the self-assessment turned into a torrent.

PRESIDENT THEODORE ROOSEVELT
ATHLETIC SELF-ASSESSMENT

- "I have never fenced, although this winter I have done a good deal of broadsword and singlestick work with my friend, General Leonard Wood and other Army officers."
- "I was fond of boxing and fairly good at it."
- "Of late years, since I have been Governor of New York and afterwards President, my life has necessarily been very sedentary; but I have certain playmates among my friends here in Washington and with them I occasionally take long walks, or rather scrambles, through the woods and over the rocks."
- "My ability to take violent exercise has been much diminished by the fact that when I have leisure I like, so far as possible, to spend it in doing something in company with my wife or children."
- "Of late years I have gone back very much in physical prowess, tending to grow both fat and stiff. I could not begin to walk or run for the length of time or at the speed of old time."
- "I have had to abandon wrestling because I found that I tended to lay myself up; and I do but little because it seems rather absurd for a president to appear with a black eye or a swollen nose or a cut lip."

"The fact remains," Roosevelt argued, turning toward the end now, "that in our modern highly artificial, and on the whole congested civilization, no boon to the race could be greater than the acquisition by the average man of that bodily habit which you describe—a habit based upon the having in youth possessed a thorough knowledge of such sports as those you outline, and then of keeping up a reasonable acquaintance with them in later years."

As Roosevelt signed off, the change in his demeanor toward Pierre de Coubertin was unmistakable. While earlier calls to endorse the Olympic movement had been quickly brushed off with excuses of decorum and conflict of interest, Roosevelt liked this idea man. "When are you coming over here?" Roosevelt asked. "I would like you to pay me a visit here in Washington." And then, as if stimulated by his own ideas and the kinship of a fellow athletic evangelist, Roosevelt laid out his playdate plan. "We will take some walks and rides together." Or something else, something robust regardless of the circumstances. "If you come when I am in the country we will row or chop trees or shoot at a target, as well as ride and swim."

* * *

St. Louis, with tacit support from Roosevelt, ended up stealing the Olympics from Chicago. Roosevelt knocked over the first domino of doom for Chicago when he issued a decision to delay the Louisiana Purchase Exposition by one year—until 1904. This delay, which seems strange given the centrality of a date to an anniversary celebration, was necessary to allow completion of the 1500 new buildings (most of them temporary, meant to last for a year or two) for the exposition.

As it became clear that holding a massive event in Chicago and another in St. Louis, in the same year, would threaten the success of both efforts, Chicago's leadership floated a series of suggestions. What if the Olympics were delayed until 1905? What if Chicago and St. Louis put aside their longstanding rivalry and shared the hosting duties of a 1904 Olympiad? There were no easy answers. As things intensified, Coubertin began pointing toward Roosevelt. It would have to be President Theodore Roosevelt that made the final, difficult call between two of his country's most prominent (and rival) cities.

"I believe it is appropriate to rely on the judgement of President Roosevelt who wishes to demonstrate constant interest and who is very competent in all sport questions." The wording here was informative. Coubertin viewed Roosevelt both as a trespasser of sorts, a political leader who *wished* to demonstrate constant interest, but also as a clear leader in the world of athletics. The IOC Board, however, missed the subtext. All seven members of the board urged Roosevelt to make the final decision.

Instead, Coubertin just decided himself.

Although Coubertin would contend years later that he had left the final decision up to Roosevelt, no evidence exists to suggest that Coubertin actually asked Roosevelt his opinion—either informally or in some binding fashion. Instead, Coubertin simply decided himself. St. Louis was in; Chicago was out. "Transfer approved," Coubertin wrote to Chicago's disappointed leaders.

* * *

The Louisiana Purchase Exposition (aka St. Louis World's Fair) opened to the first of its nearly twenty million guests on April 30, 1904.

For those Americans looking forward to the Olympics, they would have to wait for three months. But there were plenty of athletic appetizers. The expo's Department of Physical Culture, led by New York City's PSAL founder Luther Gulick, planned dozens and dozens of competitions as well as lectures on physical health and training. Visitors to the exposition could observe college gymnastics, a Missouri State track meet, a track championship for schools of the Louisiana Purchase Territory, AAU Championships, interscholastic baseball, college baseball, lacrosse, swimming and water polo, "Olympic Basketball Championships," college basketball, Irish sports, a World's Regatta, bicycling, bowling on the green, and "YMCA athletics." It was a smorgasbord of sports; very few things were left out.

The Olympic Games finally began on August 29, 1904. Roosevelt had eventually given in and accepted the Honorary Presidency of the Olympic Games. That was as much as he could offer. "I cannot accept the actual *working* presidency," he made clear.

Strangely, while Roosevelt was in, Coubertin ended up boycotting the Games he had worked so diligently to organize. Frustrated at seeing the Olympics basically folded into the exposition, Coubertin refused to even make the trip to St. Louis. It was a sign that in the eyes of the IOC, the 1904 Olympic Games had been conquered by the United States.

Three thousand spectators sat in the stands to watch the track-and-field competition get underway. The first day's slate of events included races at 60 meters, 400 meters, a 2590-meter steeplechase, and competitions in the hammer throw (16lbs), standing broad jump, and running high jump.

The track-and-field competitions took place immediately adjacent to the Citadel-looking Physical Culture Gymnasium on Washington University's campus. The stands seated 25,000 spectators. There was no shade. Fans and athletes alike had to suffer in the intense humidity of the Midwest summer. A wood-slated boardwalk butted up against the cement bleachers allowing competitors and spectators alike to move from one end of the facility to the other without getting muddy. The dirt track, wide enough for about fifteen athletes to stand shoulder to shoulder, encircled a patchy grass field. The rough track-and-field implements of the day—shin-bruising hurdles, a long jump pit, a shot put ring, and high jump and pole vault mechanisms—cluttered the space.

Unlike the modern track, the St. Louis oval was a third of a mile, rather than a quarter, around. And it was actually closer to a trapezoid in shape. Both the one-hundred- and two-hundred-meter sprints were contested on the straightaway. Still, when compared to the Paris track (1900 Olympics)—which was constantly soggy and required shot putters and hammer throwers to avoid trees with their heaves—St. Louis provided an athletic-facility upgrade.

The marquee event of the St. Louis Olympic Games was the twenty-four-plus mile marathon. The race started at 3:00 p.m. on August 30. The weather was what it usually is on a late August day in St. Louis—hot and humid, about "90 degrees in the shade." Thirty-one competitors toed the starting line. "Probably no race ever run in the history of athletics ever presented a more international character," reported Charles Lucas, a coach and scribe who wrote a firsthand account of the Olympic Games.

To start, the marathoners circled the track for a few laps. A sizeable crowd, about 10,000, looked on with interest, and probably empathy, at the small field of endurance warriors. The runners were mostly lithe and compact. They came clothed in a variety of running attire. Many wore thick trunks that covered most of the runners' legs above the knee. Chafing apparently had not been invented yet. Most of the men had flimsy footwear. Others started out the contest with shoes best described as work boots. A few runners wore long pants and long shirts. Several others wore floppy canvas hats.

Thomas Hicks, a British-born runner representing the Cambridge, Massachusetts, YMCA, settled in among the early leaders. The five-foot-six, 133-pound runner wore slippers, tight black shorts that stretched from midthigh to well above Hicks's navel, and a white singlet. He looked like he knew what he was doing. And having raced in the Boston Marathon and several other similarly lengthy races before, Hicks indeed had more experience than most of his competitors.

There were two principal problems for Hicks and the rest of the field. First, the St. Louis course was much more difficult than those of Athens or Paris. Hills (seven significant ones), dust, heat, humidity, and automobile exhaust combined with the usual pains of running twenty-plus miles to make the St. Louis event one that bordered on extreme. Second, the understanding of endurance competition itself was rudimentary. The problems became evident before the race was even halfway over. Runners cramped up and dropped out. A competitor from New York "was seized with a fit of vomiting" and forced to quit. Most seriously, William Garcia, a competitor from San Francisco, collapsed at the sixteen-mile mark. Spitting up blood, Garcia had suffered a stomach hemorrhage.

As runners dropped off one by one, Hicks and a handful of other competitors, including Albert Corey (Chicago), Sam Mellor (New York), and Felix Carvajal (Cuba) pressed on. The runners stopped at the one water stop on the course at the twelve-mile mark and greedily slurped down cups of water. "The streets were inches deep in dust," and the unregulated flow of cars along the course kept the runners from establishing a fluid rhythm. Carvajal seemed, however, to be suffering less than his competitors. He stopped to chat with spectators along the course. He stole a couple of peaches to eat as he ran. He did not particularly concern himself with getting all the way to the front. The leaders ran seven-minute miles as they made their way through St. Louis and its outskirts.

As the race moved into its third hour, Hicks took over the lead. "Never showing any desire to abandon the race," Hicks plugged away. Looking behind him, Hicks saw no other runner in sight. He allowed himself to slow to a jog;

then he walked for a bit. Always though, he kept moving. On the backsides of the hills Hicks tried to put some distance between himself and his competitors. Then, at nineteen miles, out of nowhere, Lorz blew past Hicks. And that was almost it. "For several minutes," his coach remembered, "it did appear as if the Cambridge man would collapse." To be passed so definitively robbed Hicks of his remaining hope.

But then new information trickled in; Lorz had ridden for several miles in one of the many automobiles on the course. Could this be right? Keep running, Hicks was told. Certainly Lorz would be disqualified, although the officiating certainly left some doubt.

Hicks's handlers did everything they could to keep him moving. Riding alongside their weary athlete, and at times walking and jogging at his shoulder, Lucas kept close tabs on Hicks. With three miles to go, Hicks's color was gone. He was "an ashen white." So the team jumped into action. Hicks forced down a tablet—"one-sixtieth grain strychnine"—and then ate two eggs. This was chased by a sip of brandy. Then Lucas gave Hicks a warm sponge bath, "the water having been kept warm along the road by being placed on the builder of a steam automobile." Strangely, as Hicks stumbled forward, he kept demanding more to eat.

The last two miles meant more hills. And more brandy. And two more eggs. "Hicks walked up the first of the last two hills, and then jogged down on the incline. This was repeated on the last hill." Then he was there, back to the Olympic stadium at Washington University. Hicks tried valiantly to sprint, or at least pick up the pace from his shuffle, as he made one culminating lap around the track, but he had nothing left. The crowd had already cheered the first man to cross the tape. Lorz had arrived minutes earlier, considerably fresher given his run-ride routine. In the end though, it was sorted out. The Olympic Committee awarded Hicks the marathon trophy. Sullivan's Amateur Athletic Union (AAU)—a regulatory body especially important in track and field—banned Lorz from future competition for perpetrating an athletic fraud.

The running of the marathon—chaotic, unorganized, but strangely compelling—fit the 1904 games perfectly. So too did the final medal count. The United States dominated. In these games, which had been overwhelmed by a celebration of American conquest (the Louisiana Purchase), Americans played the role of conqueror. England and France decided not to send its athletes. Only twelve nations sent teams. Six women, all of them American, participated—and all in the archery competition. Of the 651 athletes, 523 were American. As a result, the United States won seventy-eight gold medals. Germany and Cuba tied for second most with four. When considering gold, silver, and bronze medals, American athletes went home with 85 percent of the available hardware. Future American Olympic teams would never have it so good.

* * *

On November 8, 1904, Roosevelt won his own historic victory. He would not be another Chester Arthur. His waiting—as frustrating as it had been during the 1904 campaign season—paid off. "Victory. Triumph. My Father is elected," Alice wrote in her diary. When the votes were finally tallied, Roosevelt had won 336 electoral votes to Parker's 140. Roosevelt's 7.6 million popular votes bested his opponent by more than 2.5 million, making it the largest margin in history to that point. "It was a famous victory," the *Los Angeles Times* concluded. The electoral map looked like Roosevelt had hoped it would; red from West Coast to East Coast, with only the stubborn South tinged blue. The presence of Eugene Debs (Socialist Party) and Tom Watson (Populist Party) had made things a bit more interesting, but overall the election had played out without much stress for Roosevelt's Republicans.

Curiously, Roosevelt celebrated his victory by declaring that it would be his last. He released a statement to reporters at 10:30 p.m. on election night. "On the fourth of March next I shall have served three and a half years, and this three and a half years constitutes my first term. The wise custom which limits the President to two terms regards the substance and not the form. Under no circumstances will I be a candidate for or accept another nomination." The *New York Times* shared the news related to the 1908 election right alongside that of 1904: ROOSEVELT. SWEEPS THE NORTH AND WEST AND IS ELECTED PRESIDENT. SAYS HE WILL NOT RUN AGAIN.

The victory sealed and delivered, Roosevelt was free to roam about the country again. On November 26, 1904, Roosevelt finally visited St. Louis and the World's Fair. The Olympics had long concluded.

Roosevelt saw the fair in a fashion that could have only satisfied him. He moved from one gleaming, white, columned building to another. He covered as many of the seventy-five miles of walkways and roads within the grounds as possible. It was five minutes here, ten minutes there. All with a mob following behind. The "throng of more than 200,000" that had amassed in anticipation of his visit "surged hither and thither, like an unorganized army, but on the conquest of a glimpse of the President and Mrs. Roosevelt and Miss Alice." Edith and Alice themselves scurried to keep up. The schedule was ridiculous: the liberal arts building, the government building, a reception, a review of a parade of troops, the National Pavilions (starting with the German building and ending with the Japanese), lunch in the West Pavilion, the agriculture building, the stadium to watch a few minutes of the Carlisle–Haskell football game, the machinery building, the electricity building.

At least once, Alice, twenty years old, lost contact with the group. She got cut off and had to make her case, as the president's daughter—and something of a celebrity herself—to reenter the protective circle surrounding the presidential party. Alice had actually already been to the fair. She'd visited in May and June, accepting an invitation from James Sullivan to award medals at the AAU Championship games. She'd stayed in St. Louis for nine days.

The trip allowed Alice to put some distance between herself and the White House, as father and daughter struggled to be civil to each other. Alice's status in the family had always been somewhat difficult since she had a different mother than the rest. During her years living in the White House she proved to be a bit rebellious, smoking and going out with men unchaperoned. Roosevelt probably did not know how to connect with his oldest daughter. She, unlike Ted, did not bend to her father's constant prodding. Roosevelt had famously remarked of Alice: "I can do one of two things, I can be President of the United States or I can control Alice. I cannot possibly do both."

Regardless, Sullivan recognized that Alice was nearly as good for promotional efforts as her father. He was glad to have her on hand for several days of the athletic competitions. As a thanks, Sullivan and the AAU sent Alice a girdle, "composed of Exposition colors, with a buckle that is emblematic of the AAU of the US."

During his flash tour through the fountains, buildings, and exhibits of the fairgrounds, Roosevelt struggled to conceal an injury from his fighting habit. He confessed as much to Kermit. "A few days ago while boxing with Ted and the boys," Roosevelt wrote upon returning from St. Louis, "I strained one leg...I must have broken a little vein or something, because there is a huge black and purple place on the inside of my thigh literally as big as two dinner plates." Roosevelt had probably suffered a minor muscle tear. He complained of stiffness. But there was still pride involved in a good injury for Roosevelt. "I walked up through the Exposition grounds without any of the reporters getting any idea that I was at all lame."

Roosevelt bookended his 1904 boxing spree by sparring for ten rounds with Mike Donovan in the White House basement on March 3, 1905. "The day before the inauguration, between five and six o'clock, the President and I had a 'go,'" Donovan recalled, clearly relishing the memory. The streets of Washington, DC had been transformed. "Everywhere decoration abound," the *Washington Post* reported. Tens of thousands of electric lamps stood waiting to illuminate the city. The District police force, augmented by 450 additional officers, made last minute preparations. Officials worried about the weather. None of it concerned Roosevelt. He was apparently unfazed about the prospect of a loose blow giving him a black eye for the inauguration. Instead, he was "happy as a schoolboy as he stripped for the fray." Physical distraction always seemed to do the president good. "We boxed the ten hard, long rounds," Donovan, approaching the age of sixty, remembered, though he wanted out after five rounds. But he knew the rules. "I did not want to appear to be a quitter." The night before he was to be sworn in again, Roosevelt knocked Donovan down at least once. The two men struggled desperately, joyously. "At the close he was perspiring profusely, but seemed fresh enough to go much longer," Donovan recalled. In pugilistic triumph, Theodore Roosevelt ended his last day in the White House as an unelected president of the United States.

SEVEN

TED'S DANGEROUS FOOTBALL ADVENTURE

*The "Teddy" is the highest honor the NCAA may confer on an individual.
It is named after Theodore Roosevelt, whose concern for the conduct of
intercollegiate athletics led to the formation of the NCAA in 1906.*

—NATIONAL COLLEGIATE ATHLETIC ASSOCIATION,
Theodore Roosevelt Award

On August 16, 1905, Theodore Roosevelt, working from his summer head-quarters at Sagamore Hill on Long Island, wrote a letter to Harvard University President Charles W. Eliot. While the two men corresponded frequently, often discussing world politics or great literature, this letter was more personal. His son Ted was enrolling at Harvard as a freshman. Roosevelt wanted to explain to Eliot what kind of young man he was getting. "Ted is an average outdoor boy," Roosevelt began. "He has sense, and this means that he will study hard and not permit athletics to interfere with his studies."

These two presidents had a long, tangled, contentious relationship. Their letters back and forth (they exchanged more than fifty during Roosevelt's time as president) were more intellectual jousting than pleasant exchanges of information or news. The two leaders had recently gone several rounds on the issue of independence for the Philippines. Eliot had signed onto a petition calling for the United States to grant the island nation, which the US had gained control of through the Spanish-American War, political independence as soon as possible. Roosevelt disagreed. But rather than leaving the matter there (after all, did it really matter if the president of the United States and the president of Harvard agreed on the issue of Philippine freedom?), Roosevelt wrote a lengthy letter to Eliot, working to convince the man who had presided over his own time at Harvard of the errors of his ways. "It seems to me," Roosevelt wrote, that "the actual facts in the matter" nearly demanded that the thinking man "would not sign such a petition." Detail upon detail, point upon point followed. Roosevelt always piled on.

"Roosevelt's ways often excited antagonism in Eliot," one Eliot biographer noted, diplomatically. Perhaps, though, Eliot was used to dealing with fathers who were anxious about sending their oldest sons off to Cambridge. Roosevelt's August 1905 letter continued: "[Ted] is not an athlete of the first, or even the second, caliber; but I suppose he will try out for the freshman eleven this fall with the hope of becoming a substitute or something of that kind." Roosevelt wanted balance for his son. "I should not want him to give up all athletics and do nothing but study, any more than I should want him in any way to subordinate his studies to athletics."

One might credit the letter for its honesty. But it wasn't a particularly generous introduction that the president gave for his son. Ted was "average" and "had sense"; he was "not an athlete of the first caliber." Or the second caliber, for that matter. But what the letter did accomplish was to establish the fact that Roosevelt was very concerned about his oldest son's upcoming athletic experience at Harvard.

Ted, the oldest son and first offspring of the TR–Edith marriage, was born September 13, 1887. His birth took place at Sagamore Hill, the family home that the Roosevelts had moved into only a few months before. Ted experienced a childhood of wealth, nurturing, ideas, and very high expectations. Books abounded. Ted grew up steeped in the lore of American conquest and adventure. "Robin Hood, Daniel Boone, Custer's Last Stand, Gettysburg, The Battle of Mobile Bay, and The Alamo" were among the tales in the Roosevelt family library. Animals nearly overran Sagamore Hill. During his childhood, Ted had dogs, cats, ponies, chickens, and guinea pigs. These were the normal pets; the family also took in, at one time or another, an eagle, bear cub, coyote, horseshoe crab, flying squirrels, and a mountain lion.

By all accounts, Ted impressed no one with his appearance. He was—as Edmund Morris put it rather cruelly—a "small, nervous, grim, pug-ugly" boy. Ted also suffered from asthma and vision problems. Fortunately, though, the extent of these ailments for the son was not nearly as extreme as for his father. Ted struggled with asthma, but mostly it remained just an irritant. A Long Island doctor fitted young Ted with glasses at age five; he had corrective eye surgery at nineteen. So Ted did not linger in a blurry haze during his formative years as his father had. And he avoided the spectacles as a young man that had come to define his famous father.

Roosevelt demanded near-perfection from his oldest son. He wanted Ted to be erudite, tough, and compassionate. "My father believed very strongly in the necessity of each boy being able and willing not only to look out for himself but to look out for those near and dear to him," Ted remembered. "This gospel was preached to us all from the time we were very, very small."

Fathering Ted meant giving directions and doling out advice. Roosevelt rarely held back. Roosevelt did not subscribe to any parenting theory that involved standing by quietly and letting one's offspring make their own decisions—all with the knowledge that their parents stood behind them in resolute support. Roosevelt instead parented through constant suggestion and appeal. The pressure on Ted had been unbearable at times.

For Roosevelt, to be a "real boy" one needed to be nearly the opposite of what Roosevelt himself had been as a child. Roosevelt's version of proper boyhood included physicality, moral character, and education. He approved of some measure of troublemaking and violence, as long as it was in the interest of adventure. One Sunday afternoon, relaxing at the family's home near Oyster Bay, Roosevelt expanded on his ideas on boyhood with Pulitzer Prize winning journalist John J. Leary. The topic came up when Roosevelt asked Leary about how his own son was doing.

Leary: All right. Only a little too much football and swimming and not enough schoolwork—almost too much boy.

TR: That's all right. Don't let that worry you. Do you know you are fortunate in having a real boy?

Here it was. To Roosevelt—the father of four sons—there were "real boys" and, well, less-than-real boys.

TR: Some of the most splendid fellows I know have boys that if they were mine I'd want to choke them—pretty boys who know all of the latest tango steps and the small talk, and the latest things in socks and ties—tame cats, mollycoddles.

As was often the case when they spent time together, Leary let Roosevelt keep rolling. Leary simply took notes for a book that would be released the year Roosevelt died.

TR: Mine, thank God, have been good boys, a bit mischievous at times, all of them, but every boy is. Honestly, if I had to take my choice, I'd rather have a boy that I'd have to go to the police station and bail out for beating a cab driver or a policeman, than one of the mollycoddle type. He might worry me, but he wouldn't disgrace me.

When Ted was ten years old, he had collapsed under the weight of his father's expectations. Over a period of months in 1897 and 1898, Ted suffered from debilitating headaches. The pain bore down on young Ted so acutely that he remained bedridden. His daily routine halted completely. A host of physicians visited the sick boy, but none could identify the cause of his intense pain. Finally, in March 1898, Theodore and Edith took Ted to New York City for treatment. There he received a diagnosis from a family friend, Dr. Alexander Lambert. Lambert's assessment? Ted was suffering from an acute case of overparenting.

"Dr. Lambert reported that the boy was suffering from nervous prostration brought on by the way Teddy constantly drove him to perfection and Ted's desire to live up to his father's expectations." The diagnosis stunned Roosevelt. He apologized to Lambert. "Hereafter I shall never press Ted either in body or in mind," Roosevelt wrote to Dr. Lambert, making a promise that he would not, could not perhaps, keep. "The fact is that the little fellow, who is peculiarly dear to me, had bidden fair to be all things I would like to have been and wasn't, and it has been a great temptation to push him."

In 1900, the family enrolled Ted at the Groton School, an exclusive Episcopal boarding academy for boys located forty miles northwest of Boston. Kermit would join him on the rural campus in 1902. Archie and Quentin followed in 1908 and 1909. Groton became Ted's home as his own family relocated from Albany to Washington, and then as his father made his startling ascension to the presidency. It wasn't an easy way to spend one's adolescence. Groton's founder and headmaster, Endicott Peabody (a cousin of Roosevelt's first wife Alice, and groomsman at their wedding), believed in a type of Spartan monasticism. Cold showers, early wake-up calls, rigorous academics, mandatory physical fitness testing, and corporal punishment took the prevailing ideas of muscular Christianity and made them into a curriculum at Groton.

Ted hated Groton at first. Intense homesickness plagued the thirteen-year-old during his first months away from home. He was waiting for a growth spurt that never seemed to arrive. He also suffered for his father's fame, fighting with other boys who singled him out for being the son of a notable politician. Slowly though, Ted found his way. He took up singing in the choir and made headway academically. "He has won his place in his own little world and he is all right," Roosevelt reported in November 1900.

Ted also joined the football team. And through football, Ted found a way to diverge from his father's path—to earn his father's respect and admiration.

Of course, almost all boys played football at Groton. Headmaster Peabody saw to it that the game was woven into the school's fabric. "His favorite game was always football," wrote a Peabody biographer. "Football he privately admired because it is a game that is rough and hard, requiring courage, endurance, and discipline. Instinctively he trusted a football player more than a non-football player, just as the boys did."

For the less talented Groton boys, there were "elevens" associated with the school's forms (classes basically) and dorms. The boys joined teams with classmates of a similar size and age. These squads drilled and scrimmaged mostly, although occasionally an outside challenger could be rustled up for an actual game. Boys shifted up and down through the school's various squads based on their performance. Kermit, two years behind Ted at Groton, seemed to take such movements in stride. "I was dropped from the second Wachusetts to the third and was elected captain of the third yesterday," he wrote TR in 1903.

For those with more skill (and size), Groton's interscholastic squads loomed as enviable prizes. The vaunted Groton Varsity competed against nearby schools: the likes of Milton, Worcester Academy, Lowell Textile, and Rindge Manual. St. Mark's School of Southborough, Massachusetts, was Groton's main rival. The two schools began playing an annual football game in 1886.

So like his classmates, and like his younger brother, Ted played. But for Ted, an intense desire existed to move up through Groton's football hierarchy, despite his size. Ted was a striver; he played with reckless abandon. In 1901, he suffered a broken collarbone and chipped teeth while playing football. Headmaster Peabody dashed off a quick letter to the president assuring him that his son would fully recover. "I have great confidence in the diagnosis, and the general skill of our physician," Peabody wrote to Roosevelt on January 11, 1902. As for the teeth, Peabody promised to send Ted to a dentist immediately, "in order to prevent that dead tooth from losing its original beauty."

Ted wrote regular, newsy, usually rampantly positive, letters to his father. Talk of football often filled the pages of these letters. In an undated letter, probably written in 1902, Ted urged his father to both step in and butt out of his football life. "Football is going on splendidly and I have not been hurt a bit," Ted wrote in careful cursive script, on Groton School stationery. Then he got to his point. "Could you please in your next letter give me permission to play on the 3rd eleven? You know I would not do anything foolish about hurting myself," Ted reasoned. "So please do, as it will be very discouraging to have to play on the 4th please do and don't put in any conditions the boys won't be any heavier than me." Just to make sure his father had not missed the reason for the letter, Ted signed off, "So please do—Your loving Ted."

The next year, in 1903, in what would be his last year at Groton, Ted made another push to move up the ranks. He was stronger. He had spent part of the previous summer working as a cowhand in the Dakota Territory. During the fall tryout period, Ted proved himself worthy of a slot on Groton's second eleven. While not the school's top squad, obviously, the second eleven was populated with accomplished players, most of whom were a year or two ahead of Ted in school. Real athletic achievement seemed on the horizon. But then Headmaster Peabody intervened.

TR heard Ted's side of the story through a letter sent to the White House with "Hurry! Hurry!" on the outside of the envelope. "I have made the second eleven but on account of the foolish prejudices of the Rector against my playing against heavier boy[s] he had ordered me put down," Ted began.

Position wise, Ted was an "end," meaning the he played on the end of the line—both on offense and defense. Most everyone played both ways. End was a position that reformers saw as key to cutting down on player injuries. Requiring more players to line up in a stationary position, along the line of scrimmage, was thought by the Intercollegiate Football Rules Committee as a means to make the game a bit safer.

"The boys are some a good deal heavier than I," Ted confessed to his father, "but there are some which are my size." He continued on, passionately making his argument, laying out the quick case for why his father should allow him (a player who had recently suffered a broken collarbone after all) to play up several classes:

"Mr. Ayrault says he personally thinks I could stand it perfectly."

Peabody is an outlier.

"I have played three games against the first and not been hurt in the least."

I can do this; I've already been doing it in fact.

"[I] twice saved touch downs by tackling the first star quarter back."

I'm good at this.

"If you want to put any limitations...I will obey them."

I'm not unreasonable...let's compromise.

"Kermit is playing foot ball but he does not seem to the spirit of it much."

I'm really your only chance at having a football-playing son.

"It would be awfully discouraging to have to play where I did last year and me 12 lbs heavier."

Don't do this to me.

Ted proposed a compromise. He would agree to whatever stipulations his father mandated, if he could still be allowed to move up the ranks. What he did not want was his father—the president of the United States for goodness sake—to simply accept the recommendations of the Groton administration. "If you want to put any limitations please put them on a separate paper and I will obey them to the letter," Ted wrote. "But do not put them on [the] sheet you give permission as I will have to show it and the rector would readily construe them so that I could not play." The matter was urgent. "Please write right off," Ted urged. The letter sign off took a melodramatic tone—Ted was sixteen after all. "There is nothing else to say good by [sic] your loving Ted."

TR's response to Ted in 1903—as his eldest boy stood on the brink of manhood and wanted football to be part of his evolution—mirrored the sentiments he would convey in 1905 while intervening in a national football crisis that threatened the organized existence of the game. Roosevelt had mixed emotions on football; yes, he respected the game and admired its rugged qualities, but he struggled with what to do about its damaging side effects.

"In spite of the 'Hurry! Hurry!' on the outside of your envelope," Roosevelt wrote Ted on October 4, 1903, "I did not like to act until I had consulted Mother and thought the matter over; and to be frank with you, old fellow, I am by no means sure that I am doing right now." Roosevelt admitted that he leaned toward protecting his son and keeping him on a lower team. But he worried about breaking his son's spirit, causing him to feel "so bitterly disappointed" at the prospect of nonprogress.

The parenting pendulum swung back and forth in Roosevelt's letter.

"Now I should not in the least object to your being laid up...**But** I am by no means sure that it is worth your while to run the risk of being laid up for the sake of playing in the second squad when you are a fourth former, instead of when you are a fifth former."

"I have told the Rector that as you feel so strong about it, I think the chances of your damaging yourself in body is outweighed by the possibility of bitterness of spirit if you could not play...**But** in this case I am uncertain, and I shall give you the benefit of the doubt."

"I am delighted to have you play football. I believe in rough, manly sports. **But** I do not believe in them if they degenerate into the sole end of any one's existence."

"I am glad you play football; I am glad that you should box...I should be very sorry if you did not do these things. **But** don't ever get into the frame of mind which regards these things as constituting the end to which all your energies must be devoted."

"I am proud of your pluck, and I greatly admire football...**but** the very things that make it a good game make it a rough game."

As if all this equivocation wasn't enough, Roosevelt closed by trying to use Greek mythology to make sense of the situation. Because, you know, that's usually how teenage sons are most readily convinced that their fathers know best. "Did you ever read Pliny's letter to Trajan, in which he speaks of its being advisable to keep the Greeks absorbed in athletics, because it distracted their minds from all serious pursuits, including soldiering and prevented their ever being dangerous to the Romans?" TR asked.

Roosevelt conferred with officials at Groton on the situation. He and Edith held a series of parental huddles. In the end, despite Ted's protests, the adults in Ted's life, including his father, saw to it that he played with the third squad during the 1903 season. It was a risk versus reward situation. Ted was too small to risk his health for such a small prize. TR repeated himself in a second letter to Ted, sent a week after the first. "As I think I wrote you, I do not in the least object to your getting smashed if it is for an object that is worth while...but I think it a little silly to run any imminent risk of a serious smash simply to play on the second squad instead of the third."

Ted made the best of the disappointing situation. He earned some time during the 1903 season at back and center, which provided new opportunities. Even as he played with boys his own size, the football injuries continued to pile up. As winter approached, Ted was hobbled by an ankle injury. "If I were you I should certainly get the best ankle support possible," Roosevelt advised his son. "You don't want to find next fall that Webb beats you for end because your ankle gives out and his does not." In the same letter, Roosevelt again sought broader context. "I wonder if you are old enough to care for a good history of the American Revolution...I think I shall give you mine by Sire George Trevelyan."

* * *

Ted skipped his final two years at Groton. He spent 1904 living at the White House preparing for college entrance exams. He flourished as an independent scholar. He gained admittance to Harvard—a task made easier by his family connections but nonetheless an achievement. Ted walked onto Harvard Yard for the first time as a student in September 1905. At the time, Ted stood five-foot-six and weighed 130 pounds. He was athletic, but small. He was determined, but often outclassed. Still, the boy that TR had described as a "regular bull terrier," who had "broke his collar bone, but finished the game" with grit. Or perhaps Ted was chasing what TR described in 1905 (just before Ted left for Harvard) as the second kind of greatness: "to do that which many men could do, but which as a matter of fact none of them actually does."

Although it seems in hindsight like it was always going to be Harvard, Ted had seriously considered taking a different path. During his last year at Groton, Ted began pursuing admittance into the United States Military Academy and the Naval Academy. Ted desired to serve his country and take a path that might end the daily comparisons to his father. While Roosevelt valued his Rough Riding days above almost everything else, he did not approve of Ted's alternate route. He sent Ted a "long business letter" detailing his concerns about Ted becoming a professional soldier. Roosevelt worried that Ted was pursuing West Point and the Naval Academy less for their own merits than the fact that they represented something different. "It seemed to me more as if you did not feel drawn in any other direction, and wondered what you were going to do in life or what kind of work you would turn your hand to, and wondered if you could make a success or not; and that you are therefore inclined to turn to the Navy or the Army chiefly because you would then have a definite and settled career in life."

Shortly after arriving at Harvard, Ted joined the freshman football team. In doing so, he became a part of a unit that Harvard's new football coach, Bill Reid Jr., planned to make the bedrock of his program. "We are going to have first rate material for a freshman team, and properly handled ought to yield us some first-class varsity material next year," Reid wrote in his coaching diary on September 26, 1905. Perhaps this would be the key to balancing out the rivalry with Yale. Harvard needed a program, rather than just an occasionally talented team. Whatever Harvard's approach before Reid, it had not worked very well. In the twenty-five Harvard–Yale contests so far, Yale had seventeen victories to Harvard's four and four ties. And the games had rarely been close. Yale had scored 250 points to Harvard's 73 over the course of the rivalry up to 1905.

During his first year at Harvard, Ted gradually increased his playing time. And he did so in the midst of college football's "death harvest" crisis. During the 1905 season, eighteen high school and college players died due to injuries they sustained on the gridiron. Another eighty-eight college players suffered serious injury.* The *New York Times* and *Chicago Tribune* attempted to splice out the casualties, creating categories like "body blows," "injuries to the spine," and "concussion of the brain," but the reality was rather simple: football was maiming far too many American boys. Boys like Ted.

College football had been around for nearly three decades at this point. The game's popularity led schools to invest heavily in stadiums, coaches, and scholarships. Harvard not only participated in the athletic arms race, it was at the front of the pack. In 1903, the university completed construction of its massive Har-

---

* Whether eighteen is the actual, correct number remains a matter of debate. *Deadspin's* 2014 piece puts the number of deaths at twenty but then immediately calls into question its own finding. See, https://deadspin.com/did-football-cause-20-deaths-in-1905-re-investigating-1506758181. See also, John Watterson, "The Gridiron Crisis of 1905: Was it Really a Crisis?" *The Journal of Sport History,* Vol. 27, No. 2 (Summer 2000), 291–298.

vard Stadium. For a cost of $320,000, Harvard created a powerful mix of nostalgia and technology. The stadium mimicked Greece's iconic venue at Olympia in appearance. But the insides were all about innovation. Harvard used "steel-reinforced cement" to control costs while still creating a venue that could hold more than thirty thousand fans for big games. Harvard's willingness to create a venue dedicated to football opened the floodgates for other schools. Princeton and Yale certainly couldn't allow Harvard's achievement to go unmatched.

Countering fan and institutional support, there had also arisen an increasingly vocal antifootball crowd. There was even a fringe abolition movement. Harvard's own Charles Eliot was among this group's leaders.

When considering the life and career of Eliot, his opposition to college football ranks far down any list of his priorities. Eliot served as Harvard's president for a today-unfathomable forty years. He had accepted the position in 1869 but only after several other candidates turned down the position. At the time, Eliot was a thirty-four-year-old fledgling scholar. Adding an emotional burden to his challenging new career, Eliot's wife died after a long illness on the day after he accepted the Harvard presidency.

Despite the odds against him, Eliot flourished. He changed the shape and mission of higher education in the United States in ways that still reverberate to this day. It was Eliot who gave students a choice in their classes, arguing "the young man of nineteen or twenty ought to know what he likes best and is most fit for." Eliot created the secular university, pushing Harvard away from its religious roots. He created graduate and professional programs and technological training. He more closely tied research production to the mission of faculty and the university. In short, Eliot ushered American higher education into a position where it could complement the industrial revolution that occurred in the United States rather than being rendered obsolete by it.

So when Eliot took the side of abolition on the matter of *college* football (this was, after all, a university activity), it mattered. He was not completely anti-sports; he had rowed on the crew team during his own student days. Still, Eliot joined Burt Wilder of Cornell in the difficult position of criticizing an activity that his own institution profited from greatly. He wrote letters to the presidents of other New England universities on limiting games and outlawing coaching salaries. Then in 1894, Eliot took his first aggressively public swipe against the game. In his annual report on the activities and well-being of Harvard, Eliot attacked football games for monopolizing student time and encouraging deception and cheating. Football pushed universities to focus on outside constituencies (fans and boosters) rather than its own students. Eliot certainly had no patience for the unquantifiable idea that football somehow turned physical toil into moral improvements. He saw the opposite occurring; why wouldn't a football player who undercut his opponent on the field act similarly in other situations? And then of course, there was the violence.

In response, Walter Camp—Yale's football advisor (paid coaches were just coming on the scene) and "the father of modern football"—issued *Football Facts and Figures* in the same year. This book made the counterargument that football, while rough, hardly descended into the kind of unrestrained violence that its critics portended. The "experts" assembled by Camp for the task concluded, among other things, that football was roughly as dangerous as crew. So the debate was on.

In 1894, Eliot believed that reform for football was possible. "If the evils of athletic sports are mainly those of exaggeration and excess," he challenged, "it ought not be impossible to point out and apply appropriate checks." He proposed seismic changes: banning freshman, no off-campus games, and only bi-annual intercollegiate contests. Eliot won some victories, but by 1905, as Ted was fighting for a spot in Harvard's football community, Eliot doubted that any reform could really work. He viewed abolition as the only viable option moving forward.

The pressure to do something about college football increased radically at the same time Ted made his rather humble entry into Harvard's football machine. In the summer of 1905, *McClure's Magazine* (this was a muckraking periodical that took on the Standard Oil and US Steel monopolies) printed two scathing articles on college athletics. Written by Roosevelt's friend Henry Beach Needham, the articles emphasized that corruption, cheating, academic fraud, and violence were systemic problems in college football. These were the norms, not the exceptions. And the ills of the college game were trickling down to younger players as well.

This is why Endicott Peabody (remember Ted's good times at Groton?) got involved. Peabody believed that football stood at a critical juncture in 1905. This game which he had nearly mandated for every boy at Groton—both Ted and Kermit included—had become something different, something more violent and less pure, than it had been in decades prior. It was time for a serious change and serious change-agent.

Peabody wrote to President Roosevelt on September 16, 1905.

Using three pages in what might have been said in couple of paragraphs, Peabody's rambling letter still contained a clear request: "A complete revolution could be worked if we could get the coaches of Harvard and Yale and Princeton together, and persuade them to undertake to teach men to play Foot-ball honest. You are the one man, so far as I know, who could accomplish this without much effort." Roosevelt had to intervene.

To be clear, Peabody wanted little to do with Eliot and the abolition crowd. "You and I believe in the game, and in its beneficial effects upon boys and young men when it is carried on fairly," Peabody clarified, "and this is the point of my letter." Reform had to happen. "The teaching of Foot-ball at the Universities is dishonest. There are all kinds of abuses connected with the game which should be remedied." And for Peabody, it was not even the injuries and violence that were at the core of the issue. It was the ethical and moral decline that troubled him most. Football was corrupting America's youth. While some reforms could wait, Peabody reasoned, "this fundamental dishonesty calls for immediate treatment."

*   *   *

Having recently brokered peace between Russia and Japan, an effort that would win him the Nobel Peace Prize, Roosevelt seized upon Peabody's challenge. He dashed off personal invitations to the football leaders of Harvard, Princeton, and Yale. The matter could not wait; Roosevelt wanted the meeting to occur at the White House as soon as possible. Perhaps if the coaches got in the same room, a series of reforms could be agreed upon.

There was no thought of saying no to the president's invitation. On October 9, 1905, the coaches and their seconds gathered at the White House. The day was clear and pleasant, the temperatures in the mid-sixties with nary a hint of rain in the forecast. Fall was in the air. Walter Camp, Yale's longtime football man, and John Owsley, the Bulldogs field coach, came down from New Haven. Princeton sent the head of its athletic committee and its field assistant, John Fine and Arthur Hillenbrand. Bill Reid, Harvard's twenty-six-year-old coach, made the eight-hour train ride from Boston and brought team doctor Edwin Nichols along as well, as requested by the president. "Today I see the football men of Harvard, Yale, and Princeton," TR wrote to Kermit.

Roosevelt saw himself as a fixer. The aim, he told Kermit, was "to try to get them to come to a gentlemen's agreement not to have mucker [dirty] play."

At 1:30 p.m., the group sat down at a rectangular table in the White House dining room for what had to have been the first White House summit consisting of the president of the United States, the secretary of state, and six football coaches. Roosevelt came to the meeting directly from a reception for the justices of the United States Supreme Court. Reid, on the other hand, spent the morning looking over scouting reports on Yale's offensive schemes and taking in the tourist sights of DC (Reid and Nichols had trudged to the top of the Washington Monument, "where we took in the view," before heading for the White House). Yet, there they all sat.

Roosevelt claimed the center of one side of the table; Secretary Root sat directly across from the president. Camp managed to commandeer the seat at the president's right hand. Princeton's John Fine took the seat to the left of TR. The other men found their places in the remaining chairs.

Roosevelt began this White House summit on football by clarifying the situation in which the game found itself mired: "Football is on trial," Roosevelt began. "Because I believe in the game, I want to do all I can to save it. And so I have called you all down here to see whether you won't agree to abide by both the letter and the spirit of the rules, for that will help."

From there a wide-ranging conversation transpired, the exact transcription of which the press never obtained. "So far as could be learned," the *Philadelphia Inquirer* reported in its front-page, top-left story, "the President was very earnest in his desire to have as much as possible done to eliminate all unnecessary roughness" and "was particularly anxious that there be as little possible of the heavy close formation plays."

To make sure that each of these elite institutions understood that they were part of the problem, and thus must lead the way in reform efforts, Roosevelt laid out an informal list of offenses committed by each team. "The President discussed the question of football in general and made a few remarks on unfair play," Reid recorded in his diary for October 9. Then things got uncomfortable. TR proceeded by "giving an example of what he remembered of each college's unfair play from several things that had happened in previous years."

For more than two hours, the men talked football reform. Since Walter Camp had long controlled the football rule making process, he had the most to lose in the process. In fact, Camp had good reason to resent the president of the United States, and a noted Harvard man to boot, for interfering in his life's work. Camp's fingerprints were on nearly every aspect of the game of football. Camp had played and coached at Yale. But more than that, he was football's architect and theorist. Camp wrote 30 books (*Walter Camp's Book of College Sports; Football; How to Play Football: A Primer on the Modern College Game; The Substitute: A Football Story; The Book of Foot-ball; Football for the Spectator; Football without a Coach*; etc.) and 250 articles. From 1883 until 1924, Camp authored the annual *Spalding's Official Football Guide*, the most indispensable publication for those involved or interested in football.

And now the president, prompted into action by the headmaster of his children's school, had something to say about the safety and future of the game?

So as Roosevelt pontificated, Camp nodded along. "Camp appeared to listen intently," wrote one Camp biographer. But really Camp just wanted to push his current agenda; he had little interest in the president's ill-informed plans. For more than a decade Camp had suggested that football need just one major fix to stabilize the sport. By changing the yardage needed for a first down from five yards to ten, Camp contended, the action would open up. This amendment—and not the gimmicky forward pass that John Heisman (coach of Auburn and Georgia Tech among other schools) and others were advocating—would move football back onto a healthy path.

Camp did not cede an inch. Harvard's Reid captured the dynamic in his diary, that of Camp playing along and passing the time. "Camp made some considerable talk but was very slippery and did not allow himself to be pinned down to anything." Both Camp and the Princeton men denied that outright violence for violence's sake had ever taken place under their watch. Their games had never featured wanton brutality. Never. "The Princeton and the Yale men," Reid wrote, "both disclaimed *any* knowledge of *any* man's having been hurt purposely in *any* of its games." This was strange to Reid; he remembered an incident in a Yale–Princeton game where Princeton had savagely targeted one of Yale's All-American De Seaulles brothers (either Charles or John) because he had an injured ankle.

Eventually, Roosevelt had to get back to work, but even still he wanted the "football confab" to continue. He sent Camp and Owsley, Fine and Hillenbrand, and Nichols and Reid to the White House porch. They kept talking. When the men finally exited the White House, shortly after 4:00 p.m., they did so with a nebulous, we're-supposed-to-do-what? assignment for the train ride home. Roosevelt sent the men out the White House door with instructions to "draw up some kind of an agreement on the matter."

The coaches did just as much as they had to. The product matched the prompt in terms of its specificity. Here's what the Ivy League football men crafted:

At a meeting with the President of the United States, it was agreed that we consider an honorable obligation exists to carry out in letter and in spirit the rules of the game of foot ball related to roughness, holding and foul play, and the active coaches of our Universities being present with us pledge themselves so regard it, and to do their utmost to carry out these obligations.

It's possible the men could have done less, but it's difficult to conclude how. The statement contained no real concessions, no specific policy changes, and no admission that football had any structural problems at all. As long as games were played respecting the already established rules, "in letter and in spirit," everything would be fine.

Camp for his part realized that the group had been treading water. After scratching out the quick agreement on their northbound train ride, he sent the president the statement, asking for his approval. "I take pleasure in sending you herewith the results of the little meeting you called were good enough to bring about today." *The little meeting.* One has to wonder: how often does a meeting convened and attended by the president of the United States and the secretary of state, covered on the front page of the *New York Times,* get characterized as a "little meeting?"

Camp's sincerity—to Roosevelt, to his fellow Ivy League coaches, about creating actual reform in football—is difficult to gauge. Reid doubted Camp wanted change at all. In his diary entry from the day of the football summit, Reid noted that the president had not changed many minds. Reid's optimism was limited. When Reid, during the train ride, proposed working together to detail more closely exactly what separated good, rough play from excessive violence in football, an unease settled over the group. The persuasive powers of the White House were fading with each passing mile. "I must say that I do not feel that Yale and Princeton were wholly in sympathy with the idea, although they professed to be."

And so Reid, Harvard's football coach first and foremost, remained on the fence as well. He would not be a reformer at the expense of his own team. "I shall not be willing to stand by any agreement with them which I cannot feel certain that they intend to carry out in spirit and in faith...After all," Reid concluded, "the way which the game is played depends largely on the way in which the coaches take hold and the way in which the officials rule, and I think a good stiff official would do more in regard to this matter than anything else."

Reid echoed the broader Harvard community in suspecting that Yale had no intentions of backing true change. After all, Yale University had used sports to advance its institutional profile. "Harvard and Yale" became a "happy coupling" due to meetings not in academic settings but rather those on athletic fields. "Why compare standards of scholarship," the *Harvard Graduates' Magazine* satirized, "when at the boat-race or the football game Yale met Harvard as an equal?" While one might have suspected that Yale would join Harvard in the athletics reform movement, Harvard did not see much goodwill from their New Haven counterparts. "It would have been natural to expect cooperation in this imperative from the authorities of Yale—Harvard's chief competitor in sports," the *Graduates'* continued. "But from that day to this Yale has never made any spontaneous advance to meet Harvard halfway; on the contrary, Yale persistently opposed every attempt to curb, or regulate, or purify athletics."

John Owsley, Yale's field instructor, clarified to a local reporter following the White House meeting that the president of the United States had no real jurisdiction. Even as the *Hartford Courant* printed "Walter Camp's Statement," it carried this equivocation: "John Owsley, coach of the Yale eleven, said the suggestions made by the president would have no effect in modifying the game this year, but intimated that there *might* be change in the rules next year."

Still, Roosevelt believed he had done his part. He trusted football's leaders—even the Yalie Camp—to find a path forward. "I cannot tell you how pleased I am at the way you have taken hold," Roosevelt wrote to Camp on October 11. "Now that the matter is in your hands I am more than content to abide by whatever you do."

* * *

As newspapers across the United States covered the White House football meeting, a handful of dailies published an image of Ted, caught by a photographer for the first time on Harvard's football field. "President's Son in Foot Ball Armor," outlets from the *Spokane Press* to the *Wilkes-Barre Times Leader* blared. The coverage was grossly unfair to Ted; the picture captured a dour, fragile looking boy who could have easily passed for twelve years old.

The syndicated story contained enough information to satisfy those interested in the president's oldest son and enough gossip to provide bulletin board coverage for anyone concerned about defending Harvard's honor. According to the unnamed reporter, Ted made his freshmen debut on Harvard's football field along with 150 of his classmates. At first, the curious onlookers couldn't find Ted, after all he wore the same regulation red jersey and canvas trousers as all the other boys. "There were no glasses," the account rued, trading on what was perceived as a Roosevelt standard bearer.

The assessment of Ted's gridiron prospects bordered on cruelty. "Teddy Jr. does not impress one as being a candidate of promise for football honors." This characterization came from but a glance and an image in a sea of other nervous college freshman. "He does not look rugged nor does he appear to be of the thin, fast type." *Not tough, not speedy. Got it.* Then the most damning: "His movements were characteristic of a nervous temperament."

Nervous Temperament: this was an early twentieth-century catchall diagnosis that used questionable (even at this time) phrenological methods to sum up a state of physical and mental fragility. "The nervous temperament is recognized by fine thin hair, thin skin, small thin muscles, quickness in muscular motion, paleness of countenance, and often delicate health," explained George Combe, the author of 1894's *System of Phrenology*. Not one of the 150 young men on Harvard's football fields wanted to be described as possessing a nervous temperament.

Roosevelt wished Ted could avoid the press and the public clamor ("the newspaper men, camera creatures, and idiots generally") altogether. When Ted sat out a late September practice, Roosevelt appreciated that the press had been thwarted. "I saw that you were not out on the football field on Saturday and was rather glad of it," Roosevelt wrote, "as evidently those infernal idiots were eagerly waiting for you."

But Ted was not to be deterred. As the fall wore on, he worked his way through the gauntlet of classmates competing for playing time on Harvard's freshman football team. Roosevelt paid close attention, waffling between a sense of blossoming respect for his oldest son and a lagging concern that Ted didn't quite have the physical tools necessary for football success. Certainly not all the press coverage of Ted cut so sharply. The *Boston Globe* printed an image of Roosevelt on the field looking engaged and intent. The paper reported that "Roosevelt looked pretty small to be competing with the men on the squad, but he went about his work in a determined fashion."

The advice and encouragement, and the fatherly worrying, moved between Washington and Cambridge steadily, usually with letter swapping several times each week.

October 2: "Do not let these newspaper creatures and kindred idiots drive you one hair's breadth from the line you had marked out in football or anything else."

October 11: "I expected that you would find it hard to compete with the other candidates for the position of end, as they are mostly heavier than you... the fact that you are comparatively light tells against you and gives you a good deal to overcome."

Roosevelt was sure that Ted would fail on the football front—at least as a freshman. "He is not going to make the freshman eleven," Roosevelt wrote to Kermit on October 17, 1905. But instead, Ted broke through. After not playing in the freshman team's losses at Groton, Exeter, and Andover, Ted made it onto the field when Harvard traveled to Worcester Academy on October 28. He played well, making a touchdown-saving tackle and distinguishing himself as "one of the star performers for the crimson." The *Boston Globe's* title for the story was an exercise in preemptive praise. "No fault of President's Son that Harvard Freshman Are Beaten," read the widely distributed story.

"Good for you!" TR wrote to Ted four days after the Worcester game. "I was mighty glad you were put on the team for the game, and I judge from the accounts of the tackle in which you got hurt that you upheld the honor of the family all right!"

Ted cemented his spot on the team, playing well in another defeat, versus Dean Academy, and then in the eleven's first victory. Playing in Harvard's massive new stadium on a breezy November day, Ted and his teammates defeated Cushing Academy, 14–0. Finally, a win. The triumph showed, according to the *Harvard Crimson,* "a marked improvement in defensive as well as offensive play."

TR celebrated with Ted as his oldest son earned a measure of athletic success so long fought for. The letters that came regularly provided a new version of the praise and prod formula. A new conquest also emerged: Yale. Might Ted become the first Roosevelt to make it onto the field of athletic battle with Harvard's hated foe? TR hoped so, and he couldn't help but express this hope to Ted. Repeatedly.

November 6: "Good work! I was much pleased by what I read of your playing on the eleven. Of course I hope you will get in the **Yale** game..."

November 7: "We should be overjoyed to see you, but I don't want you to leave if it is going to interfere with your football; still more with your studies... As I say, don't come if it will interfere with either the football or the studies. You must not lose the chance of getting into the **Yale** game, even if it is only a small chance..."

November 11: "I was glad to see you played on your eleven on Saturday, and apparently did well. Of course I hope you get into the **Yale** game, but it doesn't make much real difference for you have been on the team and at the training table and you have evidently shown that you are a game player."

With the Harvard–Yale freshman game on the horizon, Ted (who had been chastised by TR for not writing weekly) provided a football status update. "Dear Father, I am still playing football with the first freshman but I really don't think I will stay there long," Ted opened, worrying from the start. Like almost every college football player—whether he made the competitive squad that took the field versus an opposing school on Saturday or just toiled against his own classmates—Ted battled an increasing number of injuries as the season wore on. Ted had "not been hurt much," but he had suffered enough. "Last Saturday I tore one rib a little loose and yesterday I dislocated my thumb," he wrote.

Yale was on Ted's mind too. The game loomed, and Ted worried he might not play. "The Yale game comes a week from Saturday but our team is not decided on at all yet," he informed his father.

Still, Ted again exceeded expectations. On Yale game day, the *Crimson* provided the roster of the Harvard squad that would play in the rivalry game. Roosevelt was listed second: "T. Roosevelt, left end, prepared at Groton

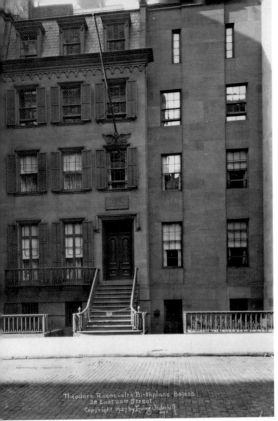

Theodore Roosevelt's birthplace: 28 East 20th Street, New York, NY. *(Library of Congress)*

MEMORANDA.

Measurements T. R. Jr.
Nov 1st 1875

Chest   34 in
Waist   26½ "
Thigh   20 "
Calf   12½ "
Neck   14½ "
Shoulders   41 "
Arms up   10½ "
   " straight   9¾ "
Fore arm   10 "

Weight   124 lbs
Height   5 ft 8 in

A tale of the tape, from Roosevelt's 1875 diary, which he entitled "T.R. Jr. Sporting and Collecting." *(Theodore Roosevelt Collection, Houghton Library, Harvard University)*

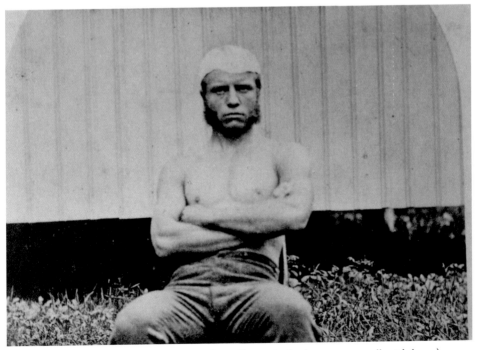

Roosevelt at Harvard, c. 1877, sporting his sculling attire (and some pretty stellar side burns). *(Theodore Roosevelt Collection, Houghton Library, Harvard University)*

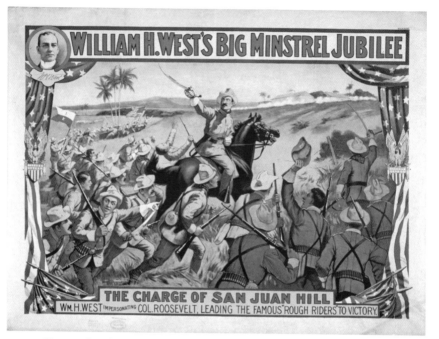

The Rough Riders' capture of San Juan Hill was celebrated in a performance by William H. West's Minstrel Jubilee, c. 1899. Roosevelt is shown leading the charge in this advertisement. *(Library of Congress)*

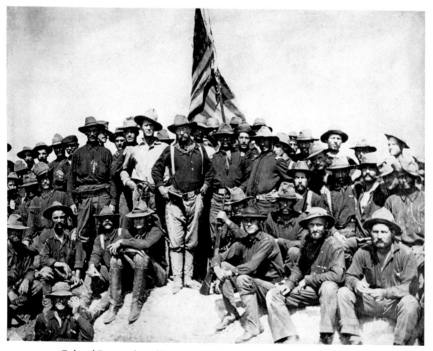

Colonel Roosevelt and his Rough Riders pose at the top of the hill they captured during the Battle of San Juan, July 1898. *(Library of Congress)*

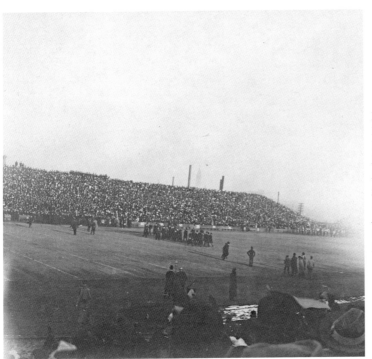

President Theodore Roosevelt crosses Franklin Field at halftime during the Army v. Navy football game on November 30, 1901. *(University Archives and Records Center, University of Pennsylvania)*

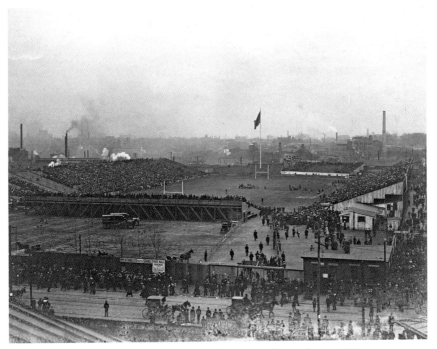

Another view of Franklin Field, University of Pennsylvania, 1901.
(University Archives and Records Center, University of Pennsylvania)

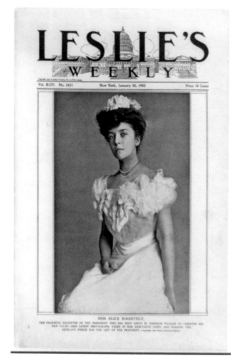

Alice Hathaway Lee Roosevelt, TR's eldest daughter by his first wife, appears on the January 1902 cover of *Leslie's Weekly*. *(Library of Congress)*

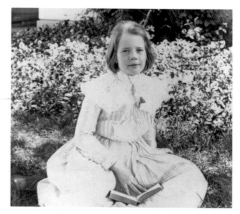

Ethel Roosevelt, 10, in the garden with a book, 1902. *(Library of Congress)*

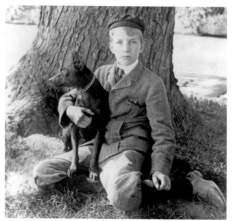

Kermit Roosevelt, 12, poses with his dog, Jack, in June 1902. *(Library of Congress)*

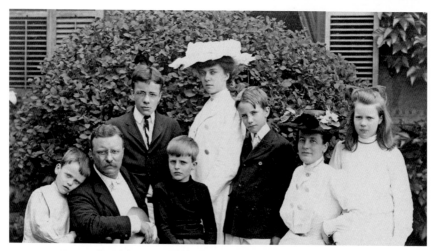

Roosevelt and family in front of their summer home near Oyster Bay on Long Island, NY, 1903. From left to right: Quentin, TR, Ted Jr., "Archie," Alice, Kermit, Edith, and Ethel. *(Library of Congress)*

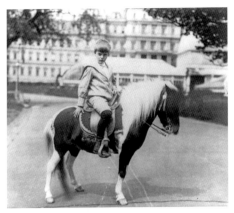
Archie Roosevelt, 6, rides Algonquin, the Roosevelts' pet pony, in 1902. *(Library of Congress)*

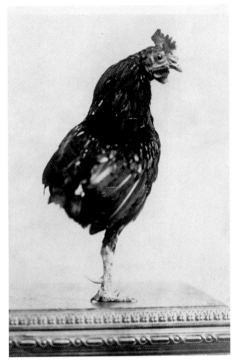
The Roosevelt children's one-legged rooster. *(Library of Congress)*

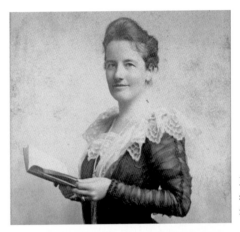
Edith Kermit Carow Roosevelt, TR's second wife, 1902. The pair had been friends since childhood. *(Library of Congress)*

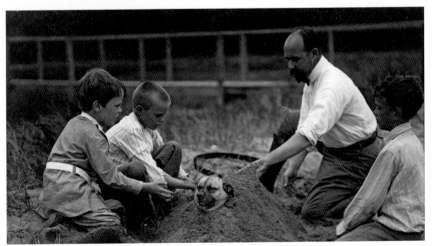
Quentin, Archie, and Nicholas (a cousin) Roosevelt at Sagamore Hill in 1904. Newspaperman Walter Russell has been cajoled into helping bury one of the family's pets. *(Library of Congress)*

Poster for the 1904 Summer Olympics and World's Fair, held in St. Louis, Missouri. *(Public Domain)*

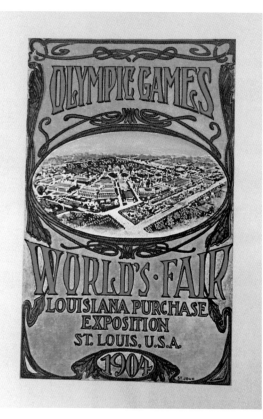

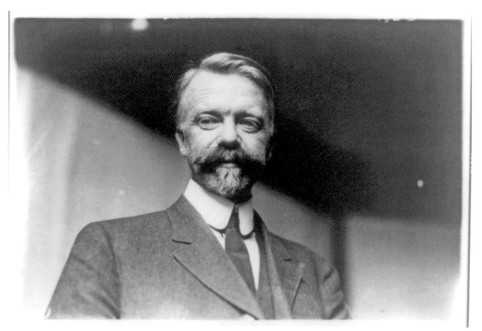

Luther Gulick: athletic evangelist, prodigious asker of questions, and forefather of the PSAL. *(Library of Congress)*

VOL. LV. No. 1422.   PUCK BUILDING, New York, June 1, 1904.   PRICE TEN CENTS.

Copyright, 1904, by Keppler & Schwarzmann.

"What Fools these Mortals be!"

Puck

Entered at N. Y. P. O. as Second-class Mail Matter.

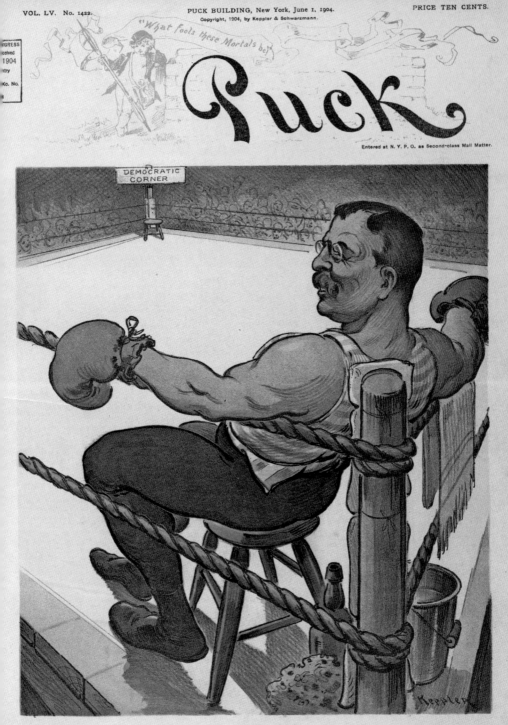

"TERRIBLE TEDDY" WAITS FOR "THE UNKNOWN."

"Terrible Teddy" waits for "the unknown" Democratic
candidate, *Puck Magazine*, 1904. *(Library of Congress)*

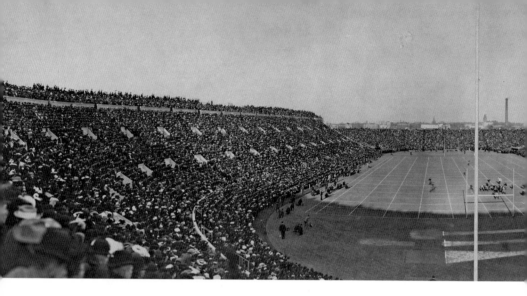

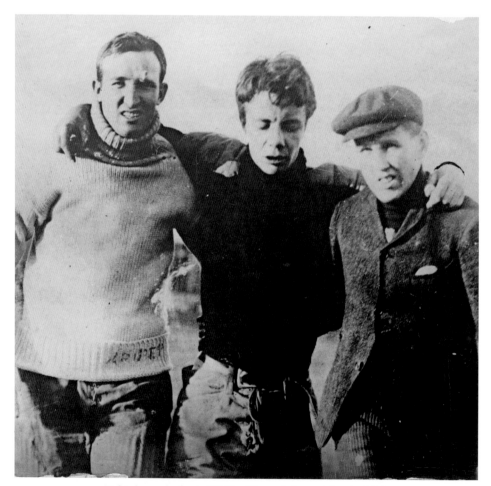

Ted Jr. leaves the football field at Harvard after an injury in 1905.
(Theodore Roosevelt Collection, Houghton Library, Harvard University)

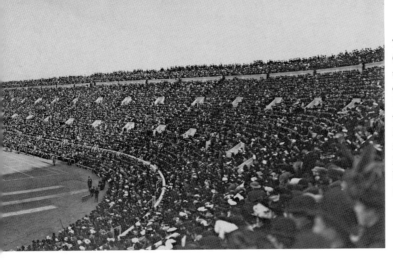

The Harvard Crimson play the Yale Bulldogs on November 25, 1905. The contest—which took place at Harvard Stadium in Cambridge, MA—was attended by 43,000 fans. *(Library of Congress)*

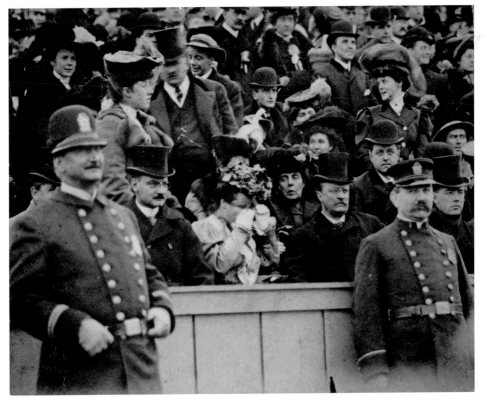

TR attends the 1905 Army v. Navy football match at Princeton University, accompanied by his wife and secretary William Loeb Jr. (front row, second from left).
(Theodore Roosevelt Collection, Houghton Library, Harvard University)

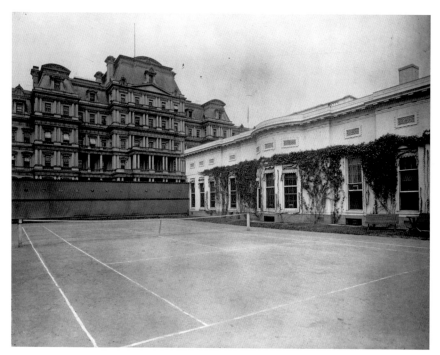

The White House tennis court, 1905. TR was always just
steps away from a match. *(Library of Congress)*

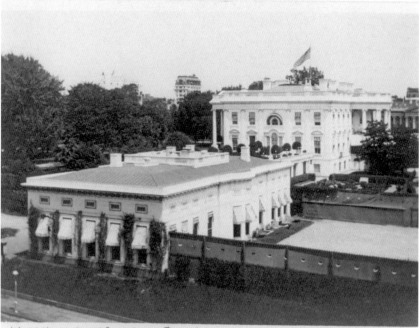

WHITE HOUSE, OFFICE BUILDING, AND TENNIS COURT — WHERE THE ROOSEVELT TENNIS CABINET MET.

Another view of the tennis court in 1909, shortly before it was bulldozed to make
room for the West Wing expansion during Taft's administration. *(Library of Congress)*

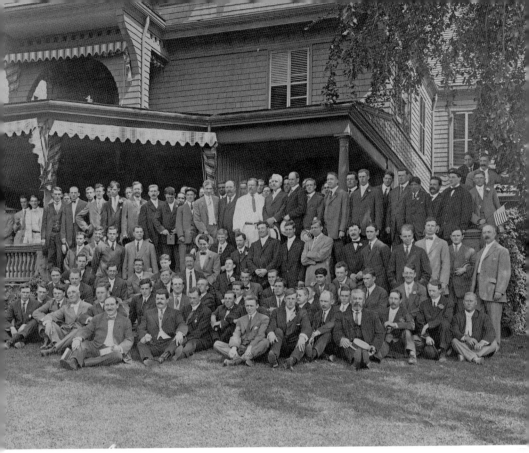

Roosevelt with members of the 1908 Olympic
team at Sagamore Hill. *(Library of Congress)*

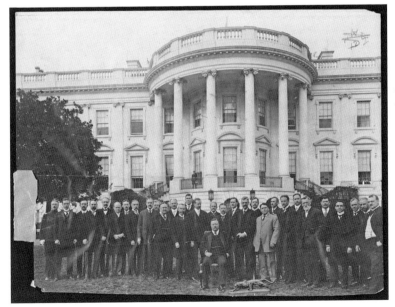

TR and his
Tennis Cabinet
saying farewell,
1909. Notice the
bronze cougar at
Roosevelt's feet.
(Library of Congress)

TR chops a fallen tree in the summer of 1905 near his Sagamore Hill home. Chopping wood was one form of exercise he undertook during and after his presidency. *(Library of Congress)*

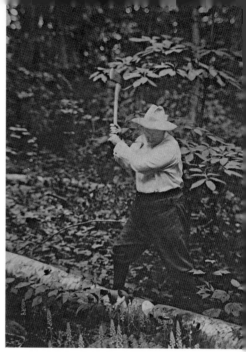

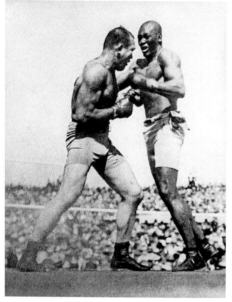

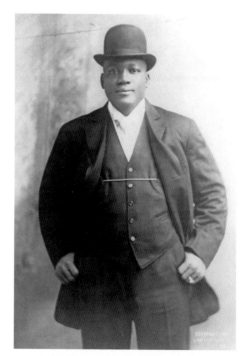

Jack Johnson battles "The Great White Hope" Jim Jeffries in the racially charged and highly publicized 1910 "Fight of the Century." Leading up to the fight, Johnson suggested TR serve as referee. *(Public Doman)*

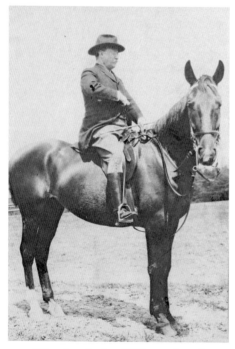

TR on horseback, c. 1909, near the end of his presidency. *(Library of Congress)*

Jack Johnson, Heavyweight Champion of the World, 1909. *(Library of Congress)*

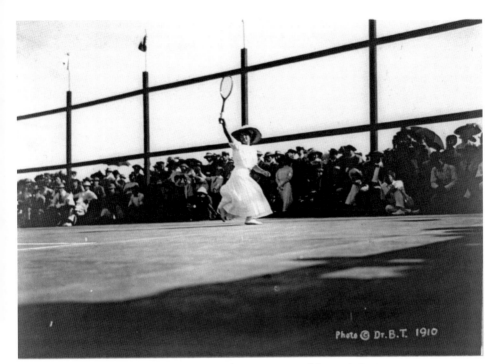

Hazel Hotchkiss Wightman, tennis trailblazer, 1910.
(Library of Congress)

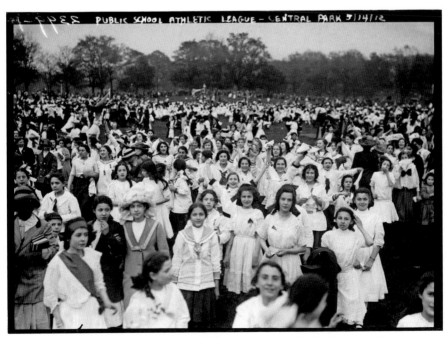

A gathering of the PSAL Girls Branch, 1912, in Central Park, New York City.
Activist Grace Dodge spearheaded the branch's founding in 1905, and by 1910,
20,000 girls were participating in PSAL activities. *(Library of Congress)*

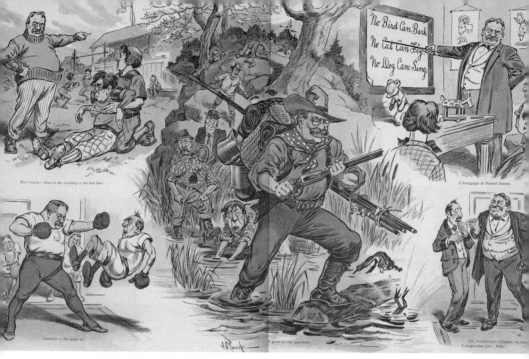

This 1907 edition of *Puck Magazine* imagines future occupations for TR after the presidency, including: rugged sporting guide, Natural History teacher, instructor in the "manly art" of boxing, athletics coach, and physician. *(Library of Congress)*

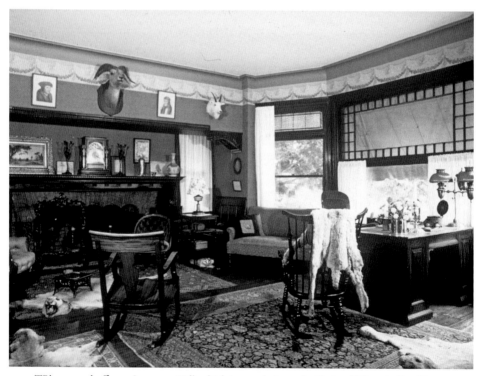

TR's personal office at Sagamore Hill, which is now designated a National Historic Site. Notice the animal skins from his many hunting expeditions strewn about. *(National Park Service)*

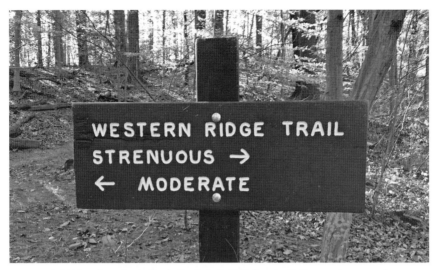

A 2019 trail marker in Rock Creek Park, TR's favorite D.C. tramping ground. When in doubt, pick "strenuous." *(Author's Collection)*

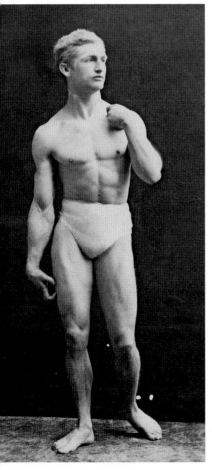

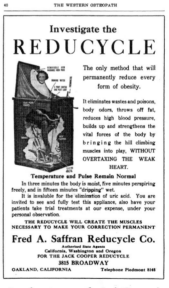

An advertisement for Jack Cooper's patented "Reducycle" machine, a sadistic combination of exercise bike and sauna. As TR's personal trainer, Cooper kept the ex-President on a challenging customized exercise regimen in 1917. *(Public Domain)*

Eccentric fitness advocate Bernarr Macfadden poses as the statue *David* in a photograph for his *Physical Culture* magazine, c. 1905. *(Public Domain)*

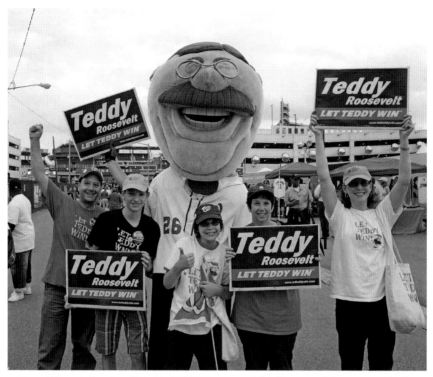

Scott Ableman, founder of *blog.LetTeddyWin.com*, and family pose with longtime underdog "Teddy" at Nationals Park. The Presidents Race, in which mascots of former US presidents square off during the fourth inning of every Washington Nationals home game, is a fan favorite. Between its inception in 2006 and 2012, Teddy failed to win a single race. *(Scott Ableman)*

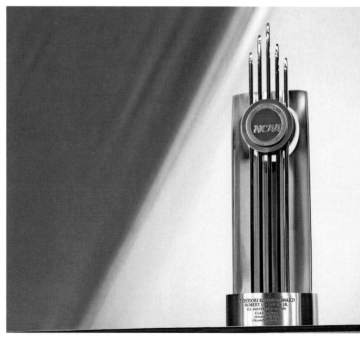

The NCAA's highest honor, The Theodore Roosevelt Award (aka "The Teddy") is given annually to former college varsity athletes who went on to become distinguished citizens of outstanding national reputation. Past winners include former US Presidents Eisenhower, Ford, (H. W.) Bush, and Reagan. *(NCAA/ NCAA photos)*

School, where he played on the second eleven. He is 18 years old, 5 feet 8 inches tall, and weighs 145 pounds."

Roosevelt weighed twenty-seven pounds less than the average of the other lineman on the squad. He was the shortest man on the team. He was the only player whose bio mentioned that his high school football experience had been as a member of a "second eleven."

But on the team was on the team. The decision to include Ted on the roster "caused no little stir among the Harvard undergraduating." According to a broadly syndicated article, "All the season it was known that Roosevelt had been putting up a great fight, but the feeling everywhere prevailed that he was too light to be chosen for the final team...This, however, is not the case." The headline from a nonlocal newspaper (about a freshman football game) said it all: YOUNG ROOSEVELT WILL BE AT LEFT END FOR HARVARD FRESHMAN.

* * *

The biggest game of Ted's life occurred on a practice field. Since Harvard's varsity was hosting Dartmouth (playing to an uninspired 6–6 tie) in Harvard Stadium at the same time as the freshman game, Ted's squad was relegated to Soldier's Field—the place where the team conducted most of its practices.

The president of the United States did not attend.

Nevertheless, the Harvard–Yale freshman football game became one of the most infamous games in college football history. Certainly it holds the distinction of being the most widely remembered non-varsity college football game, held on a practice field, ever. The Yale freshmen entered the Harvard game with a 4–2 record. Harvard was 1–5, having managed a victory only over Dean Academy. In four of its six previous contests, Harvard had failed to score.

Yale kicked off to start the contest. Harvard's offense got going right away with its plight for the day: an almost complete inability to move the ball. "Harvard was extremely weak on both offense and defense," the *Boston Globe* explained. So Harvard punted the ball back to Yale. Starting at its own twenty-five-yard line, Yale simply pushed the smaller, weaker, less-talented

Crimson players backward. Time after time, Yale rushed the ball straight through the line. No finesse, no trickery. Yale ended its first drive with a touchdown and extra point. 6–0.*

The difference between the teams was obvious. The student journalist of the *Harvard Crimson* could not (or did not want to) cover up the deficiencies of his classmates: "Throughout the game the Harvard players were clearly outclassed, and were unable to make any consistent gains. On the defense the Harvard team was weak."

In this situation—facing a hated rival, burdened by his father's constant hope that he would take part, and with the nation's press paying attention to a game it would otherwise have ignored completely—Ted fought savagely against wave after wave of attackers. He helped stem the tide and turn a whupping into a, well, less worse whupping.

Playing at left end, Ted repeatedly slid between linemen who outweighed him by forty pounds to get at the ball carrier. Yale's coach took notice: "How that little player was able to get into so many of our plays and break them up I don't know." R.B. Buren, the Yale player who played directly opposite Ted, declared him one of the finest players he'd ever seen. Was this pandering toward the son of the president? Perhaps. But Ted's play undoubtedly earned his opponent's respect.

Yale led 10–0 at halftime. Harvard managed only three first downs for the entire game. In the second half, Ted's body language seemed to change, even if his spirit seemed as resolute as ever. He was "staggering" and "groggy." His tackling shifted from "low and hard" to a more primitive approach. "He held gamely to his work, and kept getting the man with the ball," reported a journalist who seemed genuinely touched by the effort, "but they just dragged him along with them."

---

* Football's basic scoring at this juncture: touchdown–5, field goal–4, and extra point–1, slightly different than the 1901 (5, 5, 1) rules witnessed by TR at Army–Navy. Also during TR's era, some schools simply negotiated their own modified scoring system before a game. The current scoring model (6, 3, 1) was rolled out in 1912. In 1958, the NCAA adopted the two point conversion option following touchdowns.

As the game clock wound down, the repeated blows took their effect. Ted kept getting "battered and smashed by end plays, in which he was trampled down and stepped upon." The Yale coach certainly recognized that, despite his tenacity, Ted's build represented an opportunity for his squad. An undersized lineman simply meant less poundage for his boys to have to overcome. And so the Yale attack veered toward Ted repeatedly. "We planned to circle plays at end, knowing that he was very light," Yale's coach McClintock admitted after the game was over. After one play, Ted stayed down as another pile nearby unraveled itself. "He was knocked out and lay on the ground for some time," wrote a reporter for the *Washington Post*. But then he arose and played on.

Finally, it ended. Late in the second half, with Yale leading 16–0 and pushing forward again, a massive pile-up occurred. One by one, the boy-gladiators found their feet. All except for Ted. "When the whistle blew and the men were pulled off the heap, there, underneath everyone else, lay young Roosevelt, cut, bruised, and bleeding, unable to stir." His nose had been broken. He was unconscious.

At this point, his much-discussed weight (*Washington Post*: "Too bad he's so light. He's the pluckiest man on the team, and if he had a little more beef he'd make things just a little more interesting.") finally worked in Ted's favor. Several Harvard teammates helped Ted up. When it became obvious that he could not support himself, the Harvard boys carried the son of the POTUS to the locker room. He was done for the day.

* * *

"Good for you!" TR wrote to Ted on November 19, the day after the Harvard freshmen lost to Yale, 0–16. "Of course I am sorry that Yale beat us, but I am very glad that you made the team and I am not merely glad but very proud that you should have played as you evidently did play in the game." There was no holding back here. Roosevelt swelled with affection for his namesake, who had accomplished something that TR had always wanted for himself. TR may have had the Rough Riding experience, but he never took the football field versus Yale. While Roosevelt missed this seminal game in Ted's life, he did attend the varsity Harvard–Yale game one week later.

Roosevelt was proud, but he wasn't satisfied. In his same letter: "Incidentally I very sincerely hope that now that football is over you will be able to do better in your studies. A record of C's with an occasional D does not allow much margin for accidents, and while I think it was entirely satisfactory during the time you were playing football, I hope you can improve upon it a little now."

In the days that followed, speculation arose about whether Yale had unfairly targeted Ted. Was this another example of football's tendency to push beyond physical play and embrace brutish violence? After all, Yale's game plan seemed to target Harvard's smallest player. But it wasn't that simple, as evidenced even by the reactions from within the White House. "Mother and Ethel were very indignant about Yale, and Mother especially was inclined to take a very dark view of the conduct of the Yale team in playing at you," TR wrote.

TR, not surprisingly, saw it differently. "I think it was rather a compliment," he wrote to Ted. But regardless, it was imperative that Ted not make a fuss. "You are the last man in the world that would squeal about it," Roosevelt wrote. "I am very proud of what you have done and I feel that you have lived right up to the doctrines you have preached and that you have upheld the family credit in great shape."

The *New York Times* found the silver lining as well. ROOSEVELT NOSE STRAIGHT, the paper reported in the days following Ted's violent game with Yale. "Theodore Roosevelt Jr. has Yale to thank for a nose set straight. While boxing several years ago he got a blow on his nose which resulted in a slight crook at the bridge." Fortunately, football's violence took care of the problem. "In Saturday's game a Yale man's fist—or foot, maybe—took out the crook." So there was that.

Everyone could exhale with the season over. "I am mighty glad you played football this year," TR repeated, in case Ted had somehow missed the sentiment. "And I am not at all sorry that you are too light to try for the varsity, so that this will really be your last year hard at it." Ted had made no such decision, but apparently his father had.

Three times during the 1905 football season Ted appeared on the "Details of the More Serious Injuries" list kept by the *Chicago Daily Tribune*. The day after Yale, he had his broken nose set, a procedure that "caused me scarcely any pain at all," he told his mother. After resting for a day at his grandmother's house, he returned to campus a hero. "I never thought he would do it," one Harvard senior gushed. Ted was the "sandiest" freshman Harvard had seen in years. His fellow freshmen immediately moved to consider Ted for the position of class president.

The national press lauded him as well. The headlines signaled that his football career, wherever it might go from here, had been a success:

YOUNG ROOSEVELT HAS ALL HIS FATHER'S GRIT.

YOUNG ROOSEVELT: GRIDIRON HERO.

PRESIDENT'S PLUCKY SON SOMEWHAT
DISFIGURED, BUT THAT'S ALL.

When asked to weigh in on the still-flurrying football debate—the White House conference had yielded nothing yet, although the beginnings of the NCAA would be in place shortly—Ted refused to comment. "If silence means consent, however, and if his swollen face signifies anything, the President's son has learned by this time that football is strenuous," the press reported.

Despite his injury history, Ted signed on to play a second year of football at Harvard. Early in the 1906 season, Ted sprained his knee. Then in subsequent action Ted broke his ankle. Initially misdiagnosed as a sprain, the ankle never healed properly. Ted finally, mercifully, gave up football.

* * *

Just as Ted was limping away from the game of college football, the National Collegiate Athletic Association was coming to life. The organization would help cement the strange bond between athletics and higher education in the United States for the century to come, and the NCAA's birth came from a place of fear and resignation on the part of football advocates. The October

1905 White House football summit had accomplished little in terms of immediate change. The attention surrounding college football increased but so too did the numbers of injured players. At the end of the 1905 season, a Union College football player, Harold Moore, died due to a blow to the head during a game at New York University.

Moore's death set off a series of events. NYU's Chancellor Henry MacCracken wrote to Charles Eliot suggesting that Harvard host a conference to, once and for all, reform—or abolish if need be—college football. MacCracken was concerned about not only the violence in the game but also how football made American universities look to the rest of the world. Eliot, recognizing he might not actually have the power to change the game played out so spectacularly on his own campus, refused.

MacCracken forged ahead anyhow. On December 8, 1905, the "MacCracken meeting" brought together thirteen schools to discuss the future of football. Harvard did not participate, nor did Yale or Princeton. The outcome of this meeting was the call for another meeting; on December 28, sixty-eight universities sent representatives to New York City for the founding convention of the Intercollegiate Athletic Association of the United States (IAAUS).

Meanwhile, Harvard was running its own football inquisition. At issue was a particular violent play during the Harvard–Yale varsity game from a few weeks before. During the contest, Harvard's Francis Burr had called for a fair catch on a punt. Yale's defenders on the play either didn't notice the fair catch call, or they ignored it all together. And to make matters worse, one of the defenders, Jim Quill, struck Burr in the face on the tackle, breaking Burr's nose. The official for the game, Navy's Paul Dashiell, neglected to call a penalty.

This time Roosevelt decided to conduct his own investigation. He summoned Reid back to the White House. The two met on December 4, 1905. Just Reid this time; just two Harvard men talking football. Roosevelt also corresponded with Eliot, who provided sworn statements from spectators who attested to the overt brutality of the play. Roosevelt then gave Dashiell, a Navy man who happened to be waiting on a promotion from the commander in chief, a chance to tell his side of the story.

Roosevelt concluded that indeed a line had been crossed. He, for once, agreed with Eliot's criticism of football. Dashiell had blown the call (or no-call in this case), and the outcome of this contest between Yale and Harvard had been decided by wanton violence rather than skillful athletic performance. This was not football as Roosevelt conceived of it. After sharing his conclusions with all parties involved—this was a case of presidential influence through the means of simply expressing his sincere disappointment—Roosevelt withdrew again. He would take his football intervention no further. He requested that his correspondence on the Quill–Burr matter be kept confidential.

Harvard devolved into a state of a bureaucratic civil war—all over the issue of football. The day after his meeting with Roosevelt, Reid accepted the chairmanship of a Harvard Athletic Association Committee on reforming football. A few days later, the Committee on Athletics for Harvard's Board of Overseers voted to abolish football. At this point, Roosevelt jumped back in. "I do not agree with you that the game should be stopped," he wrote to Eliot on December 21, 1905.

As the new year dawned, the football debate roared on. At Harvard, the Board of Overseers issued a temporary stay of execution: no football would take place at Cambridge until a new set of reform rules was in place. Harvard's faculty, responding late to the matter but nevertheless eager to conduct a vote on something that someone cared about, voted simply to abolish the game.

Fortunately for football advocates, reform efforts began to take hold. The IAAUS worked diligently to craft a new set of rules. Led by Reid (who was leading the football cause at Harvard and more nationally), the IAAUS wrested the reform process from the Football Rules Committee that had been long controlled by Walter Camp. On March 31, 1906, the IAAUS announced its changes. The new rules mandated a neutral zone between the offensive and defensive lines before the snap of the ball, six offensive linemen, ten yards for a first down (in three downs), and the introduction of the forward pass. The changes meant to open up the action and limit mass-momentum collisions.

The changes muted some of the criticism. Based on the new rules, Harvard's Athletic Association voted to allow football to continue at the university. The

Board of Overseers, over President Eliot's objections, followed suit. Football had been saved at Harvard.

The tidal wave of injuries, not unlike those that ultimately drove Ted from the game, continued in 1906 and beyond. Reformers continued to call for changes long beyond the first decade of the twentieth century. Columbia, Stanford, Georgetown, and Cal Berkley all banned football from their campuses—until they reinstated the game at a later time. A movement by Progressive reformers to replace football with rugby on the West Coast gained some momentum before eventually subsiding. By the 1920s rumblings about sharing some of the gate receipts from big games with the players, in this university-directed "amateur" sport, began to appear in the press. But the overarching question—the question of whether football should be a part of university life in the United States—had been answered. Yes. For all its collateral damage, for all its competing interests, for all its predatory impulses...Yes. Roosevelt through his concern for Ted had pushed this argument toward a definitive answer. He was, basically, satisfied with the result.

In 1910, the IAAUS changed its name to the National Collegiate Athletic Association.

EIGHT

"WALKING"

*Walk out your troubles. There is no malady of mind or body that you
can't walk away. Not one person in ten has exercised enough. Inaction gives
you the blues and a poor stomach. The two together make bad nerves,
bad tempers, and bad characters. Walking will cure all.*

—Edward Payson Weston

Roosevelt woke up alone on his forty-ninth birthday. It was Sunday, October 27, 1907, and clouds and drizzle hung over Washington, DC. Roosevelt dressed, ate breakfast (always an event at the White House), and then headed to see Ethel and Edith at the Episcopal Eye and Ear Hospital. Ethel, sixteen years old, had undergone a minor nasal surgery. Edith stayed by her daughter's side around the clock, leaving Roosevelt without his closest companion.

Roosevelt knew better than to come empty-handed; he brought a gift for his "poor girlie." Or a regift actually. Roosevelt had received an early birthday present from Quan Yick Nam, a New York businessman who often mailed gifts to the White House. Nam had sent a jade charm to the president a few days prior. Roosevelt took this "treasure" and presented it to his bedridden daughter.

From the hospital, Roosevelt, alone save for his protection, walked to Grace Reformed Church on Fifteenth Street, near Rhode Island Avenue, where he attended the weekly service. The spired, stain-glassed, "very churchly" church was TR's worship home for all of his presidency. He attended regularly. If he had to miss, he sent Rev. John Schick a note by courier an hour before service time explaining his absence. Roosevelt took notes on the sermon, received communion, and sang along to the hymns. His pew was the third from the front, on the left side.

In addition to his daughter's health on this day, Roosevelt might well have offered up a prayer for the American economy. Wall Street teetered on the edge of total collapse. New York's Knickerbocker Trust, the city's third largest bank, had suspended operations due to insolvency five days earlier. The value of the American stock market had fallen by 50 percent from the previous year's high. The press made no bones about the culprit, labeling the crisis, "The Roosevelt Panic of 1907."

After the service, Roosevelt returned to the White House. He spent some time on his correspondence. There were dozens of birthday wishes to peruse. Roosevelt rarely went a day without writing to one of his children; he wrote Kermit on this Sunday afternoon. He did not mention his birthday. Instead, the financial crisis had his attention. "We have had a stormy week in the New York financial circles," Roosevelt wrote to his son. "I hope but am by no means sure that the worst is now over. Of course it has produced the usual paroxysm of screams and yells about me."

Roosevelt's only visitor for the day was George Cortelyou, the secretary of the Treasury. Cortelyou had spent the previous week in New York City attending to the financial crisis by extending $25 million in government deposits to floundering banks. The president received an update.

Finally it was time for the day's main event, the only happening during the day that hinted at a celebration: a long walk.

The president needed the workout. The *Washington Post* and *New York Times* had decided that the president's birthday was a fitting time to talk about Roosevelt's double chin. The newspapers feigned defense of the president: "The 'double chin' allegation" (or #TRHasADoubleChin, as we'd call it today) was actually old news, they pointed out. But still, the conversation about Roosevelt's "superfluous avoirdupois" suggested once again that Roosevelt was losing ground in the fight against extra pounds.

Just before 5:00 p.m., with the temperature dipping below fifty degrees Fahrenheit and the rain spitting, Roosevelt left the White House. The sun dipped toward the horizon. TR headed in the direction of Rock Creek Park in Northwest Washington, DC. Unlike most days, Roosevelt walked alone. He did not have Jusserand or Garfield. Pinchot must have been busy. Ted and Kermit were away at school. The Secret Service agents stayed within sight, but they too left Roosevelt alone to his walking.

The rain intensified. The last of the sunlight filtered away. And somewhere the walk turned from exercise to something of the "I've-still-got-it" ilk. Roosevelt used no umbrella; he wore no topcoat or raincoat. "During his trip, the rain at times came down in torrents," the *Washington Herald* reported. Still Roosevelt pressed on. Finally, having covered ten miles or so, Roosevelt felt fatigue set in. The president turned back; he made it to the White House at 8:00 p.m., drenched but "apparently satisfied that he had done himself good physically by the trip."

The press dutifully reported on Roosevelt's strenuous behavior and his good health. "Being only forty-nine years young yesterday," the *Washington Times* reported, "Theodore Roosevelt, President of the United States, limbered up his physique with a three-hour tramp through the rain."

The Washington papers especially were keeping a close eye on Roosevelt's health. Everyone could see the president aging. The press observed the strain of the White House. While he wasn't prewar Lincoln versus postwar Lincoln quite yet, Roosevelt's mustache was graying. He had fuller cheeks. His 1907 portrait revealed the buttons on his suit vest doing yeoman's work. And yes, there was a bit of a double chin.

The fact that Roosevelt's secretary of state had collapsed from exhaustion in August probably also heightened the health watch. Elihu Root had buckled during a visit to Sagamore Hill. "He had broken under the strain and seemed to have been robbed of his power of speech." Roosevelt immediately intervened and ordered Root off to the Muldoon Institute—a health and physical training sanitarium in Purchase, New York, run by former wrestling champion William Muldoon. For three weeks, Root rode horses, boxed with Muldoon, and took long walks in the open, country air. The United States' diplomatic work could wait.

Roosevelt did what he could to allay fears and control the message regarding his own fitness. When a photographer wanted some pictures of the president on horseback, Roosevelt agreed but then kept rejecting the proofs. *That's not how I look* seemed to be the crux of Roosevelt's objections. When rumors circulated in May 1907 that Roosevelt had "broken down physically," TR addressed the issue head on. First there was a show: "The President stretched out his arms, threw out his chest, and walked up and down his office in a way to indicate that he felt full of vigor." Next came the statistical breakdown: "They say in Wall street that I am breaking down. I weighed in this morning and touched the beam at one hundred and ninety odd pounds. I am able to take a hurdle five feet four." And then the closing: "I have never felt better in my life."

*   *   *

"We have a delightful thing at home called a 'point to point' walk," Ted remembered of his childhood. "It was really an invention of my father's." The rules were simple. "What you did was this: You took a starting point, let us say by the old barn. Then you picked up another point, perhaps two miles away, a big tree or a house or the top of a house." Then—and surely there was a great lesson at play here—you stuck to the course, no matter what. "You went directly from one point to the other, without turning aside for anything. If you came to a barn, you couldn't go around the barn—you had to go through it or over it. If you came to a pond, you couldn't go around the pond—you had to swim it."

The point-to-point walk seems endearing when thinking of a father with his children; it sounds bizarre when it involves the president of the United States and unsuspecting diplomats. "His walking has become one [of] the recog-

nized terrors of White House hospitality," was how one contemporary described it. "Often," Roosevelt recalled, "especially in the winters and early
springs, we would arrange for a point-to-point walk, not turning aside for anything—for instance, swimming Rock Creek or even the Potomac if it came in
our way."

Getting an invitation to walk with Roosevelt was both highly prized and
strangely casual. Jusserand was the best-case example. He represented France
better because he trudged through trails and streams of the mid-Atlantic region
with the president. Upon arriving in Washington, DC, Jusserand had feared
that his own relationship with TR might never equal that of the well-established
ambassadors of Britain or Germany. Fortunately for Jusserand, Britain's man
could not keep up with Roosevelt. Britain's ambassador, Mortimer Durand, fell
apart in his one attempt to walk with Roosevelt. "We drove out to Rock Creek,"
Durand recalled, "and he plunged down to the *khud* and made me struggle
through bushes and over rocks for two hours and a half, at an impossible speed,
til I was so done that I could hardly stand." Down went Britain.

Germany's man, at least during the middle of Roosevelt's presidency, fared
better. Baron Hermann Speck von Sternburg was initiated by Roosevelt right
away. Sternburg presented his credentials to Roosevelt in August 1903, at Sagamore Hill. Roosevelt liked this "first-class little fellow" right away. So much
so that Roosevelt insisted he stay with his family for a spell. "I kept him for a
couple of days as a playmate," Roosevelt confessed. "He is very fond of tennis,
of chopping, of walking, riding, etc."

The baron's fitness for scrambling declined, however, as he struggled with
lupus. For a time, Roosevelt asked tentatively for the baron to come out for a
walk. "I want you to show this letter to your wife [American Lillian Langham]
before answering," he wrote in 1904. "I am going to take Durand for a mild
scramble down Rock Creek today…If she thinks it is all right, then will you
join me at the White House in rough walking clothes…" But as the rejections
piled up, Roosevelt stopped asking altogether. Down went Germany.

Jusserand proved to be the steadiest walking mate of the ambassadors. Vive
la France!

Regardless of the company, Roosevelt loved Rock Creek Park. Located five miles to the north of the White House, it was another world. Exertion, opportunity, challenge—these things confronted a man in RCP. Nuances receded and literal cliffs loomed for the climbing. Roosevelt had learned the park with Leonard Wood when Wood was stationed at the White House and Roosevelt worked as the assistant secretary of the Navy. The two had named certain passages and rock formations. The "seal's walk" and "the chimney," the former requiring passage via a slide on one's stomach, were two favorites. "We liked Rock Creek for these walks because we could do so much scrambling and climbing along the cliffs," Roosevelt said. Roosevelt seemed to want to remind himself daily that his body still provided a congruent partner for his mind. He needed to remember that his efforts while sitting at a White House desk were not the sum total of his abilities.

Even TR's Sabbaths seemed aggressive. "Sunday is President Roosevelt's day of rest, although many people who have been invited to help him in taking his rest are inclined to think his rest and recreation are what would generally be called hard work or violent exercise," wrote one White House reporter. Roosevelt walked and climbed and romped in the District and Virginia and Maryland throughout his presidency. His favorites—Garfield, Pinchot, and Jusserand—often tagged along.

Lawrence Murray too, who had fared poorly on his first excursion with Roosevelt, kept at it as he stayed in Washington. He marveled at the president's desire to challenge himself and his natural surroundings. Crazy as he thought Roosevelt was, Murray jumped at the president's invitations. Then as now, few turned down the president's call.

"On Saturday afternoon the President loved to drive out in the country eight or ten miles with three or four others," Murray remembered, "dismiss the carriages and walk back along the most difficult route he could possibly find." Roosevelt also favored the sheer rocks of Rock Creek Park, some rising more than seventy-five feet above the water, for challenging climbing assents. "He made these walks and climbs so often that he knew exactly where the niches were, and where to look for the finger holds, and never made a mistake." Or at least rarely. "But once…he missed his footing on a rainy day and fell about fifteen feet into the water and on some sharp rocks in the bed of the creek."

For Murray, Roosevelt's pace was always the worst part. "What the President called a walk was a run: no stop, no breathing time, no slacking of speed, but a continuous race, careless of mud, thorns, and the rest." Murray always brought up the rear. On this particular day, when Murray caught up to the rest of the presidential group, they stood at the foot of a rock wall staring up. *Seriously?* After a short deliberation on best routes, the group began scaling upward. Murray watched carefully for the optimal foot- and hand-holds as his colleagues went first. Then he lifted off, barely keeping up. "Everything went along all right until we came to a place along the back where the rocks went up perfectly straight for about fifty feet." There was no turning back. Roosevelt led, as usual, from the front and determined the group should proceed upward. "Be careful," the president yelled. TR went first and "made the climb all right but after a hard struggle." Gifford Pinchot and Knox Smith summited with impressive strength and precision.

Only Murray remained on the rock face. He made slow progress initially. Then all at once Murray found himself stuck in a humiliating climbing purgatory. "I got half way up and then for the life of me I could not see or feel on this bare wall of perpendicular rock a place for a toe or a finger." Murray probed in all directions. Then to his increasing panic, he discovered that he could not descend either. "And," Murray recounted years later, "to fall was serious injury at the least."

From the top, Pinchot, Roosevelt, and Smith provided a torrent of advice. Nearly paralyzed in his position, Murray edged a bit in one direction, then in the other. Finally he admitted defeat. "At last I said that I could not possibly get up." Death on the side of a Rock Creek cliff was indeed a sad way to go out. But then his walking partners sprang into action. Roosevelt probably (Murray did not admit as much) leaped at the chance to make a rescue. Climbing, hiking, and now saving a perilously perched, civil servant climber. What a day!

Quick as a wisk Roosevelt fell on the ground, grabbed a small scrub oak tree, and told Pinchot to put his arm around Roosevelt's body and lower himself over the cliff as far down as he could and possibly his leg would come down so I could reach it. This Pinchot did, and I was able to get a firm hold with one arm and then steadied and reassured, with the other I was able to get up after a few anxious moments. Pinchot and Smith who are great jokers told everyone that I was a good climber, and made a fair showing in the opening trail, only seemed to feel safer hanging on a rope even if made with human legs.

This image, too, is almost too much to believe. The US president and his esteemed director of forestry laid on the ground, held on to a shrub, and made a human ladder. Then a fellow government employee climbed to safety.

Like Murray, Jules Jusserand became a regular walker. "After a while," Jusserand said, "President Roosevelt gave me that unique proof of trust and friendship: he asked me to a 'walk.'" Thus began the US–Franco Rock Creek Summits that provided Roosevelt and Jusserand with great pleasure over the course of Roosevelt's second term in the White House. For Jusserand, the walks always meant a forfeiture of an outfit. "Put on your worst clothes," Roosevelt would mention casually to Jusserand as they planned for an afternoon walk. He did it so often that Jusserand's answer eventually shifted from one of casual accommodation to a joking, "But, Mr. President, I have no worst clothes left."

As Murray recounted, Jusserand recalled the walks as excursions that involved very little walking at all. The cardinal rule involved *not* avoiding the obstacles in one's path. "My first experience...not knowing the rules of the game, which were never to go around an obstacle, I went around several." Roosevelt provided a quick, friendly correction. "But the moment I knew, I stuck to the rule, greatly helped by my youthful climbings in the Forez mountains." The pace these middle-aged men kept is difficult to calculate despite the many memories of Roosevelt's brisk speed. We can guess that they were not moving much faster than a fifteen-minute mile. Roosevelt was, after all, a rather stocky, completely ordinary athlete nearing his fiftieth birthday. There were not records being won.

* * *

While everything that Roosevelt did garnered attention (he was the president of the United States after all), he was not the nation's most famous walker. Not even close. That designation belonged, in 1907 (as it had for the past four decades), to Edward Payson Weston. A "craggy, white-haired gent with a walrus mustache," as one historian put it, the sixty-nine-year-old Weston was an evangelist of "the gospel of walking."

In 1907 (as Roosevelt was torturing civil servants in Rock Creek Park), Weston was at the tail end of a career that stretched back to the election of Roosevelt's hero, Abraham Lincoln. In 1860, Weston lost a bet and as a consequence walked 478 miles from Boston to Washington, DC. He just missed arriving in time to see the inauguration itself but enjoyed celebrating with the new president at an inauguration ball. After serving in the Union Army during the Civil War, Weston made walking his career. He became a high-stakes pedestrian. He moved from one challenge to the next, pushing the bounds of what Americans deemed possible. Over the next six decades, as railroads expanded and the first prototypes of automobiles appeared, Weston made the case that walking had hardly been explored as a true means of transportation.

His feats were legendary. In 1867, Weston walked from Portland, Maine, to Chicago. He covered the 1,326 miles in thirty days. In 1874, Weston walked five hundred miles around a track in less than five days. During the second half of the nineteenth century, Weston participated in more than one thousand endurance contests. Twice he walked across the United States. In 1885, Weston dueled with Daniel O'Leary in his last head-to-head contest. The two men battled in a 2,500-mile match race, walking around arenas across the eastern half of the United States, in a sort of roving walking circuit. Over the course of fifty-four days, Weston averaged forty-six miles per day. Weston surged from behind to win. Weston trekked from Manhattan to Albany, New York, in the dead of winter, battling ice and snow to cover the 160 miles in less than sixty hours. Weston held the records for 200, 250, and 300 miles.

The press referred to him, simply, as "The Pedestrian." And Weston was a showman. He loved to interview. He glad-handed every potential business partner and publicist within reach. When Weston completed a 5,000-mile trek around Great Britain in one-hundred days (Sundays excluded), the whole world heard about it.

Occasionally, Weston failed in his high-profile challenges. Roosevelt had attended one such event. In 1896, Roosevelt, then police commissioner, looked on (he was slated to be the honorary starter, but he arrived too late) as Weston attempted to break his record of 112 miles in twenty-four hours. Starting at 10 o'clock on Christmas night, Weston walked around a track built over the ice at the Skating Palace on Lexington Avenue. The track was eight laps to a mile. For the first nineteen hours, Weston was a "well regulated machine." He clicked off one mile after another. Then he began to fall apart. His stride hitched, and then Weston became too dizzy to walk. He had to rest for a few minutes. Just a few minutes. Doctors intervened, however, and insisted that Weston remain down for nearly an hour, ruining any chance of breaking the record.

Even with 112 miles out of reach, Weston demanded that he be allowed to do everything that he could. He got back on the track and walked until the final minute. Then he trudged an extra lap just to be sure. When it was all over, and only 103 miles had been covered, Weston broke down in tears. "I am a fool," he apologized to his onlookers.

In 1907, just two days after TR took his soggy birthday walk, Weston set out from Portland, Maine, for Chicago. He departed too at 5:00 p.m. with Mayor Clifford and more than five thousand well-wishers sending him off. "Three rousing cheers were given to Mr. Weston when on the exact stroke of 5 he started on his long tramp to Chicago," the *Boston Globe* reported. His first stage consisted of a measly twenty-eight miles, just something to limber up the legs. Unfortunately for him, the weather did not hold up. Rain fell; roads became muddy quagmires. But as always, Weston continued to walk. He arrived shortly after midnight. Weston retired, asking that he be woken after four hours rest. Then the quest continued.

Brazenly enough, Weston intended not just to complete the same course in 1907 that he had walked forty years ago in kicking off his pedestrian career, he actually intended to better his time. He believed his sixty-nine-year-old legs, with literally thousands of miles on them, could deliver him to the Windy City faster than his much younger ones could. "My first few miles," Weston told the people of Kennebunkport who were there upon his arrival, "convinced me more than ever that I can beat my former record."

Weston's walks were in part a health crusade. At each major stop along his route, fans and reporters converged upon the perambulator. Over and over, Weston gave his version of a stump speech, with slight modifications depending on his audience. His advice was relatively simple: Get moving. "Walk out your troubles," Weston advised. "There is no malady of mind or body that you can't walk away. Not one person in ten has exercised enough. Inaction gives you the blues and a poor stomach. The two together make bad nerves, bad tempers, and bad characters. Walking will cure all."

Weston shared Roosevelt's belief (and that evidenced by groups like the PSAL) that athletics were for the masses—for every man, woman, and child, regardless of whether they had the skill to throw a ball or a predisposition toward competition. All Americans, according to Weston, needed to exercise. In a lengthy interview given in Buffalo during his 1907 trek, Weston proffered all sorts of advice. "Eat nothing but wholesome, digestible food and plenty of it." Eggs, apples, steak, cocoa, oatmeal, rice—these were among Weston's favorites. Then there were the habits to avoid: tobacco, beer, stuffy rooms, tight collars, restrictive shoes, and tonics. "Remember," Weston preached during his precious hours of rest, before he returned to his westward walking, "every man can be an athlete if he tries." In short, Weston subscribed to Roosevelt's idea that for some men, greatness came simply through doing those things that normal (using the term loosely here) men could do but rarely did.

When Weston crossed over the boundary of the City of Chicago at 1:00 a.m. on November 26, three thousand people were waiting for him. A squadron of policemen cleared the way, making sure that Weston would not be tripped up as he neared his finish line. Weston, for his part, understandably, was getting a bit chippy. "The old man plodded on, seeming unmindful of the attention he was receiving, or, more properly, rather scornful of it as putting further difficulties and distractions in the way of an already difficult task," the *Chicago Tribune* reported. Weston retired for a few hours of sleep rather than arriving at his finish line in the middle of the night; such a feat of elderly athletic accomplishment could not happen without a fitting celebration.

The next day, Weston finished the job. Arriving at the federal building at Jackson Boulevard just after noon, Weston knocked three times on the door. When it opened, Weston made certain that his record would stand. "You are my witness that I tapped 'home,'" Weston said. Confirmed. Weston had broken his old record. He arrived in Chicago, having covered 1,235 miles in twenty-five days. He shattered his previous record by one day, three hours, and twenty-five minutes.

With thousands of fans swarming the area, Weston retreated to the Illinois Athletic Club on Michigan Avenue. Certainly he deserved a nap, or a bath, or an unrushed meal by this point. But the masses would not be dissuaded. The mob blocked traffic. Men yelled for Weston to make a speech. Finally, realizing he had no other option, Weston appeared on a balcony above the building's entrance. "This is the most enjoyable occasion of my life," Weston said. And it was not just about him. "I walked to Chicago for glory. I wanted to do my part," Weston clarified, "to show all Englishmen, Frenchmen, Germans, Australians, and other nations that Americans can beat them at everything." Then the old, tired walker went back inside.

*　　*　　*

The fact that Edward Weston had a nickname for Roosevelt in the first place was coup. That the nickname Weston came up with was "Mr. Strenuosity," and that Weston used it when talking to reporters during his walk from Portland to Chicago in 1907, well...Roosevelt probably enjoyed that. It made Roosevelt an honorary member of the serious pedestrian class.

With a country to run, and a family to attend to (Weston had virtually abandoned his own), Roosevelt did nothing close to what Weston did as a walker. Roosevelt marked his walking by hours, not by days. He completed tens of miles in a given week, not hundreds. But always Roosevelt's walking was made more notable by the fact that it was the president who was doing such things. Even as Roosevelt entered into his last full years in the White House, the public loved stories of the president's unpresidential behavior. Often passersby spotted the commander in chief and all his men climbing, or romping, or swimming in Rock Creek Park, or elsewhere around the District. They gathered to watch. Some even attempted to join in.

In such cases, Roosevelt respectfully asked for a bit of athletic freedom. He requested that he be allowed to act as any other citizen could—although few wanted to crash through the wilderness the way Roosevelt did. "Once or twice, as we had begun our 'walk' before dark, people on the other side of the river, excusably curious to watch what the chief of the State and his friends were doing, alighted from their carriages and followed us from a distance," remembered Jusserand. Roosevelt always balanced diplomacy with self-preservation. "The President walked toward them, raised his hat, and politely bowed, and asked them to kindly desist, which they all did."

If there was one walk that captured what it meant to *walk* with Roosevelt— the strain, the camaraderie, the craziness—it was the one Roosevelt saw fit to include in his autobiography.

It transpired on a humid May evening in the last years of his presidency. Roosevelt led a cadre of walkers out into the wilds of Virginia. The group featured three regulars: Jules Jusserand, Robert Bacon (then assistant secretary of state), and General Thomas Barry (in command of the US Occupation of Cuba). Two other guests (left unnamed in Roosevelt's autobiography) rounded out the walking force. The Secret Service delivered the men to their starting point, traveling five miles northwest of the White House, along the Potomac

River and C & O Canal, to the Chain Bridge. There they crossed into Virginia. Once over the old iron truss passageway, the walkers were deposited onto the rocky shoreline of the Potomac River.

The dominant feature of the landscape here was rock. Geologically speaking, Virginia could not be less hospitable to visitors entering from the District. Deposits of shale, sandstone, quartz, amphibolite, and granite created a craggy, sharp shoreline. Jusserand found it abrupt. Did they really want to walk here, a place "lined all along with rocks and cliffs?" While it was not nature undisturbed—active quarries scarred the area—the dislocation of this place from the creature comforts of the White House could not be missed. No road existed near the Virginia shoreline, just a narrow path. The men could see the Little Falls rapids a half mile upriver. Jusserand and the others eyed the terrain "with horror." Then they were off.

Right away, the walk turned into a climb. The men navigated a "very steep and slippery" rock face using a rope tied to a tree, the handiwork of quarry men who worked the area. Roosevelt took the lead. The regulars expected nothing less from their enthusiastic, if increasingly pudgy leader. "We prudently proceeded to ascend separately, one by one, the President, as always, leading the way." The men certainly had a wonderful canvas upon which to work. This was the region were the Potomac River had cut through landscape most dramatically, creating cliffs and crevasses along the tree-covered shorelines and dramatic twists and rapids in the river itself—most famously at Great Falls ten more miles upriver.

After the initial ascent, the men worked their way across the top of the cliffs. Roosevelt pushed the pace. The men trotted through the ups and downs. Thick underbrush filled in the gaps between the stone. For Jusserand, the challenge centered on the "thorns, stones, and rivulets." Avoid the first two; charge through the third. This was not the day to care about the lifespan of one's footwear. Try to keep up.

The men were all about the same age. Jusserand and Barry were in their early fifties, a few years older than Roosevelt. Bacon was the youngest of the group. He had graduated from Harvard with Roosevelt, in 1880, but had been just nineteen at the time. While at Harvard, Bacon rose to god-like status as an athlete. Walter Camp described Bacon at Harvard as "a tall crinkly haired blond giant, handsome as an Adonis," who captained the Crimson's football and baseball teams and reigned as "one of Harvard's great athletes."*

"We shall never see his like again," Camp concluded.

The men worked their way through the Virginia landscape. Roosevelt's point-to-point mentality, though not directly in effect for this workout, drove the experience. "When a fine steep cliff was found," Jusserand wrote of this famous walk, "it was taken by storm." No one looked for easier paths around. Those in the back had to watch for falling stones unloosed by the men clamoring up first.

It did not take long for the climbing to take its toll. Up and down, over and through made for exhausting, sweaty work. Even though the summer heat had not yet engulfed the capital region, there was still the requisite humidity. "We were on the shady side of the river but were soon dripping with perspiration," Jusserand remembered.

Roosevelt never, never got over the idea that he was outclassed physically. "Most of the men who were oftenest with me on these trips," Roosevelt wrote, before mentioning Barry and Bacon specially, "were better men physically than I was; but I could ride and walk well enough for us all to thoroughly enjoy it."

---

* Roosevelt had introduced Bacon to Washington romping in 1905, when Bacon left his post working for J.P. Morgan and accepted a position at the State Department. "Put on some old clothes," Roosevelt had told several members of his usual crew, "for I intend to initiate Bacon." That Bacon showed up for the walk in his best suit and a fine pair of shoes, as rained poured down, only added to Roosevelt's excitement over the process. The group headed to the canal near Georgetown. Then TR tested his new man. Seeing no bridge, Roosevelt tried to separate the nattily attired Bacon from the rest of the group. The veterans would wade through the canal; Bacon was asked to hold everybody's stuff. "Bacon, you take our watches and pocketbooks; Pinchot and I will wade across. You go down to the bridge yonder and meet us on the other side." Fortunately for Bacon, he recognized what was happening. Roosevelt had issued a challenge. "Not by a darn sight," Bacon responded, "I came out on this walk with you and I am going where you go." This act of gameness—the ability to set aside one's sensibilities in order to revel in a physical challenge—solidified Bacon's position as part of the Tennis/Romping Cabinet. *Chicago Daily Tribune*, October 21, 1905.

The physical exertion, and the camaraderie, and breathtaking natural scenery were a powerful brew. And as often happened, Roosevelt pushed the envelope further.

How about a swim? Like right here, in the Potomac River, Roosevelt suggested.

By this point in his Washington, DC tenure, Jusserand knew just how to deal with such Roosevelt overkill. Go with it. "An excellent notion," Jusserand responded. So the men stripped off their clothes. The president of the United States, the assistant secretary of state, a major general in the United States Army, the French ambassador—and those two other guys—got naked. Once in that bare state, the men inched toward the river. Jusserand recounted the scene. "A passerby with a camera might have taken a picture worth having: the chief of State and his friends, alined, stark-naked, along the bank."

As the men pushed into the swirling waters (the Potomac River near Little Falls today is dotted with "If you enter the river, you will die" warning signs), Roosevelt shouted at Jusserand.

"Eh, Mr. Ambassador, have you not forgotten your gloves?"

To be clear, these were not French gloves. The gloves in question were worn for protection. Jusserand had suffered from scratched and bleeding hands on previous excursions. He learned his lesson; the more protective clothing one had on a Roosevelt walk, the better. But Jusserand saw the humor in TR's strenuous craziness. The gloves were staying on. "We might meet ladies," Jusserand shouted back to the president, ever the French gentleman.

The men swam for a bit in the cold river. Then Roosevelt was ready to continue the walk. No one had towels. Thus each man had to wrestle back on his already sweaty clothes over his wet limbs. The socks-and-shoes situation made Jusserand grimace. All the men really. "We slipped on our garments," Jusserand recalled, "and introduced into our socks feet covered with a layer of greasy mud."

The walk resumed. By now, the temperature had dropped significantly. The men kept moving to avoid a chill. The group climbed several more rock faces until they reached an appropriate climax for the adventure. This edifice stopped Jusserand and Barry cold. Too much. Can't do it. Roosevelt, of course, and Bacon gave it a try. "It was interesting to see Mr. Roosevelt slowly ascending, trying every little protuberance in the cliff, showing the clever patience and composure of a bear," Jusserand remembered.

At least one member of the group had the sense to question the endeavor. "This should not be allowed." Just watching the president of the United States take such risks made him dizzy. But Roosevelt proved up to the task. He reached the top safely. Bacon suffered the indignity of ripped pants on his ascent, but he too summited the rock edifice.

Then it was time to return to civilization. The group made its way to a rendezvous point. There the Secret Service reemerged. "We were driven back in our open carriages and should have got pneumonia, but did not," Jusserand said.

After the walk, Jusserand cleaned himself up and went to dinner with Senator Henry Cabot Lodge. There, Jusserand regaled the assembled group details of the late afternoon scramble. He described the terrain and the climb. He mentioned the men involved and how they fared. But that was all. Jusserand mentioned nothing about the skinny dipping.

Roosevelt, on the other hand, spared no detail. He told the story of the "walk" that night too—in all its glory.

NINE

BASEBALL'S GREAT ROOSEVELT CHASE

Father and all of us regarded baseball as a mollycoddle game. Tennis,
football, lacrosse, boxing, polo, yes—they are violent, which appealed
to us. But baseball? Father wouldn't watch it, not even at Harvard.

—ALICE ROOSEVELT LONGWORTH

Today's Washington Nationals may never win a World Series title, but they seem to have a knack for presidential history, at least as it pertains to their mascot race. During each home baseball game, the Nationals have a presidential mascot race after the top of the fourth inning. The Mt. Rushmore quartet—Washington, Jefferson, Lincoln, and Roosevelt—loop around the field to the delight of Nationals fans. It's good, simple fun. "The only two rules we had," said Josh Golden, the Nationals' director of marketing, "were don't fall down and Teddy doesn't win." And for the first 525 races (yes, 5-2-5), Theodore Roosevelt did not win. Ever. Payback, as they say, is a, well...it's not fun.*

---

* For anyone even remotely interested in the Teddy as struggling mascot saga, a visit to the Let-TeddyWin site (https://blog.letteddywin.com/) is a joy. Here's a site, representing a community of sorts, dedicated to justice for a mascot president running in an MLB marketing ploy. Brilliant.

Roosevelt really began solidifying his place in this baseball purgatory in 1906. During his fifth full year in the White House, his cold war on baseball could no longer be overlooked. The press picked up on the fact that Roosevelt ignored the World Series (PRESIDENT DECLINES. WILL NOT BE ABLE TO TAKE IN THE WORLD'S SERIES) and never attended Major League games in the District. "The fact is," the *Baltimore Sun* wrote in 1906, "that Mr. Roosevelt is not greatly interested in the national game nor has he ever been."

Baseball's leadership could have just let it go. Roosevelt's time in the White House was dwindling; there would be a new president to win over in a couple of years. But no. Rather than minimizing Roosevelt's slight, baseball's leadership launched an all-out assault to win over Roosevelt. *Oh yes, he will like us* became the (unstated) rallying cry. It seems clear now that baseball had hit its adolescence. The game was at once confident in its newfound strength and desperately insecure about where to sit in the cafeteria that was America's Strenuous Life paradigm.

"We first learned to admire Mr. Roosevelt while we were on the editorial staff of the Outing Magazine in the early '80s," wrote Henry Chadwick, the self-proclaimed "Father of Baseball," in 1903. "'We the people' should feel happy, indeed, by reason of the fact that our President combines with his 'strenuosity for the right' and enlightened conscience and a large measure of brains." Such statements by baseball leaders became commonplace. Chadwick, along with the editors of the *Sporting Life* (known as "The Paper that made Base Ball Popular"), sporting goods magnate Albert Spalding, and American League President Ban Johnson all did their parts to get Roosevelt on board with the National Pastime. Still, the president did not attend a game during his first term, despite the fact that the Senators' ballpark sat just two miles from the White House.

The realization that TR remained MIA from MLB launched baseball's Great Roosevelt Chase. Baseball leaders set their sights on Roosevelt in earnest in 1906. The chase continued through 1907.

It began with Ban. Ban Johnson, president of the American League, called at the White House in early April 1906. That Johnson could gain access to

Roosevelt was a less an indication of Johnson's standing than Roosevelt's open-door policy toward visitors to the presidential mansion. Still, the two dignitaries sat down to talk. Johnson told reporters proudly that he and Roosevelt "had a very interesting talk of probably ten minutes' duration."

Johnson wanted Roosevelt's support, and what Johnson wanted he usually got. He was a ruthless business man, the veritable "Czar of Baseball." Johnson had reveled in taking on the National League and poaching away its best players. Johnson was so cold and unsympathetic when it came to business matters, that his contemporaries joked that he had probably been weaned on an icicle. Such emotionally detached tactics, however, didn't really work with the president of the United States. So to the White House Johnson brought a gift. Perhaps he could woo Roosevelt to the ballpark.

With as much ceremony as he could muster, Johnson presented Roosevelt with "a Golden Pass." The pass entitled the president to complete access of the District's American League stadium. He could attend any game at the stadium, which sat where Howard University's hospital is today, and with any number of companions. The doors were always open, Johnson emphasized, to the president. If he wanted, Roosevelt could even "adjourn the Senate and both houses and take the whole bunch to the game." Seriously, just come.

The golden pass was just what it sounded like—a pass laced with gold.

According to Johnson's suspiciously self-serving report, Roosevelt "expressed regret that he had never been able to play the game of baseball." But it wasn't for lack of affinity: "He had always been an admirer of the game, but on account of his poor eyesight had never been able to take an active part in the game." The conversation, according to Johnson, ended with a promise. "The President assured Mr. Johnson that in [the] future he would attend many of the games played at the grounds in the capital."

The reporters of the *Washington Post,* perhaps knowing Roosevelt a bit better than their out-of-town competitors, took a pessimistic view of the effectiveness of the pass in changing Roosevelt's behavior. While the *Sporting News* exuded hope, the *Post* remained skeptical. The stakes were clear. WANT PRESIDENT AS FAN, read the *Post*'s headline covering the Johnson visit. "Washington Club aims to have Mr. Roosevelt attend Games." But the District paper also acknowledged that Roosevelt had rather conspicuously avoided the game to this point in his presidency. This seemed unlikely to change. Still, representatives from the AL and the Washington Senators pulled out all the stops. "One of the most costly and artistic annual passes ever issued by a baseball organization has been made for presentation to the President of the United States," the article made clear. "This pass, embossed in gold, is enclosed in a seal case, on the outside of which is a monogram of the President, 'T.R.,' in solid gold."

Who could resist such a flattering gift? Baseball assumed Roosevelt had been won over and would beat a path directly to the ballpark. So, prior to Opening Day of the 1906 season, the Washington Club constructed a "special box for the personal use of the President and his party" at American League Park. Just to be ready.

Maybe baseball had the moral high ground in this pursuit. After all, Roosevelt in 1906 again agreed to serve as the Honorary President for the Olympic Games, this time of the American committee, since the ill-fated, off-year Olympic Games was held in Athens, Greece. Roosevelt provided a message of congratulations for the American Olympians, one that James Sullivan paraded around as an official endorsement. "The President again showed his deep interest in the success of the team," Sullivan crowed. Why couldn't baseball get a bit of this presidential affirmation?

While getting Roosevelt to actually attend a game emerged as baseball's Holy Grail, the effort anchored a broader plan meant to link the president to baseball. An issue of the *Spalding's Official Base Ball Guide,* which happened to feature a provocative essay on baseball's origins (Was it possible the game was not uniquely American?), tried a Rough Rider-baseball connection. "Wellington said that 'the battle of Waterloo was won on the cricket fields of England,' and President Roosevelt is credited with a somewhat similar statement that 'the battle of San Juan Hill was won on the base ball and foot ball fields of America.'"

The next year's publication of the popular *Guide* shifted tactics slightly. What if baseball was actually best understood as an embodiment of Roosevelt's "Square Deal?" The Square Deal was the phrase that Roosevelt had co-opted to describe his domestic agenda. While broad, it included aspects of consumer protection and corporate regulation. "If there is one thing that I do desire to stand for," Roosevelt explained, "it is for a square deal, for an attitude of kindly justice as between man and man, without regard to what any man's creed or birthplace or social position may be."

What could be more square than a pitcher and batter facing off? Certainly the ball did not care about a man's station in life. "When two contesting nines enter upon a match game of Base Ball, they do so with the implied understanding that the struggle between them is to be one in which their respective degrees of skill in handling the bat and ball are alone to be brought into play." To baseball purists, Roosevelt's Square Deal, which had become a "new National Phrase," was essentially the "Love of Fair Play" that had always guided baseball's development.

Alas, the 1906 season came and went without Roosevelt attending any baseball games, personalized AL pass or not.

Undeterred, supporters of baseball tried again as the 1907 season dawned. Perhaps recognizing that a grassroots campaign might help, the *Sporting Life* worked to point out that Roosevelt was one of the few important people in Washington, DC *not* interested in baseball. Even the stuffy Supreme Court got it. CHIEF JUSTICE HARLAN, OF THE NATION'S HIGHEST COURT, PLAYS BASE BALL AND MAKES A HOME RUN IN HIS 74TH YEAR, trumpeted one headline. "Far from distracting from the dignity of the distinguished incumbent of the Supreme Court seat, the ability of Harlan as a hitter will add to it. That home run is a human touch, a specimen of Americanism that will go far toward popularizing the venerable judge." Then, just so its readers would not miss the point, the writer posed a rhetorical, shaming question. "How Theodore Roosevelt, who instinctively seems to know how to do the thing that pleases the people, came to overlook the diamond and its opportunities is a mystery."

Baseball was on its knees now. There was no sense of shame when it came to chasing down a US president. Having given TR a pass that went unused in 1906, the National Association of Professional Base Ball Leagues (NAPBBL), which became known as baseball's minor leagues, decided to step up the pressure on Roosevelt significantly. Rather than just awarding the president a pass to one particular league, for a given season, the NAPBBL invited the president to attend baseball games forever. The pass presented to Roosevelt on May 16, 1907, at the White House transcended almost every conceivable baseball boundary. The "President's Pass" covered thirty-six leagues and 256 cities; it bestowed upon Roosevelt "life membership in the National Association of Professional Base Ball Leagues, with the privilege of admission to all the games played by the clubs composing the association." The size of a normal baseball ticket, this honorary pass was made of solid gold.

The ticket itself drew press attention. The ticket "doubles in two on gold hinges to fold, so that it may be carried in the vest pocket." The ticket had an engraved picture of the president and the date of presentation on its front. "The photograph of President Roosevelt is beautifully enameled on the fold. The rim is intertwined with delicate chase work. This remarkable card was engraved by Mr. Arthur L. Bradley...It is pronounced by all who have seen it to be a fine piece of artistic workmanship."

As had been the case the year before, Roosevelt welcomed baseball's leadership at the White House to present its self-serving gift. The president of the NAPBBL, P.T. Powers, led a small contingent of baseball lifers into Roosevelt's office. Powers did not let his chance at an audience with the president of the United States go by without taking an aggressive swing at getting Roosevelt's support. For a few minutes, Powers had the floor as Roosevelt listened. Then Powers introduced J.H. Farrell, secretary of the league, to make baseball's case. "Mr. President," Farrell began. "A nation is known by its sport, and that nation that fosters and encourages manly sport is the one that will produce manly men with rugged constitutions and perfect physical development.

"The sport of this country, above and beyond all others is base ball. It is rightly called the national game, and its right to be so called is undisputed." Roosevelt listened attentively; he knew how to give his visitors their moment in the White House. Farrell pushed on. "We all gain strength, courage and much moral growth from the national game." Finally, Farrell moved toward his climax. "To its devotees all over this fair land from ocean to ocean there is nothing more gratifying than the fact that the present executive head of this great nation is an ardent champion of the national game." Roosevelt was not an ardent champion of the game, of course, but Farrell was rolling by this point. Baseball deserved Roosevelt's support; after all this was a "game that nourishes no 'molly coddles.'"

To Farrell's and the National Association of Professional Base Ball Leagues' credit, the short speech ended with a flourish of honesty. Why had the group come? "We desire to make you one of us as much as we can," Farrell said. "We desire to make you one of us as much as we can by tendering you a life membership card to any and all games of this, the largest Association ever organized in base ball history." Roosevelt accepted the gift, and the speech, with his typical good graces. He did not make any promises, but he examined his new golden ticket closely. He "expressed his warm thanks" and remarked that baseball had particular potential because "men of middle age" could participate. Roosevelt also, according to the baseball men, "said he regarded Base Ball as the typical game for Americans." These ranked as compliments, sort of.

Roosevelt never used his solid gold, National Association of Professional Base Ball Leagues ticket. In fact, Roosevelt did not take in a single professional baseball game during his time as president.

*   *   *

Why? Why did Roosevelt give a cold shoulder to the game that boomed in America during his presidency? Sure, the Roosevelt family fled the District for Sagamore Hill for much of the summer, but a game here or there was not too much to expect from a sports fan like Roosevelt.

The answer might indeed be as simple as Roosevelt's poor eyesight. It is difficult to think of an American more famous for wearing eyeglasses than Theodore Roosevelt. After all, Roosevelt's pince-nez glasses are literally carved in stone at Mt. Rushmore. But still, go ahead. Give it a try. Maybe Woody Allen? Benjamin Franklin? Ruth Bader Ginsburg?

Now, try to picture a baseball player—any ballplayer at all—wearing glasses. It's not so easy. That's because, to put it simply, the game of baseball favors the strong-sighted. Visual acuity ("the clarity or sharpness of vision") undergirds baseball success, perhaps more so than any other sport. And the higher the level of baseball play, the better the vision of the players involved. Among Major League Baseball players, in fact, 20/20 vision is hardly enough. Big-league ballplayers tend to have what neuroscientists Aaron Seitz and Jenni Deveau call "super vision."

Looking back, many of baseball's best players have had extraordinary eyes. Babe Ruth reportedly possessed 20/8 vision (meaning that what others would see with clarity from eight feet, Ruth could see from twenty). Barry Bonds, according to Dr. Bill Harrison, baseball's preeminent vision specialist, scored the highest sight scores ever recorded. That (plus extensive steroid use, allegedly) made Bonds one of the game's greatest hitters. The US Navy found that Ted Williams had 20/10 vision when he enlisted during World War II. So perhaps Roosevelt, who had -8 D myopia, and baseball were an unlikely mix from the start.

Researchers have argued over the role of myopia in shaping an individual's preferences and habits. The so-called "myopic personality" tends to be introverted and studious. That does not sound much like Roosevelt. Whether or not there is a causal relationship between TR's eyesight and his rejection of baseball is, of course, difficult to prove. Certainly Roosevelt struggled with his eyes throughout his life. Even after receiving corrective glasses, Roosevelt remained constantly aware of his vision problems. In Cuba, he had sewn several extra pairs of spectacles into the liner of his Rough Rider uniform. He could not charge if he could not see. Later, Roosevelt reported to his eye doctor, Dr. William Wilmer, that he suffered with floating and black spots, and haziness during his presidency. So when Roosevelt said, upon observing Quentin effortlessly tossing a baseball around, "I don't think that I should be afraid of anything except a baseball coming at me in the dark," he might have been speaking literally rather than metaphorically.

For TR, there were other strikes against baseball. Baseball lacked an obvious physicality. Roosevelt preferred athletic pursuits that caused its participants physical discomfort. The collisions and striking of boxing and football; the physical fatigue of tennis or a long tramp through a forest—these were the types of activities that Roosevelt favored. Alice, Roosevelt's oldest daughter, always free with her opinions, cased the matter in such terms. "Father and all of us regarded baseball as a mollycoddle game. Tennis, football, lacrosse, boxing, polo, yes—they are violent, which appealed to us. But baseball? Father wouldn't watch it, not even at Harvard."

The mollycoddle threat always loomed for Roosevelt. "As I emphatically disbelieve in seeing Harvard or any other college turn out mollycoddles instead of vigorous men," Roosevelt said at a Harvard speech in 1907, "I may add that I do not in the least object to a sport because it is rough."

In case it needs saying, there was no group or individual in the pro-mollycoddle camp. Charles Eliot, Roosevelt's longtime foe, for example, did not champion the idea of his institution turning out these mollycoddles that Roosevelt so feared. Nevertheless, Roosevelt fought vigorously with his strawman. The press noticed. THE PRESIDENT ON MOLLYCODDLES, the *Atlanta Constitution* headlined a few days after Roosevelt's Harvard Union speech. What did Roosevelt mean exactly with this term, the article asked? "College professors, café chefs and deep-sea fishermen have been called upon for a definition of the word, and their respective opinions as to the prevalence of the species." But nobody really used the word quite like Roosevelt. The basic definition: "an effeminate man."

Roosevelt also objected to baseball's overt professionalism. And this critique had deep roots for TR. Professional baseball received Roosevelt's scorn a decade before ballplayers had their first World Series. "When money comes in at the gate [specifically at baseball games], sport flies out the window," he said. In an article written for the *North American Review* in August 1890, entitled "Professionalism in Sports," Roosevelt framed professionalism as the sludge created by America's athletic engine. "Of course any good is accompanied by some evil," Roosevelt rationalized. "A small number of college boys... neglect everything for their sports, and so become of little use to themselves or any one else...The amateur not the professional, is the desirable citizen, the man who should be encouraged," Roosevelt preached. Roosevelt further warned America against the "national decadence" of professional sports.

It was true that as baseball had developed during the late nineteenth century, it came to embrace a particularly corrosive version of capitalism. In order to control labor costs, baseball owners put in place the simple but devilishly effective "reserve clause" in 1869. This anti-competition, anti-capitalist measure allowed each baseball club to "reserve" or control five players each year. The reserved players could not be offered contracts by any other teams in the league. What started out as means to control a few high-profile players on each team expanded to become a universal rule covering all players on all clubs. Control salaries to boost profits; the idea is practically timeless. It was a ruthless way to conduct capital-labor relations. "The reserve clause exists for two reasons," Curt Flood would explain a century later as he fought to break the clause. "One, to cut down the money the ballplayers get, and two, to give a feeling of power to men who like to play God over other people's lives."

It should be noted that Roosevelt did not go so far as to limit his boys from playing baseball. He did not worry that the game would somehow ruin the boys for manhood. In fact, Roosevelt even had hopes that Quentin, who turned ten in 1907, might change the family's growing reputation as baseball boycotters. "I like to see Quentin practicing baseball," Roosevelt wrote. "It gives me hopes that one of my boys will not take after his father in this respect, and will prove able to play the national game." Quentin—a rather infectiously joyous child, especially within the confines of the White House—played with a group of boys who called themselves "The White House Gang." The team preferred the White House lawn as the site for their practices and games, even going so far as to begin carving out a diamond in the otherwise-fine Executive Mansion lawn.

*　*　*

Despite Roosevelt's consistent pattern of either belittling or ignoring baseball, the game grew in significant ways. Perhaps most significantly, in 1903 baseball had held its first World Series. For the first time, the champion of baseball's American League faced off with its counterpart from the National League. This started the tradition of America's "Fall Classic."

Now it should be noted that the historian is often like the dog and the squirrel when it comes to historical firsts. He or she will be working away, researching and writing diligently when a first—out of nowhere—emerges. *Squirrel! First!* This "discovery" then derails what had previously been a well-planned paragraph or chapter or book. Or career. Just in case dogs and squirrels undersell the idea, Marc Bloch termed this tendency the "Idol of Origins." Every historian has worshipped this deity occasionally.

In the case of the first World Series, however, a turning of the head is appropriate. The nine-game series, initially referred to as the "Baseball Championship of the World," pitted the Boston Americans of the American League against the Pittsburgh Pirates of the National League. The series drew nationwide press attention from the start. The *Boston Globe* had so much coverage that it printed a special edition, "Baseball Extra," after each game. The series did not mean professional baseball outside the AL and NL shut down for the season, but it did focus the nation's attention on the two World Series clubs. The series made baseball more national than ever before. Newspapers from Steven's Point, Wisconsin, to Louisville, Kentucky, to San Francisco, California, reported daily on the games between clubs from Pittsburgh and Boston.

The two rival leagues had only recently come to a monopolistic agreement to stop poaching players away from each other, a timely development given that Roosevelt had established the US Department of Commerce at about the same time to facilitate such business enjoinders. Indeed the series reveals baseball's movement toward more cohesive business practices, mirroring the organizational efforts unfolding in American business at the time.

In terms of future Hall of Famers, the first World Series featured Cy Young and Honus Wagner, two of the most popular baseball players in the nation. In a way, the men were caricatures of two versions of America colliding at the time: the farmer and the industrialist. Cy Young, born Denton True Young, grew up on a farm in Gilmore, Ohio, a small hamlet about one hundred miles south of Cleveland. He attended school through just sixth grade before turning full-time to farm work. And there Young would have stayed had it not been for a lively arm and a ruthless competitiveness. Young honed his pitching skills at the expense of farm varmints. "I usta kill squirrels when I was a kid," Young recalled years after the fact. From squirrel killer to pitcher, Young began a Major League Baseball career that would span twenty-one years and result in 511 career pitching wins—a record total so far out of reach that baseball experts predict it will never be broken. By the 1903 series, as he closed out his fourteenth big-league season, Young had a thick midsection and darkening circles under his eyes. He was not a picture of athleticism; he was simply a master pitcher.

Wagner on the other hand grew up in the Pittsburgh metropolitan area, in a neighborhood that would later be renamed for steel magnate Andrew Carnegie. Wagner was the son of German immigrants. Like Young, Wagner did not make it to high school. Instead, at age twelve he joined his brothers and father, and almost all the men from his neighborhood, working in the coal mines. These were the men that gathered the fuel necessary to run Superior Steel & Union Electric Steel. Mining offered relatively high wages and predictably deplorable working conditions.

That Wagner managed to escape from the region's coal mines to its ballfields made him a hero to Pittsburgh's working classes. Wagner certainly looked like he could have wielded a miner's pick with ease. He was a bigger version of Roosevelt—stocky, almost six feet tall, thick chested, and heavy for the times. He tipped the scales at two hundred pounds, looking more like a football player than a man who could gobble up grounders and fire them to first base with surprising nimbleness and fluidity.

The first World Series games were hard fought and remarkably quick—the final contest took only one hour and thirty-five minutes. The crowds were drunkenly boisterous. "They'd pour right out onto the field and argue with the players and the umpires," remembered Tommy Leach, an infielder for the Pirates.

The first World Series was also a testament to twentieth-century mass transportation. Here was a world that allowed a competition to take place in two cities that sat some 575 miles apart. The series bounced back and forth between Boston and Pittsburgh. In Boston, the clubs played at the Huntington Avenue Ballgrounds, a venue that sat in an industrial part of town (where Northeastern University is today) and featured a covered grandstand behind home plate and stands behind first and third base. Advertisements (suspenders, hatters, whiskey, sporting goods, etc.) adorned the outfield fence. The field dimensions at Huntington were ridiculous: 350 feet down the left field line, a mere 280 feet to the right corner, and 530 feet to center. In Pittsburgh, the clubs faced off at Exposition Park, a tidy venue that sat on the banks of the Allegheny River.

The 1903 series played out as a back and forth affair. The Boston and Pittsburgh clubs had compiled basically the same records (Boston 91–47; Pittsburgh 91–49). The eight games in the series, with exception of Game Five, were all decided by four runs or less.

Boston lost Game One at home. Then it came back with a gem in Game Two. Riding a three-hitter by pitcher Bill Dineen, Boston got itself back in the series. Patsy Dougherty, the Americans' leadoff hitter, smashed a ball toward right field just moments after the game had commenced. Guessing that the ball had gone far enough, Dougherty rounded third and headed for home as the throw came from the outfield. He slid into home plate safe for a leadoff, inside-the-park home run. It was just the start of the Dougherty show. In the sixth inning, Dougherty made it easier on himself, "driving the ball over the left-field fence, an extremely long distance on the Boston grounds."

Game Three of the series went to Pittsburgh, 4 to 2, giving the Steel City players a two games to one lead in the series. But the most notable aspect of the third game was the enormous crowd that showed up once again at Boston's ballpark. This time nearly 19,000 spectators descended upon a park with seating for roughly half that many people. As a result, the line between the fan and the player was blurry. With nowhere to sit, the throngs pushed onto the field. Writing of the record assemblage, the *New York Times* marveled at the turnout and commented on the difficulties of mass-spectator events during a time when stadiums were poorly designed. "[The crowds] were massed from just beyond the outfielders' regular positions to the fences and all around the diamond inside the stands." With people scattered everywhere, rules had to be modified. "Fair hits into the crowd went as two-baggers." While Boston police did their best to keep the throngs under control, their effectiveness ebbed and flowed depending on the mood of the crowd. Never before had a baseball game been so closely affected by fans watching a contest. "The police had considerable difficulty in clearing the field for play, and later in keeping the people from encroaching onto the field. Thus the playing conditions varied somewhat from inning to inning." Concluding somewhat hopefully, the *New York Times* reporter assured readers that the crowds had enjoyed the game, "probably without influencing the result."

After intense games on Thursday, Friday, and Saturday, the clubs rested and traveled on Sunday and Monday. When the Pirates arrived back in their home city, five thousand supporters greeted them at Pittsburgh's Union Station. The series resumed on Tuesday, October 6 at Pittsburgh's Exposition Park. On consecutive nights, the clubs played Games Four, Five, Six, and Seven. Pittsburgh took the first of the four, giving the club a commanding 3–1 lead in the series.

Modern baseball fans, especially those in the sabermetrics crowd, know that such a series lead is usually safe. But Boston romped to an 11–2 Game Five victory behind the pitching of Cy Young. The men from the Hub then took Game Six 6–3. Pittsburgh eked out a Game Seven victory, 1–0 before Boston secured a 3–0 victory in Game Seven. The series stood at Boston 4; Pittsburgh 3. Then the clubs traveled, again taking Sunday and Monday off, back to Boston to finish the series.

Meanwhile in Washington, DC, Roosevelt went about his business without paying any attention. As the Boston and Pittsburgh ballplayers fought it out to determine the winners of the first World Series, Roosevelt considered, again, what to do about Cuba and the Philippines, how the Yosemite region might be preserved, and how to handle ongoing labor v. capital clashes. While baseball interests had largely coalesced around the American and National Leagues and the first World Series, not all industries were so cooperative.

"Both capital and labor have gone wild," Roosevelt wrote to William Taft on the day of Game Eight.

For the final game, Boston's Royal Rooters, a wild fan group, made their presence known. And in an era long before stadium controls would disallow spectators from bringing into the ballpark certain loud or dangerous items, the Rooters brought their own band. The group hired the Boston Letter Carriers Band (it was a crazy group, really) to play the club's unofficial theme song, "Tessie," over and over.

The final game flew by in ninety-five minutes. Boston pitcher Bill Dineen, who was making his fourth start in the series, never let Pittsburgh's batsmen get going. He fanned eight and allowed just four hits. Boston put three runs of its own on the scoreboard, two in the fourth and one in the sixth, providing all the offense Dineen needed.

The final out of the series played out a bit like "Casey at the Bat," a poem that was reprinted annually as a rite of spring in some newspapers. In the bottom of the ninth inning, with two outs and two strikes, Pittsburgh's revered shortstop Honus Wagner ("Yeah, everybody loved that old Dutchman!") stared down one final pitch from Boston's "Big Bill" Dineen.

Slowly the big pitcher gathered himself up for the effort, slowly he swung his arms above his head. Then the ball shot away like a flash toward the plate where the great Wagner stood, muscles drawn tense waiting for it. The big batsman's mighty shoulders heaved, the stands will swear that his very frame creaked, as he swung his bat with every ounce of power in his body, but the dull thud of the ball, as it nestled in Criger's waiting mitt, told the story.

The game ended. Boston's rowdy fans—never content to simply watch from the stands—erupted in celebration. They poured onto the field. The Rooters hoisted Dineen, the hero of the final game, onto awaiting shoulders and paraded him around the grounds. Then they headed off to a nearby tavern. Serious drinking awaited.

After skipping 1904, baseball made the World Series an annual affair beginning in 1905. Thus, the first five World Series were held while Roosevelt was president.

He ignored them all.

* * *

What's so strange about Roosevelt's cold war on baseball is just how lonely it was. Roosevelt acted almost as a solitary critic. The antibaseball island Roosevelt ruled had just a few cranky inhabitants. Inhabitants, ironically, like Charles Eliot, who opposed the game in a manner which seemed entirely out of touch with competitive sports. "I understand that a curveball is thrown with a deliberate attempt to deceive," Eliot had said. "Surely this is not an ability we should want to foster at Harvard."

In 1906, not only was there not a "baseball is dying" cottage industry comparable to today's, the game's popularity was basically doubling every few years. Major League Baseball attendance increased, by percentage, more during Theodore Roosevelt's presidency than any other. With a sixteen-team circuit, Major League Baseball drew 3,603,615 fans in 1901. In 1909, still with sixteen MLB clubs (although the cities had switched around a bit), attendance had ballooned to 7,236,290. In a stroke of luck that baseball's leaders could not really claim to have orchestrated, baseball became all things to all people. The game was "a source of rural nostalgia for city people," *and* "the sport of choice for farmers." It drew men and women, blacks and whites (in segregated seating arrangements), and the poor and the rich as spectators.

While Roosevelt refused to take baseball seriously, one could make the argument that baseball took itself *more seriously* than ever during this period. And that's saying something. At the same time leaders of baseball were courting Roosevelt with golden tickets, they also found the time and wherewithal to conduct a multiyear, nationwide study on the origins of the game.

The result of all this seriousness on baseball's part was the Abner Doubleday myth. This is why the Baseball Hall of Fame resides, buried under four feet of snow every January, in Cooperstown, New York.

Now just mentioning Doubleday leads one to the precipice of a baseball wormhole (people and ideas go in and never come out), but here we go.*

The question of baseball's origin had been contested ground for decades. Long before Roosevelt ignored the game, other people loved baseball enough to ask: Where did the game originate? When did baseball play start? The questions were harmless enough. It is part of being human, after all, to wonder about origins and intents. But it was during the first decade of the twentieth century that the creation questions turned from dinner table fodder to highly charged political inquiries.

Determining the simple benchmarks were fairly straightforward. Professional baseball organized in earnest in the United States following the Civil War. Beginning almost immediately after America's great North–South conflict, baseball clubs began forming by the dozens, especially in America's larger cities. The proliferation of clubs led to increased competition and the desire for codified rules of competition. Building off the groundwork done by the National Association of Base Ball Players (which held conventions to discuss baseball's rules and codes of conduct), the National Association of Professional Base Ball Players organized in 1871. The National League, with its "stringent provisions against revolving and dishonesty of players," formed in 1876.

But what about before that—what about the very, very beginning? What about creation? Or was it evolution? The tone surrounding what should have been a lively but relatively low-stakes debate changed over the course of Roosevelt's administration. Gradually disagreement on the matter became akin to disloyalty to the game and to America.

---

* One should enter into the debate over baseball origins with great caution, or at least with a lot of time to kill. I relied heavily, gratefully on John Thorn (especially Thorn, the official historian of Major League Baseball), Warren Goldstein, and David Block for this section. Their works on baseball's creation are not the only books on the topic—not by far—but they are three of the best and, in the case of Thorn and Block, most recent. See, John Thorn, *Baseball in the Garden of Eden: The Secret History of the Early Game* (New York: Simon & Schuster, 2011); David Block, *Baseball Before We Knew it: A Search for the Roots of the Game* (Lincoln: Bison Books, 2006); and Warren Goldstein, *Playing for Keeps: A History of Early Baseball* (New York: Cornell University Press, 1989).

Albert Spalding led baseball's inquisition. By the turn of the century, Spalding could no longer stomach one of the working theories—the idea that baseball descended from the European game Rounders. This simply could not be. Spalding, and America, had too much at stake.

Spalding had made his fortune from the game of baseball. He pitched brilliantly for the Boston Red Stockings and Chicago White Stockings during the 1870s, professional baseball's embryonic years. Spalding was an early adopter of the baseball glove, and he possessed a serviceable fastball and pinpoint control. In an era when teams often carried only one pitcher, Spalding proved indefatigable. In 1874, he pitched more than six-hundred innings. In 1876, in the first year of National League competition, Spalding led the league with forty-seven victories. Then, at twenty-seven years old, Spalding abruptly retired as a player. It was not that Spalding's performance on the field was dipping (quite the contrary) but rather that he could no longer wait to exploit the business possibilities surrounding the game.

Spalding went to work full-time providing baseball players, clubs, and leagues with the equipment necessary to play the game. Spalding opened, with his brother Walter, a sporting goods store in Chicago in 1874. From there an empire grew. Spalding's baseball business had every conceivable built-in advantage. Spalding remained officially connected to the National League as a part owner of the Chicago franchise. Spalding's reputation as a star player yielded fond reminisces from a generation of baseball fans. More practically, the creation of the *Spalding Official Base Ball Guide* made the Spalding company the most preeminent voice on all matters in the baseball world. Published annually, the *Guide* provided the baseball public with league standings, player profiles, and information about new rules. And each *Guide* doubled as a catalogue to order Spalding goods.

Even before the TR chase really heated up, on October 31, 1904, Spalding had written to a longtime friend—A.G. Mills—floating the idea of a special commission "to search everywhere that it is possible and thus learn the real facts concerning the development of the game." Mills liked the idea. Working from his home among the Theosophists, along Sunset Cliffs overlooking the

Pacific Ocean in Point Loma, California, Spalding began calling in the favors he had accumulated over a lifetime in the game. Things came together. Spalding had a commission in place by March 1905.

An article in *Spalding's Official Base Ball Guide* took the debate public. "There seems to be a conflict of opinion as to the origin of base ball," Spalding began. "I think the game has arrived at an age and at a point in its development when this mooted question should be settled in some comprehensive and authoritative way and for all time." Spalding's foil was Henry Chadwick. It was America versus Britain. "Some authorities, notably Henry Chadwick, claim that base ball is of English origin and was a direct descendent of the old English juvenile pastime called 'Rounders.'" Nonsense. "I am unwilling longer to accept this rounder theory without something more convincing than his oft-repeated assertion that 'base ball did originate from rounders.'"

TR himself had stumbled into baseball's paternity debate decades earlier. On April 8, 1889, Roosevelt, then working for the US Civil Service Commission, had attended a New York City reception celebrating the return of a Spalding-led baseball club from a six-month world tour. Roosevelt joined Mark Twain and 250 other guests for a nine-course meal, complete with "wit and oratory" recognizing the ballplayers, at the city's famous Delmonico's Restaurant.

As the evening wound down, A.G. Mills, the man that would take charge of the 1905 special commission, declared boldly that baseball had sprung forth in the United States. Purely and completely. Baseball, according to Mills, "in its present perfect state," was "an evolution of American genius." Then, grossly exaggerating the data available to back up his claims, Mills declared that "patriotism and research alike vindicate the claim that it is American in its origin." After Mills's speech on baseball's nationalistic purity, the assemblage broke into table pounding and feet stomping. "No rounders! No rounders!" came the chant.

The "Special Base Ball Commission" a decade and a half later began its work in March 1905. The seven commissioners had all sorts of credentials. A.G. Mills, the chairman of the commission, had served as the president of baseball's National League from 1882 to 1884 and worked in the game for most of his life. Arthur Gorman was a senator elected from Maryland and had been president of the National Association of Base Ball Players immediately following the Civil War. Morgan Bulkeley had been the first president of the National League and then had gone on to represent Connecticut, first as governor and then in the United States Senate. Nicholas Young had served as secretary and president of the National League. Alfred Reach and George Wright had been "two of the most famous ball players in their day." Finally, anchoring the group, James E. Sullivan, president of the AAU and all-around-instigator-of-trouble at the 1904 Olympic Games, agreed to serve as secretary of the Special Commission.

What about Roosevelt?

According to Major League Baseball's official historian John Thorn, Spalding actually considered asking the president to serve on the committee. As he was working to organize the committee, Spalding recalled back to Roosevelt's presence at the "No Rounders" meeting of 1889. Roosevelt had been at that celebratory evening at Delmonico's. "Clearly Spalding had given thought to naming the President of the United States to the Special commission, but we do not know if he extended a formal invitation," Thorn concluded. "Not much of a baseball fan, 'Teddy' would have been an anomaly alongside eventual appointees." Indeed.

For more than two years, from 1905 to 1907—during the same time as baseball's Great Roosevelt Chase—the Mills-led commission diligently gathered as much information as possible about the beginnings of baseball. Spalding's public call for "all possible facts, proofs, interviews, etc., calculated to throw light on this subject" cast a wide net. Advertisements went out in newspapers across the country. Spalding certainly hoped that the outcome would ordain baseball as America's undisputed pastime. Despite these leanings, Spalding let the commission do its work. Letters poured in recalling long-ago games. "The Secretary, was deluged with communications from different parts of the country, all having a more or less being on this question," *Spalding's Guide* reported later. So many letters came into the commission, in fact, that Spalding promised that he would eventually fund the production of a dedicated volume to the evidence that the commission had produced.

Amazingly, the commission settled on a story that included two Abners, Abner Graves and Abner Doubleday. Graves, a seventy-three-year-old miner living in Denver, claimed that he remembered the beginnings of baseball. And that that beginning had occurred in Cooperstown, New York.

"I notice in Saturdays 'Beacon Journal' a question as to the 'origin of base ball' from the pen of A.G. Spalding," Graves wrote to the committee. "The 'American game of Base Ball' was invented by Abner Doubleday of Cooperstown, New York, either the spring prior, or following the 'Log Cabin & Hard Cider' campaign [thus around 1840] of General Harrison for President." From there, Graves filled in as many details as he could remember. First, the boys had been playing "Town Ball," a game that involved striking a ball with a flat board and running between two goals. Fielders "scattered all over the near and far field" and could hit the running batsman with the ball. The game was something like cricket.

"Abner Doubleday then figured out and made a plan of improvement on town ball to limit number of players, and have equal sides, calling it 'Base Ball' because it had four bases." And that was it. From a moment of genius, a flash of inspiration, a new game sprung forth.

To the commission's credit, Sullivan dashed off a follow-up inquiry to Graves. How sure was Graves of his story? "You say this game of Base Ball as invented by Doubleday was undoubtedly the first starter of Base Ball and quickly superseded Town Ball," Sullivan wrote. "Could you give me the name and address of any persons now living in Cooperstown, New York City, or elsewhere, that could substantiate your recollections of Doubleday's invention or his first introduction of the game of Base ball?"

Graves could not. He had no real supporting evidence to validate his story. He was an old man. He would soon be hospitalized for mental illness. "You ask if I can positively name the year of Doubleday's invention, and replying will say that I cannot, although am sure it was either 1839, 1840, or 1841," Graves wrote back to the commission. It was simply matter of too much time passing. "It is impossible to get documentary proof of the invention," Graves reasoned, "as there is not one chance in ten thousand that a boy's drawing plan of improved ball game would have been preserved for 65 years."

Initially the committee regarded Graves's tale as a distracting rabbit trail, but the Doubleday story gained traction as pieces of the story began to surface in the press. Graves had sent his initial response to the *Akron Beacon Journal*. Not surprisingly, Cooperstown's *Otsego Farmer* picked up on the theory. So too did several other newspapers across the country.

The problem for the committee was that no other plausible history of baseball's rise had surfaced. After more than two years of searching, the committee had nothing else. Finally, fatigued of the entire matter and with the Doubleday story becoming increasingly well known, the committee acquiesced. And why not? Doubleday made a fine patriarch for the game. He had attended West Point and fired shots defending Ft. Sumter as the Civil War began. Doubleday fought with distinction at Gettysburg in 1863. Doubleday had probably spent some time in Cooperstown, although not at the moment prescribed by Graves. In short, Doubleday fit within the paradigm of the Strenuous Life.

On December 30, 1907, Mills sent a letter to Sullivan making the case for Doubleday. This became the closest thing to an official report issued by the committee. Spalding took the matter from there, publishing his own much lengthier report in the 1908 *Spalding's Official Base Ball Guide*. From there, the news of baseball's pure roots seeped out. After two years of chasing Roosevelt to no effect, baseball got its dream headline. ORIGIN OF BASEBALL: SPECIAL COMMISSION DECIDES IT IS STRICTLY AMERICAN, stories proliferated in American newspapers during the lead-up to the 1908 season. The takeaway was clear. Americans needed help from no nation when it came to sports. "Baseball is thus proved to be, like poker, a genuine American product," the New York *Sun* said.

Graves certainly understood what was at stake in the baseball origins question. Just as Neil Armstrong would claim the moon for America, Graves intended to plant the Stars and Stripes on baseball. Graves had wrapped up his correspondence with the committee in a mix of fatigue and vitriol. "My Typewriter thinks this is a pretty long letter on one subject," Graves concluded. "Your letter asked for as full data as possible and I have given you all the items I can in a rambling sort of way." Then Graves's final thought: "Just in my present mood I would rather have Uncle Sam declare war on England and clean her up rather than have one of her citizens beat us out of Base Ball. Yours truly. Abner Graves."

Some years later, Graves would shoot and kill his wife—a woman forty-two years his junior. A jury found Graves to be criminally insane. He died in an asylum in Pueblo, Colorado.

Yes, via a lunatic, during Roosevelt's cold war, baseball got its creation story— one situated in bucolic upstate New York and featuring a Civil War hero. The committee's decision was presented with no hint of uncertainty. The commission reached a unanimous conclusion: "Base Ball is of American origin, and has no traceable connection whatever with 'Rounders,' or any other foreign game."

*　*　*

Just one extra inning on all of this. The Roosevelt-baseball relationship makes clear something that hindsight tends to obscure: Presidential influence is a mysterious thing. While Roosevelt—a tremendously popular, Strenuous Life president—belittled baseball, the game expanded by leaps and bounds. The World Series got its start. Millions of Americans each year packed the country's ballparks. And if all that wasn't enough, the game took on the "America's National Pastime" badge of honor during this era as well.

"Base Ball has its patriotic side," Albert Spalding concluded. Of the Mills Commission, Spalding said, "Their decision should forever set at rest the question as to the Origin of Base Ball." It, of course, did not. A *Collier's Magazine* article began the process of debunking the story in...1909! Generations of scholars since have completely debunked the idea that Doubleday invented the game. But none of that really, fundamentally changed the narrative set in place by the Mills Commission. Baseball is still referred to as America's National Pastime. The Baseball Hall of Fame still remains in Cooperstown, New York. And amazingly, the Doubleday tale still persists. As recently as 2010, MLB Commissioner Bud Selig stated, "I really believe that Abner Doubleday is the 'Father of Baseball.'"

TEN

LEGACY

For a person may labor with wisdom, knowledge and skill, and then
they must leave all they own to another who has not toiled for it.
—ECCLESIASTES 2:21

I f the lame duck phase of a presidency were a suit jacket, it would (1) be made of polyester, (2) bunch up under the armpits, and (3) require some serious gut sucking in order to actually get it buttoned. You could wear it, but barely. No one would want to keep it on for very long.

This process of losing power due to limited time remaining in office—being a lame duck—was especially uncomfortable for Roosevelt. Roosevelt hated to say goodbye to the presidency. He, unlike some men who held the office, did not seek relief from the pressures of the office. Roosevelt had faith in Taft ("I think that he has the most loveable personality...He is going to be greatly beloved as President."), but this provided only a modicum of solace. Roosevelt would be exiting the White House at fifty years and 128 days, the youngest ex-president ever. He would miss the decisions, the power, the White House and its grounds, the endless debates and meetings, the travel—all of it, really.

This feeling of loss at leaving the White House so pervaded Roosevelt's thoughts that it even spilled over when he met his longtime political foe William Jennings Bryan: "When you see me quoted in the press as welcoming the rest I will have after March the 3rd take no stock in it, for I will confess to you confidentially that I like my job...I have enjoyed every moment of this so-called arduous and exacting task."

While serious change was afoot, other things stayed stubbornly constant. Roosevelt continued to battle his weight. Forget metaphorical jackets, Roosevelt's actual clothes were uncomfortably tight. This part of Roosevelt's athletic struggle remained constant; it never got easier. "I'm sorry to say that I have not only grown fat, but also a little gouty..." Roosevelt said in 1908. The press joked about Taft's size ("He's a great big...He's a regular floater."), but Roosevelt, too, cut a less than athletic figure.

Although his strenuous activities continued, Roosevelt could not upend the simple caloric reality that his body faced on a daily basis. He ate too much—far too much. As companion Archie Butt noted while staying with the Roosevelts in the summer of 1908: "You think me a large eater; well, I am small in comparison to him. But he has a tremendous body and really enjoys each mouthful. I never saw anyone with a more wholesome appetite, and then he complains of not losing flesh. I felt like asking him to-day: 'How can you expect to?'"

Roosevelt would have been excused for ignoring trivial matters during his final days. Many modern presidents during their lame duck days turn to legacy building (their Presidential Library, vaguely defined diplomatic forays) as their time in power dwindles. But Roosevelt remained fixated on the daily conflicts. He could no more turn off his impulse to engage in every conversation and every debate than he could let pass by a tempting dish at the dinner table. It had always been this appetite—for food yes, but also ideas, debates, conflict, knowledge, stimulation—that powered Roosevelt's engine.

And so, true to himself to the end, Roosevelt spent the summer of 1908 involved in two back-to-back episodes of athletic meddling.

The first involved a familiar and formidable foe—Charles Eliot. Once again Roosevelt saw fit to intervene regarding the role of athletics at his alma mater. ROOSEVELT IN HARVARD FUSS, the New York *Sun* explained. This time it was Harvard's crew team that caught Roosevelt's attention. The team had a crisis, and its members appealed to Roosevelt, the commander in chief of the

United States and a Harvard man after all, to intervene on their behalf to minimize a library book controversy. Two Harvard University crew team members—Sidney Fish, the number two man on the varsity, and Charles Morgan Jr.—had been suspended from the crew team just days before a June 25 competition against Yale University.

The crisis stemmed from what today the NCAA calls, "The Student-Athlete Experience." The experience of being—at the same time—a student and an athlete. While the concept seems relatively straightforward, the term "student-athlete" is actually a legally charged one. Ray Dennison died in 1955 from an on-field collision while playing football for Fort Lewis College. His widow filed for workmen's compensation death benefits. Fort Lewis and the NCAA objected: these were not employees, they were students who happened also to be athletes. A juxtaposition was born. "We crafted the term student-athlete and soon it was embedded in all NCAA rules and interpretations," said NCAA President at the time, Walter Byers. The courts bought it.

For Morgan and Fish, there was no official label, but the challenges of being both a student and an athlete at Harvard were no less significant. This was the strange brew of higher education and competitive athletics—unique really to the United States—that Harvard had helped create. For the annual regatta against Yale, Harvard's crew team decamped to a training site located along a Connecticut section of the Thames River. The facility, known as "Red Top," housed the Harvard men in the lead-up to this oldest of contests. "The race training is unique in the world of college sports," *Harvard Magazine* explains of the still-active tradition. "Harvard and Yale are the only colleges that maintain special training camps to prepare for a single athletic contest." The problem for Fish and Morgan was that they had to leave for Red Top training precisely as the year-end examination period began. There was still schoolwork to be done.

Morgan, a senior, needed to complete some required reading for an English class. His thesis remained mostly undone. Sure, it was percolating in his head somewhere, but very little of it had actually been committed to paper. So, trying to balance school and athletics, Morgan decided he would simply remove the book he needed (borrow it really) and bring it along to training. That way he could complete his assignment and, hopefully, return the book before anyone noticed it was gone.

For the extraction, Morgan enlisted Fish to help. The two smart New Yorkers could pull off something as simple as this. Morgan located the item in Harvard's Warren Library. He took the book from the shelf and casually walked toward a library window, which was conveniently open. It was nearly summer after all. Morgan then handed the book—a pamphlet really—out the window to Fish. Done. Mission accomplished.

Unfortunately, college boys are rarely as cunning as they think they are. A librarian had watched the whole thing transpire. *Stop! Unhand that book!* Flustered, Fish lied when asked to identify himself. Morgan stammered through an explanation. He was just a student, trying also to be an athlete, headed off to defend Harvard's honor against Yale. Couldn't the librarian just let them go? Bookless and reprimanded, Morgan and Fish left, headed for Red Top, never suspecting that the matter would intervene in their futures.

But a few days later, Morgan received word from Cambridge that he needed to return. Dean Hulburt wanted to see him about the library matter. Fish, sensing trouble, decided to return as well, although he "did not get any official summons." The two boys met with Harvard administrators. Two members of Harvard's Graduate Rowing Committee sat in on the proceedings. Whatever the students' explanation for the episode, it did not work. Harvard suspended Morgan and Fish "indefinitely," forcing both men to give up rowing for the remainder of the year. Most significantly, they would not be available for the 1908 match with Yale.

The petty theft, if it could even be called that, and resulting suspension of Morgan and Fish was covered by newspapers across the nation. The *Boston Globe* put the matter on its front page. Then Roosevelt got involved and things escalated considerably. "Roosevelt takes it up," was how a newspaper as far away as the *Topeka State Journal* reported it.

Unable to resist, Roosevelt telegrammed Eliot. "Is it not possible, and would it not be more fitting and just," Roosevelt wrote, "to substitute another punishment for Fish and Morgan, if, as stated, they merely took away a book which they were permitted to use in the library?" Roosevelt was planning to attend the Harvard–Yale regatta; he wanted Harvard's best team on the river. Yale, winners of the 1907 contest, needed a beating. At issue for Roosevelt was the effect that a suspension would have on everyone besides Morgan and Fish. "It is unfair and unnecessary to make all of us suffer," he concluded.

Somehow—neither side would admit to anything—Roosevelt's telegram became public. It had not been leaked by the White House, and of the possibility that someone had stolen a copy from the executive telegraph office, "I should regard as well-nigh impossible," Roosevelt concluded. Most likely, Harvard released the document to the press. It was a last swipe at a president who, while a Harvard man himself, had meddled in the school's affairs one too many times.

In the ensuing weeks, Roosevelt would write a nearly ten-page letter to Charles Eliot debating the punishment, accusing Eliot of determining to "strike a blow at Harvard athletics."

The more Roosevelt thought about Morgan and Fish, the more he deemed them victims rather than criminals. Here were two students "emphatically engaged in doing work that was of benefit to the whole college," Roosevelt wrote to Eliot. And how did their university provide support for such work? Had Harvard kept up its end of the ill-defined student-athlete bargain? Not even close. "They had to go down to Red Top just about the time of the examinations, and the college authorities, as a matter of honorable obligation, should have endeavored to give them every facility to study at Red Top to just as much advantage as if they were not at Red Top." Translation: it was Harvard's responsibility to make sure that its students participating in events on behalf of the university had the resources necessary to keep up with their schoolwork.

Eliot was severely unmoved. He not only rejected Roosevelt's suggestion that the punishment be altered; he questioned the president's very moral compass. Eliot had no patience for Roosevelt's line of reasoning. "Each man did a dishonorable thing," Eliot said.

One [Morgan] violated in his private interest and in a crooked way a rule made in the common interest. The other [Fish] gave a false name and did not take a subsequent opportunity to give his own. The least possible punishment was put on probation, but even that drops from the crews. A keen and sure sense of honor being the finest result of college life, I think the college and the graduates should condemn effectively dishonorable conduct. The college should also teach that one must not do scurvy things in the supposed interest or for the pleasure of others.

The tone of the message is stunning. The crime was *borrowing* a library book without going through the proper protocol. But the backstory—the nearly eight-year-long struggle between two presidents over the role of athletics at Harvard and for the nation—carried the day. To hell with Fish. Forget about Morgan. The president of the United States be damned. This was about Harvard's honor, at least to Eliot.

Morgan and Fish remained suspended. The press seized on the power dynamics:

HARVARD PRESIDENT FLOUTS THE BIG STICK

PRESIDENT IS SNUBBED

TEDDY TURNED DOWN BY ELIOT

"Though there is some secrecy with regard to who gave out the correspondence, it is now definitely known that President Eliot of Harvard administered a rebuke to President Roosevelt for the latter's attempted interference..." the New York *Sun* reported. The *Boston Globe* put Eliot's smackdown on the front page. ELIOT'S REPLY ENDED IT, read the headline on June 23. "President Roosevelt has discovered that it was a much simpler matter to be mediator between Russia and Japan than act as a peacemaker between the student-oarsmen Sidney W. Fish and Charles Morgan Jr. and Harvard university."

Ironically, Harvard dominated Yale when the two schools met for their regatta on June 25. The Crimson did not need Morgan or Fish. HARVARD VARsity Gives Elis Worst Beating in their History, the *Globe* reported. In fact, things were so lopsided that Yale's eight-man boat stopped midway through their race. Harvard's pace had burned out the men from Yale.

Roosevelt, chastened from the whole episode, did not even get to witness Harvard's victory. His presence was required at a funeral for Grover Cleveland in New Jersey instead.

The crew-gate of 1908 marked the last significant tussle between President Eliot and President Roosevelt. Both were in their last days of leadership. On November 23, 1908, just twenty days after the election of Taft confirmed that the White House countdown was on, Roosevelt wrote Eliot a heartfelt letter of congratulations. Eliot was retiring from Harvard. He had served the institution well. "It has been a great career, my dear President Eliot, and as an American and a Harvard man I congratulate you with all my heart," Roosevelt wrote.

The letter revealed a truth about Roosevelt that remained fixed even as he readied himself to leave the White House. Roosevelt understood that even his station had limits; he did not expect to win every debate. The president of Harvard outranked him when it came to the Harvard crew team. But that reality did not lead Roosevelt to gird his curiosity or keep his ideas to himself. He was not afraid to make an argument he might lose—even in a very public fashion. He had lost plenty when it came to advocating for athletics in the United States. So it should not surprise us that Roosevelt took the time to argue for a crew team, about a library book, just weeks before his presidency ended. Nor that he held no ill will against Eliot when the argument went in Eliot's favor.

* * *

After intervening on behalf of Harvard's crew team, Roosevelt moved right on to a debate about the proper running of the four hundred meters. He found himself engaged in a dispute involving a United States' track athlete at the summer 1908 Olympic Games.

Held in London (after Rome backed out on the bid following the 1906 eruption of Mt. Vesuvius), these Games ratcheted up the American–British rivalry. Pierre de Coubertin, ever intent on building the Olympic movement, looked on with concern. "From the very first day," Coubertin noted, "King Edward had taken exception to the American athletes because of their behavior and their barbaric shouts that resounded through the stadium." The Americans did not seem to care. They had been the only nation to refuse to wear Coubertin's costumes for the opening ceremonies and (allegedly) dip their flag in deference to the British royal family...They just came to win.*

As the United States struggled to match Britain, especially in the hotly contested track-and-field competition, controversy erupted. The event that pushed the American–British tension over the edge was one that America has come to virtually own over the course of Olympic history: the four-hundred-meter race. Once around the track. Out of a possible twenty-eight gold medals in this event, the United States has won nineteen—68 percent. Great Britain has the second most gold medals in the event: two. One of those British wins came from Eric Liddel and was such a surprise that it inspired the movie *Chariots of Fire*. The other British win in the 400 came in 1908.

The Olympic Stadium in London, known as White City Stadium, was a sight to behold. It featured a cinder running track inside a banked bicycle track. It could seat 68,000. With standing room, the venue had a capacity of 100,000. Unfortunately for the British organizers, such crowds proved exceedingly difficult to draw. But if there was a spark to the Games, it came from the festering rivalry between the United States and Britain. The US in particular, led by James Sullivan, viewed the games as less an opportunity for international camaraderie and more as the time to demonstrate just how strong (and fast and skilled) Americans were. As Olympic historian George Matthews has pointed out, the 1908 Games were an opportunity for Britain and the United States to contest their economic and cultural rivalry in a new manner. The Games were "a means of demonstrating the overall cultural superiority and promoting nationalism."

---

* The Americans could not match the athletic machine Britain had revved up for the competition. Britain won three times as many medals as the United States: 146–47. Britain's fifty-six golds far outpaced the US's twenty-three. Thus the United States received a bit of comeuppance after their romp in 1904.

The final for the 400 featured four runners: three Americans and one Brit. The Americans were a study in the Ivy League diversity possible in American sport. John Carpenter came from Cornell University. W.O. Robbins ran for Harvard University. And the third American—J.B. Taylor, a Penn man—was described as "a negro with a magnificent stride" by (deep breath!) the *Official Report of the Olympic Games of 1908, Celebrated in London, Under the Patronage of His Most Gracious Majesty King Edward VII.* While two African American athletes had won medals in 1904, Taylor had his eyes on becoming the first black American to bring home a gold.

The British runner in the final, Wyndham Halswelle, was "the athletic idol of the British." Halswelle was a lieutenant in the British Army and had won the 100, 220, 440, and 880-yard titles in the 1906 Scottish Championships. He was a compact runner with a Charlie Chaplin moustache. Expectations were that Halswelle would win a glorious victory for Britain in what would be one of the Games' marquee events.

The four runners lined up on the narrow track on July 23. There were no lanes. The rain that had hampered attendance abated. As the men took their positions, it became clear that Taylor got jobbed. As the man with the slowest qualifying time, Taylor was forced to line up on the extreme outside of the other three runners, a fatal deficit in a one-lap race. "Apparently the arranging was done by a man who did not want all the contestants to get a fair start," Sullivan explained. "Taylor's position caused him to give away yards which he could never regain."

At the gun, Robbins surged into the lead. Carpenter and Halswelle tucked in behind. Taylor lagged far behind, basically out of contention. As the runners rounded the first bend, Robbins hugged the rail while Carpenter flared out to the right. Halswelle waited in the third position. Then the straightaway was upon the sprinters. Halswelle, growing impatient, lengthened his stride and pushed to get around the two Americans.

The passing proved difficult. Carpenter, certainly conscious that Halswelle was intent upon making his move, edged further toward the outside of the track. At one point, according to one of the British officials, Carpenter sprinted along a mere eighteen inches from the edge of the running track, dangerously close to crossing into out-of-bounds territory, which in this stadium was the bike track. The men approached the home stretch. "It looked like anybody's race as they approached the last turn, the three leaders being bunched," the *New York Tribune* reported.

As the trio flew off that last turn, the group bounced further to the right. "Everyone close to this spot," Sullivan clarified, "noticed that the three men swerved toward the outside of the track." The reason behind this bounce was either (1) aggressive tactical running by Robbins and Carpenter with Halswelle caught up in the jet stream, or (2) a foul by Carpenter. Either way, it caught the attention of the officials surrounding the track. They scrambled into action.

As the runners entered the homestretch, several officials—all British—intervened. One stepped onto the track and, not quick enough to catch the leaders, stopped Taylor and pulled him off the track. Another ripped down the finishing tape. No runner would have the satisfaction of breaking the tape in this race. Meanwhile, Carpenter, Robbins, and Halswelle thundered home. Carpenter reach the end point first, crossing the finish line in what appeared to be an Olympic record. American spectators in the stands erupted with cheers.

Then confusion broke out. Obviously something had happened, but no one was quite sure what. Carpenter believed he had won. British officials thought a foul had been committed. James Sullivan celebrated but all the while kept an eye on the growing huddle of officials. Halswelle was outraged, both at the result and the Americans' tactics. "Then," as the *New York Tribune* reported, "the announcer made a brief statement through a megaphone that the race had been declared void."

An "official inquiry into the final heat of the Four Hundred Metres Race" was convened. All the conveners were conveniently British. They compared notes. Carpenter was not allowed to provide a statement in his own defense. The inquisition concluded that Carpenter had "willfully obstructed" Halswelle. The two leading Americans, but Carpenter mostly, had pushed and jostled Halswelle to the point that the race was compromised. Halswelle reported that Carpenter had done more than just "bore" outward in order to obstruct

Halswelle's stride. Carpenter had delivered two elbows, "two vigorous blows on the chest," the resulting bruising of which a doctor (British) had confirmed. Carpenter would later offer a different account, stating that he had never made contact with Halswelle.

After two hours of deliberation, the voiding was confirmed. John Carpenter: Disqualified. The Final: To be rerun, minus Carpenter, two days later.

The American team objected to the decision. Robbins and Taylor were resolute; they refused to run a redo. So Halswelle ran a final alone. His remains the only walkover victory in Olympic history. Halswelle cruised around the track in just over fifty seconds, far off his personal best. Britain won the gold medal.

As president of the United States, Roosevelt had exactly zero obligation to comment on Carpenter. When, in the 1972 Olympics for example, the US Men's Basketball team was robbed of a gold medal when Russia got to replay the final seconds of the title game not once, but twice, President Richard Nixon did not weigh in other than to say: "Well, we got screwed." He did not engage in weeks of back and forth with IOC and Soviet officials in order to set the record straight.

But perhaps this isn't a surprise. Nixon was no Roosevelt; his head isn't on a giant rock in South Dakota. The NCAA doesn't award a trophy annually in memory of Nixon.

As news of Carpenter's disqualification played out in the press—as Sullivan and other American officials ratcheted up the pressure on their British counterparts—Roosevelt stewed. He requested more information. Here was one more chance to weigh in on athletics and America's role in an increasingly international athletic arena.

Starting in August, and not wrapping up until election season in November, Roosevelt had a four-way conversation about this controversy surrounding four men circling a track for four hundred meters as fast as humanly possible. From James Sullivan, Roosevelt learned the American perspective. This was the side Roosevelt wanted to believe. Carpenter had been fast, strategic, and tough; he won. The British cheated the United States out of a gold medal. "I have read what you say with concern," Roosevelt wrote to Sullivan, after receiving Sullivan's report. "I am sorry to say that it corroborates the impression that I had already gained." Roosevelt tried to push Sullivan to be restrained ("nothing is to be gained by more talk"), but it was a difficult pill for both men to swallow. "The dignified and wise thing for us to do," Roosevelt urged (himself as much as Sullivan), "is to make not a public comment of any kind, but to content ourselves with celebrating as we ought to do the fact that no athletic team has ever won any such athletic victory as ours on this occasion."

If Roosevelt and Sullivan served to simultaneously talk each other down and work each other up, Roosevelt's correspondence with George C. Buell (an American investment banker), Theodore A. Cook (British Amateur Fencing Association, author of the Official 1908 Olympic Report), and "The Right Honorable" Lord Desborough (president of the British Olympic Council) allowed for an all-out debate. What had happened? How did the Olympics reflect the Americans and the British? What was the point of international athletic competition anyhow?

Several times Roosevelt protested that he did not have time for such lengthy exchanges...but then he would reply with a lengthy, nuanced letter. He just could not help himself from engaging.

Over the course of several letters, Roosevelt laid out his defense of Carpenter and the United States Olympic team—and by default the athletic culture of the United States as well.

Point 1: Britain had been expecting a dirty race, thereby nearly guaranteeing such a foul would be called. "The morning of the race one of your sporting papers ('The Sportsman'), and possibly other papers, appeared with the statement that foul play was anticipated from the Americans, but that care would be taken to see that it was not successful. Such a publication was an outrage."

Point 2: Whatever had happened on the track between Carpenter and Halswelle, it had not been nearly so clear as the British officials and press (with its "unmeasured vituperation") made it out to be.

Point 3: The same officials that intervened against Carpenter allowed an atrocity of rules violations in the marathon contest, the very day after the 400, which nearly cost the United States a gold medal. Roosevelt had become a near-expert on this particular irony. "When the Italian [Dorando Pietri] came on the track at the Stadium he fell; that he was stimulated by the cheers of the spectators and officials and by other forms of encouragement, and proceeded." There were "stimulants administered to the Italian in utter disregard of every principle of fair play." What's more, the runner fell repeatedly, only to be "illegally and improperly helped" back to his feet repeatedly and pushed forward repeatedly. In the end, a British official took Pietri's arm and helped him over the final yards as the American in second place closed the gap quickly. With Pietri across, the Italian flag was quickly raised, celebrating Pietri's victory. Where were the vigilant British officials in all of this? "But again the British officials decline to take the action which they are bound to take, their conduct being in scandalous contrast to the way in which the day before they broke the tape and crowded on the track in advance of any decisions as to the fouling of Carpenter."

Point 4: "Carpenter is a Cornell man." Rather than somehow, as a Harvard alum himself, holding this against Carpenter, Roosevelt explained that his cousin—George Roosevelt—had competed against Carpenter many times without a hint of scandal. "He says that he is a good, straight fellow."

Point 5: Officials refused to allow Carpenter to give a statement in his defense following the contest. Did the British have no sense of due process?

Point 6: The British runner (Halswelle) was aided by British officials, in Britain. "The judges, who were not of his [Carpenter's] nationality, but of the nationality of his opponent, held him guilty of fouling."

Point 7: Carpenter ran a faster time than Halswelle did in the subsequent, solitary race. "When the next day the competitor who had thus been handed the race as a gift, ran over the course alone and tried to make record time, he failed to come up to Carpenter's time."

Point 8: The British officials had failed to follow proper protocol. This Roosevelt added, in an agitated scrawl, at the bottom of page two of his nine-page letter to George Bruell. "Remember also that the conduct of the judges in the Carpenter race in breaking the tape, crowding the course, and declaring the race off on a foul before any investigation could possibly have been held, was in itself in the highest-degree improper and unsportsmanlike."

Point 9: The United States would not be bullied by international athletic standards. "If the attitude of mind you betray in this letter represents the general attitude of the men interested in British sport," he wrote Cook, "I most emphatically hope that American athletes will not again appear on English tracks; and I am quite indifferent as to whether they are barred out, because I should protest in any event against their going."

Point 10: It appeared the British had cheated in the tug of war competition. "The British officials permitted their team to appear with hobnails and steel plates."

Point 11: The United States had still dominated the track-and-field competition. "My idea is to refrain from every statement which will tend to cause international bitterness, and simply to congratulate the American team, which, as your correspondent shows, before an unfriendly audience and with unfriendly surroundings nevertheless score so signal a triumph."

Roosevelt, as always, connected the athletic issue back to himself. He too had experienced a Carpenter–Halswelle situation. "Thirty years ago I was in a footrace in which I was beaten, where my antagonist and I touched, and each of us frankly believed that the other had fouled him," Roosevelt remembered. What did Roosevelt do? Well, he certainly did not go calling for a new race. "Neither of us," Roosevelt clarified, "made the claim and neither for a moment supposed the other had fouled him intentionally." If only Olympic competition could play out so simply.

Eventually, the issue fizzled out. Halswelle remained the gold medalist; Carpenter remained disqualified. Roosevelt had lost his second athletic argument of the summer. Most tragically, Taylor, who had won a gold medal as a part of the 4x400 relay team, died of typhoid pneumonia shortly upon returning to the United States.

*   *   *

By October 27, 1908, on his fiftieth birthday, Roosevelt could see his post-presidential life just over the horizon. Just as importantly, the rest of Washington, DC could see it too. Before long, Roosevelt would not even be a lame duck. His work was done; the hay was in the barn. "I have had a good time in my fifty years, and have done some work," Roosevelt wrote to Kermit (who had recently started at Harvard) on his half-century birthday. Roosevelt celebrated his fiftieth quietly: lunch with Edith, a few minutes sitting under the apple tree by the fountain, then a ride on Roswell—his favorite horse.

As for the election of 1908, Taft romped to victory. Running on Roosevelt's legacy and endorsement, as well as his own record as secretary of war, Taft won 51.6% of the popular vote. He amassed 321 electoral votes to Bryan's 162, making WJB's third presidential run his most lopsided defeat.

Taft Acclaimed President by the American People, read the *Washington Post*'s headline on November 4, 1908. As a man "swept into the White House by great popular wave of approval," Taft started his tenure as president with none of the uncertainty Roosevelt had known at his outset. And indeed as the vote counters quickly pointed out, Taft had actually bested Roosevelt in New York: "Taft's plurality larger than Roosevelt's in 1904."

Roosevelt's reaction to Taft's win was a mixture of pride and grief. He wired Taft congratulations at midnight on election night ("I need hardly say how heartily I congratulate you, and the country even more,") and then, uncharacteristically, refused to give the reporters still gathered in the White House pressroom any comment. He was for once a man with nothing to say.

The goodbyes piled up as 1908 gave way to 1909. The Roosevelt family hosted fifty relatives and friends for Christmas lunch. The White House, while growing quieter as Alice, Ted Jr., and Kermit had all moved out, hummed one last time with Ethel's debut extravaganza. It was a night "ablaze with color as merry guests danced," according to the *Washington Post*. Ethel was, as the Roosevelt family prepared to leave the capitol, "the most interesting figure in Washington society." A seventeen-year-old beauty, she made her debut wearing "an Empire frock of soft white satin." Five hundred guests had been invited. White House porters served dinner at midnight; there was dancing in the East Room until 2:00 a.m. For once it was not a night about the president. In a long column on the event, the *Washington Post* had only this to say about Roosevelt: "The President was present during the evening." Alice's debut in 1902 had marked the beginning of the First Family's time in DC; Ethel's signaled its close.

During the summer and fall of 1908, Roosevelt wrote often to William Howard Taft, starting his letters with a simple, "Dear Will." In the correspondence, Roosevelt advised Taft on labor matters. He urged Taft to be careful with the Navy. "One closing legacy," Roosevelt wrote. "Under no circumstances divide the battleship fleet between the Atlantic and Pacific Oceans prior to the finishing of the Panama Canal."

Perhaps providing more finality than any other farewell was that of the Tennis Cabinet. Roosevelt hosted the motley group on March 1, 1909. The men gathered at 1:30 p.m., crowding into the White House's state dining room as the countdown toward the Taft inauguration commenced. All the fellows—well most them, thirty-one in all—were there. "Gentlemen: You are here nominally as members, or to meet the members of the 'tennis cabinet,'" Roosevelt began, strangely formal. These were, Roosevelt clarified, "men with whom at tennis or hunting or riding or walking or boxing, I have played, with whom I have been on the round-up or in the mountains or in the ranch country."

They were more than just the "men associated with him in sports," though. These were Roosevelt's friends. Especially Jusserand, Garfield, and Pinchot. The whole group had played a key role in facilitating Roosevelt's approach to the strenuous presidency. Athletics for TR had always been about people. Saying farewell to this group was difficult but filled with humor too. The *New York Times*'s sub-headline for the story captured the strange dynamic at hand: EXPRESSES REGRET AT LEAVING FRIENDS WHO HAVE LOYALLY SUPPORTED ADMINISTRATION—RECEIVED BRONZE COUGAR.

What do you get a retiring president who gave you access to the White House tennis court and an astounding appreciation for the possibilities of Rock Creek Park? The men decided on a bronze sculpture, "Charging Panther." It was handcrafted by Alexander Phimister Proctor, an American artist who was known for his ability to capture the American wilderness through his work. The names and titles of the Tennis Cabinet members were inscribed on the base of the sculpture.

Seth Bullock, a former lawman from Medora, North Dakota (and later Deadwood, South Dakota, sheriff), and lifelong friend of Roosevelt, was chosen to present the sculpture to Roosevelt. While merely an "honorary member of the tennis cabinet," given that he did not hold an official position in Washington, Bullock had the gravitas for the presentation duty. Roosevelt counted Bullock among his closest friends; Bullock loved Roosevelt. The panther sat on a nearby table, blocked from Roosevelt's view by an arrangement of roses. When it was time, Bullock moved, clumsily, to make the presentation. Nothing from this point on went right. "Toward the end of the dinner," Roosevelt recalled, "Seth got up and began pawin' among the roses and I put out my hand to restrain him, when I remembered that Set was a two-gun man, so I let him alone." The problem was emotion. Bullock could not do it. He was a self-described "poor hand at saying good-by." So rather than giving his prepared speech, the overcome lawman awkwardly pushed apart the flowers to reveal the gift. *Here—take it.* Roosevelt understood.

Then the men adjourned outside, onto the South Lawn, for a photograph. Roosevelt sat, cougar at his feet, with his favorite men surrounding him. The men were like Roosevelt. All middle-aged white men, most with mustaches. The group had the look of former athletes. The shoulders were still strong, the backs still rigid for the most part, but cheeks had grown rounder, the stomachs thicker, and hair thinner as the years progressed.

Roosevelt's last letters as president to his Tennis Cabinet were thoughtful, if understandably melancholy. To Jusserand he wrote a rambling missive admitting that "I should have particularly liked to have remained as President." He continued, searching: "We cannot any of us tell whither civilization is tending, or what may be the strength or even direction of the great blind forces working all around us. But I very cordially agree with Lord Acton [Roosevelt was reading (in French) the Italian historian Guglielmo Ferrero in his free time] that we are honor bound to do right *because* it is right."

Roosevelt wrote too to convey his deep affection to Gifford Pinchot and James Garfield. On February 24, 1909, Roosevelt wrote Pinchot a letter, "not written about you," but instead explaining his appreciation to Pinchot for Garfield. Then a week later came another letter to Pinchot, this time singling him out for a literary hug. "Just a line about yourself," Roosevelt began. "I am a better man for having known you. I feel that to have been with you will make my children better men and women," Roosevelt wrote. Then Roosevelt wrote a letter addressed to both men. Wrapping up this letter, Roosevelt zeroed in on exactly what had made their time together so special: "For seven and a half years we have worked together, and now and then we played together—and have been altogether better able to work because we have played."

Here was, perhaps, Roosevelt's most poignant athletic legacy: the bonds formed with men who took to the court, or trail, or ring with him.

ELEVEN

WAIT...JACK JOHNSON?

*It will be some time before we get a hired man in Washington to suit
down to the ground as Roosevelt does. When he retires he will be the
undisputed champion in his class, and the belt will be his for keeps,
and no champion ever retired with a belt that can show more class,
gameness, and wallopitiveness than Theodore Roosevelt.*

—John L. Sullivan

The sports world did not pause for Roosevelt to say his goodbyes. It kept
right on churning. During the period between the 1908 election (November) and the 1909 inauguration (March), Jack Johnson became the
first African American fighter to win boxing's World Heavyweight Championship. This ascension by a black man to the pinnacle of athletics rattled
white America. His reign caused race riots and lynchings. For Roosevelt,
Johnson represented a last-minute shift in the Strenuous Life experiment.
Johnson challenged the racial bias inherent in Roosevelt's ideas about athletics. And if nothing else, Johnson abruptly dethroned Roosevelt as America's
most talked about boxer.

Roosevelt, like many Americans, could maneuver his thinking to a place
where he connected boxing with racial survival. In 1895, Roosevelt wrote in
the *North American Review* about the importance of "the preservation of a
race." He expressed concern that white Americans might become a race that

did not "breed well or fight well." While breeding and fighting referenced imperialism, Roosevelt undoubtedly made a boxing connection as well.

And in terms of boxing itself, a precedent was already in place at the turn of the century—enforced by John L. Sullivan—that said only white men would be allowed to fight for the sport's highest title.

During his presidency, Roosevelt compiled a mixed record on civil rights. "His contradictory racial views were often at odds with his basic egalitarian approach to people," was how Roosevelt expert Kathleen Dalton described it. Always an admirer of Abraham Lincoln, Roosevelt gave a Lincoln's Day address in 1905 that revealed much about his own views on race. Like many of Roosevelt's speeches, this particular one was filled with substance and several beautiful turns of phrase. It meandered down several rabbit trails before concluding with a flourish. For those looking back and searching for evidence that Roosevelt was at least ahead of his own times when it comes to the promotion of racial equality, his 1905 speech provides some ample material. "Our effort should be," Roosevelt opined to a crowd of 1,300 at New York City's Waldorf-Astoria, "to secure to each man, whatever his color, equality of opportunity, equality of treatment before the law."

But for those suspicious of Roosevelt, like those who doused the TR statue in front of the New York City Museum of Natural History with "blood" in 2017, the 1905 Lincoln speech contains proof as well. While Roosevelt wanted general uplift for society, he distinguished between the capabilities of different races. "The problem is to so adjust the relations between two races of different ethnic type that the rights of neither be abridged nor jeoparded [sic]; that the backward race be trained so that it may enter into the possession of true freedom, while the forward race is enabled to preserve unharmed the high civilization wrought out by its forefathers." Here was the crux of the matter for Roosevelt: there was a forward race (whites) and a backward one (blacks). He favored the idea of equality, he even fought for it on an individual level, but he did not spend much time considering structural solutions that might ensure it.

More than anything he said, however, Roosevelt's legacy on racial matters hinges on a grievous misjudgment he made in 1906. In that year, safely in the middle of his popular tidal wave, Roosevelt made a decision that fundamentally changed his status with African Americans. At issue was the handling of an outbreak of violence in Brownsville, Texas, that occurred in August 1906.

Roosevelt received his first official report on the matter on August 16. "At a few minutes before midnight on Monday," a telegram from Brownsville's mayor informed the president, "a body of United States soldiers of the twenty-fifth United States infantry (colored), numbering between 20–30 men...begun firing in town and directly into dwellings, offices, stores and at police and citizens." The gunfire had put the town on notice. "We find that threats have been made by them that they will repeat this outrage," the mayor continued. "We look to you for relief; we ask you to have the troops at once removed from Fort Brown and replaced by white soldiers." The parenthetical (*colored*) resided at the center of the issue.

Roosevelt requested a full investigation by the War Department. He certainly recognized that the mayor of Brownsville was providing only part of the story. Newspaper reporters, too, had their own assessment of the situation. But what had really happened? According to the *Brownsville Herald,* a "mob of negro soldiers" came into town unprovoked "and opened fire on it." DASTARDLY OUTRAGE BY NEGRO SOLDIERS, read the headline. In the background, however, was the racial tension born from stationing black troops in the region. Scuffles had occurred right from the start between the black regiment (Buffalo Soldiers as they were known) and Brownsville's mostly white citizenry. A nebulous rape charge surfaced. Many whites just wanted the black troops gone from their midst.

Things got increasingly complicated. The black soldiers refused to break ranks and speak with the investigators. With good reason, they did not trust their own Army to treat them fairly. The issue festered until, believing that he had enough information—or at least all he was going to get—Roosevelt signed Special Order number 266 on November 5, 1906. He then waited until late in the day the following afternoon, which just happened to be Election Day, to announce the action. The order summarily discharged, dishonorably, all of the black enlisted men stationed in Brownsville—167 total. It cost the soldiers their careers, salaries, honors, and pensions.

Overnight, Roosevelt lost his standing among black Americans. "He shot us when our gun was empty," remarked Dr. Charles Morriss, an African American pastor in New York. "Thus shall we answer Theodore Roosevelt, once enshrined in our love as our Moses, now enshrouded in our scorn as our Judas."

Among those who would hold the decision against Roosevelt for years to come was a heavyweight boxer: Jack Johnson. Johnson found no reason to excuse such a decision. He called into question Roosevelt's entire claim to African American allegiance. "Mr. Roosevelt, he travels on one thing. He ate dinner with Booker T. Washington," Johnson would point out years later. It was not that dinner but Brownsville that formed Johnson's core assessment of Roosevelt: "When Roosevelt was in Cuba, our great black army saved him. After that he comes home and hears one man was killed in Brownsville and expels the whole army." The truth about Roosevelt came out in the time of trial. "We all know," Johnson said, sarcasm dripping, as part of a stump speech he developed, "how Mr. Roosevelt gave us colored folks a fair chance in the Brownsville affair."

*   *   *

If unloosed to consider the connection between Theodore Roosevelt and Jack Johnson, statistical satirist Tyler Vigen (see Chapter 2 footnote) might conclude that every time a sports-obsessed president leaves the White House, a revolutionary black man ascends to boxing's Heavyweight Championship. Not so much. But the timing of one man's departure with the other's arrival deserves at least a moment of consideration. During every part of Roosevelt's presidency, Jack Johnson was working his way up through the heavyweight ranks. Training. Fighting. Striving. Pushing for a chance. Then, just as Roosevelt was leaving, Johnson claimed the title.

A round-faced, thickly muscled, defensive tactician, Johnson overwhelmed most fighters who dared face him in the ring. Outside it, Johnson experienced the most unlikely of American tales. "How incongruous is that that I," Johnson said, "a little Galveston colored boy, should ever become an acquaintance of kings and rulers of the old world, or that I should number among my friends some of the most notable persons of America and the world in general!" It was indeed quite a ride.

Johnson's life started differently from that of his ancestors and most people of African descent up to that point in America. "Jack Johnson belonged to the first generation of American blacks to be born free," was how one of Johnson's biographers described this monumental change. Free. But certainly not equal—not in terms of legal or societal norms. This was Jim Crow America. Black men faced limited employment opportunities, obstacles in voting, restrictions on where they could live, limited educational opportunities for their children, and the threat of being lynched for glancing at a white woman. And not just in the South. In 1908 in Springfield, Illinois, a race riot broke out over an alleged rape. Two black men—Scott Burton and William Donegan—both elderly and neither an actual suspect in the crime, were lynched by a marauding mob.

The thing, *the* thing about Johnson—beyond even his fighting ability—was that he had this radical notion that he should actually live by his own rules. He favored white women and fast cars. Literally. The former caused him more trouble from American law enforcement than the latter. As Johnson explained it, he had been rejected by the women of his own race. At twenty, he married Mary Austin; she left him after three years. Then he fell for a black prostitute named Clara Kerr in Chicago. The two moved together to California where, according to Johnson, Kerr discarded him and ran off with a horse trainer. Johnson was done. "The heartaches which Mary Austin and Clara Kerr had caused me, led me to forswear colored women and to determine that my lot henceforth would be cast only with white women."

Johnson began his fighting on the docks of Galveston's harbor at age thirteen. He had no choice. "My associates," as Johnson called them, generously, "To them, fighting was one of the important functions of existence. They fought upon every occasion and on any pretext...It was up to me to hold me own." He did. By sixteen Johnson had begun to develop a reputation as a boxer; by twenty-one Johnson was fighting regularly in Galveston bouts and occasionally traveling to cities such as Chicago or Memphis for bigger fights.

It's an educated guess as to how many fights Johnson actually participated in during his long career—probably hundreds if exhibitions and hastily put together scraps are counted. In 1902, Johnson fought thirteen times. He faced white and black men. He almost always won. On February 3, 1903, Johnson fought Ed "Denver" Martin. Martin weighed twenty pounds more than Johnson and stood six inches taller. Martin knew how to box, too, using some of the same defensive tactics that Johnson deployed.

Johnson and Martin met at Hazard's Pavilion in Los Angeles, a venue that sat four thousand spectators and had hosted the likes of Dwight L. Moody, Booker T. Washington, and William Jennings Bryan. For twenty rounds, Johnson pounded away at Martin. Finally, in the eleventh, Johnson knocked Martin to the canvas with a right hand. Twice more during the remaining rounds, Johnson sent Martin tumbling. When it was over, the judges awarded Johnson the decision; he was now something he could never accept as enough but would take nonetheless: the "Colored Heavyweight Champion of the World."

Johnson continued to fight and win, fight and win throughout the first decade of the twentieth century. Despite his burgeoning résumé, however, the world heavyweight title remained practically, if not officially, out of his reach. Jim Jeffries, who held boxing's most important title from 1899 until 1905, simply refused to face black fighters. Tommy Burns abided by the same policy after taking over for Jeffries. It was the long-established, standard practice.

Johnson's only choice then was to continue to win the fights he could actually secure. He took to punishing those white fighters that would face him with "a shade of cruelty" while doing just enough to defeat his black opponents. Finally, in July 1907, Johnson got a fight with former heavyweight champion Bob Fitzsimmons—a badly out of shape former champ (but still a name in the boxing world) who needed a quick cash score. Johnson knocked out Fitzsimmons in round two.

The victory over Fitzsimmons seemed to shift public opinion. Johnson, despite his race, deserved a shot at the world heavyweight title. He had simply won too much to be ignored. Critics of Burns as an illegitimate champion (since he had won the title from a weak fighter—Marvin Hart—upon the

Jeffries retirement) began pushing Johnson. "Tommy's enemies," the *Chicago Tribune* reported, "continually argue that he is not champion of America until he defeats Jack Johnson."

* * *

In a small, almost imperceptible way, Roosevelt supported boxing's segregated norms. Roosevelt had befriended the fighter most responsible for creating the very specific color line that kept Johnson from a heavyweight title shot—John L. Sullivan. "He has been my friend for many years, and I am proud to be his," Roosevelt said. Nearly the same age as Roosevelt, Sullivan was among the most famous ex-athletes alive during the Roosevelt era.

Sullivan had fought during the 1880s, a time when boxing rules were minimal and "men still believed that a real fight meant a bare-knuckle one." In this savage fighting climate, Sullivan dominated for nearly a decade. Sullivan had faced Jake Kilrain in the last bare-knuckle championship fight on US soil on July 8, 1889. The fight took place in sultry Richburg, Mississippi, and lasted seventy-five rounds. Sullivan won, cementing his position as America's ultimate fighting man.

Not surprisingly, retirement proved difficult for a man like Sullivan. The police picked up Sullivan on gambling and wife-beating charges. His primary skill—brawling—did not translate well into civilian life. He remained an icon though. He took to calling at the White House. And Roosevelt never turned away interesting people. TR knew that Sullivan was struggling. "It was mighty decent of old John L. to come over to see me...I more than half suspect he needs help himself, but I would not for the life of me insult him by even a hint of an offer."

While no one, ever, accused Sullivan of being an idea man, he deserves some of the blame for creating a wrinkle in boxing's code. Sullivan readjusted boxing's racial Rubicon. He knew that interracial fights happened. They always had; they probably always would—at least in some venues. So the cause for Sullivan became protecting the Heavyweight Championship above all else from the black race. Sullivan had a sense of duty: "he felt a particular obligation to ensure that he would never yield [the title] to an African American."

Even with an athlete of Sullivan's caliber, Roosevelt could not resist a bit of the comparison game. "I do not suppose I feel quite as fit as you do, my fellow semi-centenarian," he wrote Sullivan in 1908, "but I am all right." Roosevelt admired Sullivan's strength and tenacity. He saw Sullivan as somehow connected to the United States' struggle to maintain its edge internationally. "I know that his former profession is not a very exalted one," Roosevelt said of John L., "but he was a fair fighter, and he never threw a fight, and, in his way, he did his best to uphold American supremacy."

The broader quest to demonstrate American (white) supremacy took on many forms—some more tangible than others. As Johnson probed for a title shot, the Great White Fleet, which consisted of sixteen newly built US Navy battleships, each with its hull painted a gleaming white, sailed around the world. Roosevelt had ordered the mission to demonstrate American military strength. From December 1907 until February 1909, 14,000 sailors manned the armada; the fleet covered more than 43,000 miles and made stops on six continents. There was no subtlety here. The world could not ignore the United States' new navy if that navy showed up at their doorstep.

Shortly after the Great White Fleet pulled away from Australia, Jack Johnson arrived. He had followed Tommy Burns, the heavyweight champion, to the country. Before that, Johnson had followed Burns throughout Europe. "Johnson on Burns' Trail: Colored Heavy-weight Arrives in London with manager... Fight any-where...Burns Wants $30,000," summarized one newspaper.

A fight with Burns was a possibility. To be sure, Burns was a racist ("All coons are yellow," he said), but getting rich remained Burns's fixation. Burns had grown up in Canada and in poverty just as gripping as Johnson's. Born Noah Brusso, Burns changed his name to something more Scottish-sounding for publicity reasons. He spent his whole career trying to make up for his start in life. He traveled the world looking for the best fights—not so much because he wanted to challenge himself as a boxer but because he wanted paydays. "I will defend my title against all comers, none barred," he said. "By this I mean white, black, Mexican, Indian, or any other nationality." Burns could not afford John L. Sullivan's brand of racism. For enough compensation, he would fight anyone.

The money in boxing, unsavory as it seemed to people like Roosevelt who constantly sought to separate boxing from prizefighting, sometimes transcended racial bias. For a guaranteed $30,000 (roughly $850,000 today), Burns agreed to a match with Johnson. John L. Sullivan immediately expressed his displeasure: "Shame on the money-mad Champion! Shame on the man who upsets good American precedents because there are Dollars, Dollars, Dollars, in it." But much of white America (to say nothing of black America), and white Europe, and white Australia wanted the fight. Someone had to shut Johnson up.

Burns and Johnson squared off on December 26, 1908, in Sydney, Australia. Bettors favored the smaller, less accomplished, but white fighter. The odds stood at 5–4 for Burns during the week leading up to the bout. For his effort, Johnson was guaranteed $5,000. For Johnson, the fight was one of his first in which he carried true contempt for his opponent. Unfailingly genial and cordial, Johnson rarely fueled his engine with hate. But Burns was different. Johnson heard his slurs and viewed Burns as an uncouth and illegitimate champion. After all, Burns had assumed the title only after Jim Jeffries retired.

Legitimate or not, Burns's biggest problem was his lack of size. While Johnson looked like a modern-day heavyweight fighter, over six feet tall and nearly two hundred pounds of sculpted muscle, Burns was fighting up. Burns gave up five inches and more than thirty pounds to his opponent. Although Burns had made a career of defeating bigger fighters, this gap was too much.

The bell rang shortly after 11:00 a.m. the day after Christmas—"Boxing Day" as it's known in Australia. The fight began with Johnson skipping out of his corner and unleashing a flurry of jabs at Burns. He did not let up throughout the fight. Johnson used his typical "clever way," peppering Burns with punches while never really opening himself up to take a return shot. He deftly warded off Burns's flailing charges and responded with pointed counter-blows. "The fight was one of the easiest of the more important fights of my career," Johnson said. Johnson simply wore the smaller fighter down. In the fourteenth round, Johnson knocked Burns to the canvas for the fifth time. Burns got up, slowly. Johnson wasted no time moving back in, and just as Johnson reared back to unleash another shot to Burns's head, the referee, urged by attending police officers, rushed in to stop the fight.

Johnson had won; Negro Johnson Now Champion of the World, read the next day's newspapers.

Johnson foreshadowed Muhammad Ali with his post-fight comments. Of course he had prevailed. He was the far superior fighter. And he wasn't afraid to say as much. "I never doubted the issue from the beginning," Johnson explained in a widely circulated interview. "I knew I was too good for Burns. I have forgotten more about fighting than Burns ever knew." Johnson had put his money where his mouth was, betting heavily on himself, checking in just before the fight began to make sure that his financial wagers had been booked.

* * *

We do not know what Roosevelt thought about Johnson's victory. Given the president's long connection to boxing and his voracious appetite for news, we can assume that he learned about the Johnson–Burns fight almost immediately after its conclusion. A few weeks later, TR got a chance to talk about it with a professional fighter. On that day, Battling Nelson, a lightweight boxer, visited the White House, promoting his new "75,000-word" (all the promotional materials made mention of the word count, perhaps surprised that a boxer could write so much) autobiography, *Life, Battles and Career of Battling Nelson: Lightweight Champion of the World.*

Nelson congratulated the president on a ninety-eight-mile ride he had taken the day before—a jaunt meant to demonstrate to the men of the United States military that physical fitness should be a lifelong pursuit. Then the conversation shifted to Jack Johnson. From the longtime fighter, Roosevelt harvested information. "He was particularly interested as to who would be the best man to fight Johnson," Nelson told reporters upon leaving the White House. "I gave him my honest opinion—that Jim Corbett was my choice, although if Ralph Rose would train he might have chance." Nelson told Roosevelt that Jim Jeffries would likely perform poorly if matched with Johnson. Then Roosevelt autographed a photograph for Nelson and sent the fighter on his way.

Johnson ruled the boxing world as Roosevelt left the White House. Inauguration Day for Taft came with a blizzard. As the snow piled up, the inauguration organizers were forced to move the ceremony inside the US Capitol. "The change stirred to disappointed wrath thousands of men and women who had dared the howling snowstorm and gathered on the stands and about the Capitol to witness the inauguration." But the weather left no choice.

Roosevelt departed from Washington, DC immediately after the inauguration. "Theodore Roosevelt is again a private citizen," the *New York Times* reported. Roosevelt waved to thousands of well-wishers as he boarded a train headed for Sagamore Hill at Union Station.

Once home, Roosevelt puttered around a bit, doing some writing for *Outlook* and chopping some wood. Then, after just three weeks as a relatively unencumbered private citizen, Roosevelt boarded the *SS Hamburg*, carrying a rabbit's foot given to him by John L. Sullivan, bound for East Africa. From there Roosevelt would travel to Europe. His feet would not touch American soil again for fifteen months.

On his "Expedition of Africa," Roosevelt helped gather more than 100,000 specimens for what would become the Smithsonian Museum of Natural History. He had a grand time shooting at, well, almost everything. Roosevelt's goal was to kill one of each of the five fiercest animals on the African continent: buffalo, elephant, lion, leopard, and rhinoceros. "Down he came!" Roosevelt wrote about one of the nine lions he ended up killing. By Roosevelt's meticulous count, he killed 296 animals during the safari, including nine lions, three elephants, and thirteen rhinos.

After Africa, Roosevelt moved onto a farewell tour of sorts through the capital cities of Europe. The trip was partially backed by Andrew Carnegie, the industrialist who had become an international peace advocate. Roosevelt, joined by Edith and accompanied by Ethel (eighteen years old) and Kermit (twenty), traveled to Norway in order for TR to give a long delayed Nobel Peace Prize speech. Then they went on to Rome (where the Pope refused to see Roosevelt), Paris, and Berlin. Germany was the most perplexing stop of the tour. Roosevelt spent several stimulating but deeply troubling days with Kaiser Wilhelm II. The "Germans did not like me, and did not like my country," Roosevelt said after the visit. Traveling on to London, the mood lightened. A telegram from Carnegie awaited Roosevelt in Britain: "Your future is, recent events excepted, likely to excel your past since you are a born leader of men with the sublime audacity to perform wonders." Roosevelt undoubtedly appreciated the sentiments; who wouldn't?

* * *

Meanwhile, Jack Johnson removed all doubt about his grip on the heavyweight title. He defeated Victor McLaglen, Frank Moran, Jack O'Brien, Tony Ross, Al Kaufman, and Stanley Ketchel all while Roosevelt paraded as the "World Citizen." As the ranks of challengers thinned, the white boxing public began calling for the former champion, Jeffries, to return to the ring in order to right the country's racial ship. Perhaps he could be the "Great White Hope" the nation so desperately wanted. Jack London, the celebrated novelist who covered the Johnson–Burns fight for the *New York Herald*, led the Jeffries movement. "Jeffries must emerge from his alfalfa farm and remove that smile from Johnson's face," London wrote. "Jeff, it's up to you."

The problem for "Jeff" was that he had been retired for five years. He was thirty-five years old in 1909, well past his prime as a fighter. He was soft and paunchy. But letters arrived constantly at Jeffries's home urging him to take on Johnson. What made the letters especially intriguing to the old fighter was the fact that he needed the money. Among other ventures, Jeffries had launched an athletic club in Los Angeles, and it was struggling mightily.

So Jeffries gradually began moving more. He began to consider the possibility of taking on Johnson. "Jeffries has been taking light exercise," the *Atlanta Constitution* reported. "And by this method he has reduced his weight from

270 to 230 pounds." Finally, on April 19, 1909, Jim Jeffries yielded to the pressure: he agreed to a fight with Johnson. While it would take some time to get in shape and settle the financial details, Jeffries was in. "That nigger can never lick me," Jeffries said during the lead-up to the fight.

Both men stood to make a significant fortune from the match. The fighters entered into a contract to share the motion picture rights to the contest. The men agreed to a 60–40 split of the fight proceeds with the lion's share going to the winner. The Tex Rickard promotion machine raised the fever pitch surrounding the event. Jeffries, mostly by virtue of his skin color, remained the favorite in the months leading up to the bout. Even Jeffries, though, recognized that he was smaller, older, and badly out of practice. Undoubtedly feeling the intense pressure, Jeffries faced his training tasks grimly. He closed his camp and pushed away all visitors. Johnson on the other hand acted like a politician even as he trained. He danced through his workouts with a kind word and smile for almost every man, woman, and child who descended upon his training camp.

Before too long, the "Fight of the Century" went looking for Roosevelt. Tony Gavin, a Buffalo policeman who had been a Rough Rider, wrote Roosevelt with news of the fight. Roosevelt, from Africa, responded: "That must have been a rattling fight between Ketchel and Johnson," Roosevelt wrote in what he probably assumed would be held as private correspondence. "Johnson is unquestionably a first-class fighter. I wonder if Jim Jeffries can get back into form; if he can, it will be a tremendous battle when they meet." Enclosed with the letter, Roosevelt sent a pressed flower for Gavin's wife, Alberta.

Gavin could not keep quiet; he shared Roosevelt's letter with the press. Who could keep such a secret? So, in January—with Roosevelt somewhere in Africa and the fight still seven months away—headlines of ROOSEVELT LIKES JOHNSON and COL. ROOSEVELT WONDERS IF JEFFRIES CAN GET INTO FORM, and JEFFRIES CHEERED UP BY ROOSEVELT'S FAVOR appeared in newspapers across the country. The press's pent-up demand for Roosevelt stories bubbled over.

Johnson, for his part, knew precisely what to do with the Roosevelt storyline. Where others might have stepped back in deference, Johnson surged forward. "Ex-President Roosevelt ought to be a good authority," Johnson wrote in a letter to the *New York American* (reprinted widely) in response to the publication of Roosevelt's letter to Gavin. "He has been boxing himself, and should know the merits of both men, and I think he should make a good referee, being our nation's chief life, and a great leader was he."

Johnson played politics as well as he boxed.

The referee question was actually a pressing one. Johnson and Jeffries argued back and forth during the months leading up to the fight about who might serve in the vital role. "If the club would choose [TR] as referee, it would satisfy me to a queen's taste," Johnson wrote. "He is cool and collected, and no one can rattle him and get his goat." Johnson signed off: "Your Champion, Jack Johnson."

It was a brilliant bit of theater by Johnson. His move forced Jeffries to come and say that, yes, he too approved the idea of Roosevelt serving as referee. And as important, the story, which most newspapers recognized as a promotional stunt, raised the issue of fair officiating. When the *Buffalo Commercial* reported, "And now Jeff says Teddy would make a good referee," for example, it ended the story with a comment on the fight's fairness. "Johnson will insist on a man whose honesty cannot be questioned to act as referee," the paper explained. "The negro is afraid he may be 'jobbed.'"

Roosevelt never publicly responded to the referee job offer, but Johnson had already scored his first point.

The fight promoters used Roosevelt too. Promoter Jack Gleason settled on a well-worn idea to connect the former president to his event, presenting Roosevelt with the first ticket (gold, of course) for the event. The gesture worked as well as it had for baseball; it gained attention. ROOSEVELT TO GET FIRST FIGHT TICKET, read a broadly distributed headline. "The first ticket for the fight between Jim Jeffries and Jack Johnson at San Francisco on July 4 will be presented to Theodore Roosevelt on his arrival to New York...The ticket will be made of solid gold."

The lead-up to the Johnson–Jeffries fight coincided with the countdown for Roosevelt's return from abroad. The public support for Roosevelt (evidenced through newspaper stories, letters to the editor, and speeches) while he traveled was varied and voracious and almost universally adoring. Even before he set foot back on American soil, calls came for Roosevelt to take over leadership of the New York state Republican Party, to run for Speaker of the House, and to have his own "Roosevelt Day" and a special "Loving Cup" gift (signed by the governors of every US state) presented to him upon his return.

Public interest in Roosevelt's impression of Taft grew as well. What was ROOSEVELT'S VERDICT ON TAFT, the *Washington Post* postulated just days before TR arrived in New York City. "It is expected that soon after his return Col. Roosevelt, as he prefers to be called, will let loose his pent-up view on American politics with old-time vigor and frankness..." Newspapermen stoked the idea—far-fetched as it was—that Roosevelt might arrive home and promptly start a new political movement. Or he might lead a radical new third party or he might simply reclaim what was rightfully his anyhow: the Republican Party.

Roosevelt arrived home in style. Escorted by a battleship, several torpedo boat destroyers, and a fleet of personal watercraft that came along for the ride, Roosevelt's ship made its way into New York City's harbor on June 18, 1910. The *New York Times* estimated that a million Americans jammed the Big Apple port to welcome him home. Political friends and Rough Riders forced their way onto the docked ship to greet their returning leader. Roosevelt was paraded toward downtown. "He passed through five miles of cheering crowds to the centre of the city," the *New York Times* reported, "amid thousands of his fellow-citizens, whose welcome showed him that they were as happy over his homecoming as he was himself." Curiously, and perhaps somewhat disingenuously, Roosevelt reported to the press mob covering his arrival day that he sought privacy more than anything else. The press saw through the request. Surely Roosevelt had not changed that much.

Roosevelt shook countless hands and made a few speeches before making his way to the family's retreat at Sagamore Hill. There Roosevelt went to work carrying out his duties for the *Outlook*. He used the magazine, a weekly produced in New York City, to thank his loyalists. "I am very glad to be back once more in the *Outlook* office, and from time to time hereafter I shall have certain things to say to the readers of *The Outlook*," TR announced matter-of-factly. The relationship was indeed simple. Roosevelt wrote for a salary. The *Outlook* enjoyed having one of the most popular Americans (and a prodigious author to boot) writing under its masthead. Roosevelt secured a voice for his bubbling-up ideas. It would be through the *Outlook* that Roosevelt would make his thoughts known on Jack Johnson and in doing so begin the lead-up to his eventual 1912 run for the presidency.

The same day Roosevelt's reintroduction appeared, Rex Beach, a novelist tasked by the *Atlanta Constitution* with covering the Johnson–Jeffries fight, weaved together the return of Roosevelt with the impending fight. The two seemingly disparate events had common roots. Why were Americans so interested in Jeffries and Johnson, Beach asked? Yes, there was a fight—a big fight— but big contests had come before. Subsequent "fights of the century" would proliferate for the long duration of the twentieth century. Of course the racial complexion mattered. But Beach settled on a more philosophical explanation for the fervor surrounding the Johnson–Jeffries fight. "We are hero worshippers, every mother's son of us; personal superiority is our fetish," Beach wrote. And thus Roosevelt's connection: "Only yesterday we offered such a welcome as the world has never known to a fighter. No Roman emperor," Beach explained, did "ever review such a pageant of honor as Theodore Roosevelt."

In this article about the fight, Beach focused largely on Roosevelt: "An armada met him at the threshold of his land, uncounted thousands line his route of march and rent of the skies with such a crashing uproar that the jealous heavens opened wide and let loose their warring elements to drown it." There were satire and hyperbole here to be sure (it appeared under a REX BEACH GIVES VIEWS ON FORTHCOMING BATTLE FOR THE CONSTITUTION headline), but the juxtaposition of Roosevelt's arrival home and the American public's interest in a boxing match should not be missed. "People will say that the Roosevelt demonstration was planned to celebrate his conquests..." Beach wrote, "but for every high-domed bespeckled citizen who looked upon the central figure of that pageant as a president, there were ten hoarse-voiced, big-lunged, sore-footed human beings who perched upon curb and window ledge to welcome Teddy as a man."

Such a reception would not have happened for many others, not for John D. Rockefeller nor William Howard Taft, Beach argued. "No. It was Roosevelt we admired. It was Teddy, the real, vital red-blooded, fighting human being whom we welcomed. The Anglo-Saxon loves a fighter, and we know that our most prominent citizen was one of that sort."

* * *

The "Fight of the Century" pitting black champion Jack Johnson versus the "Great White Hope" Jim Jeffries took place, finally, in Reno, Nevada, on July 4, 1910. The venue for the fight had switched from San Francisco to—ultimately—Reno when controversy arose over ties to gamblers in the Golden State. The boxers agreed to a forty-five-round contest. As the combatants made various side bets, rumors swirled that one of the fighters would take a fall. With these loose standards and with such obvious gambling taking place, Roosevelt did not attend. He did not use his golden ticket. Again. This was not his type of boxing. The *Washington Post* reported that Roosevelt, "one of the greatest exponents of civic righteousness in the world," wanted to go to the fight but had been unable to alter his busy post-presidency schedule. Doubtful.

Roosevelt, it seemed, was the only one who did not want a ticket. Three hundred reporters descended upon Reno for the fight—coming from all parts of the United States and abroad. Almost every conceivable rentable space in Reno—"hotel rooms, Pullman cars, cots, billiard tables, hammocks, or park benches," according to boxing historian Randy Roberts—was occupied the night before the contest. Workers pounded boards into place in the hastily erected bleachers until minutes before the fight. Filmmakers—and this would be important—positioned their cameras around the makeshift, outdoor arena. At 1:30 p.m., with the temperature well over one hundred degrees, twenty thousand spectators flooded into the facility rabid for a brawling spectacle.

"Hardly had a blow been struck when I knew that I was Jeff's master," Johnson said after the fact. Johnson came out talking. "Come on now, Mr. Jeff. Let me see what you got. Do something, man." That Johnson could do the joke and jab tells you something about the competitiveness of the fight. Using his superior speed and strength, Johnson warded off Jeffries's punches. Johnson countered with devastating shots of his own to Jeffries's ribs and head.

Through four rounds, things held somewhat even; Jeffries even managed to draw first blood with a shot to Johnson's jaw. During rounds five through eight, though, Johnson took control. Jeffries could see openings, but he wasn't nearly quick enough to exploit them. He could sense one of Johnson's uppercuts on the way, but he couldn't bob in time. He was stuck in old-age quicksand. "My muscles wouldn't respond as quickly to the dictates of the brain," he explained.

In the fourteenth round, Johnson broke Jeffries's nose. In the fifteenth, four Johnson shots in a row put Jeffries on the canvas. It was the first time in his career that Jeffries had been knocked down in a professional fight. After a nine count, Jeffries arose. Then Johnson moved in for the kill. A flurry of blows to the head took the last of Jeffries's strength. He fell again. Jeffries's seconds stepped through the ropes and into the ring, stopping the fight for good.

For Johnson, the Jeffries fight proved his legitimacy: "The 'white hope' had failed, and as far as the championship was concerned it was just where it was before the beginning of the fight, except that I had established my rightful claim to it beyond all possible dispute." While always controversial in African American communities because of his proclivity for vice, Johnson also personified redemption. The *Chicago Defender* put it simply: Jack Johnson was "the first negro to be admitted the best man in the world."

*   *   *

The fight was sensational; the fact that the whole thing was caught on film was a technological marvel. The footage is grainy and jumpy, but irrefutable, too. While Americans might have read about a close fight in their newspapers, with racially biased reporters propping Jeffries up, there was no denying the lopsided nature of the contest to those who watched it. Johnson was fluid and powerful; Jeffries was crouched and tentative. Johnson sent Jeffries sprawling through the ropes in the final round. The film oozed with physical domination. And these "fight pictures" made Johnson, according to one film historian, "in essence, the first black movie star."

This was too much, too dangerous for white America. Many wanted to know, *Where had the Strenuous Life gone wrong?*

Johnson's victory provided a political opening for Roosevelt. Roosevelt had always commented on the manner in which athletics *should* operate in the United States. Now, just back from what seemed like a lifetime away, Roosevelt found his voice again. "I sincerely trust that public sentiment will be so aroused, and will make itself felt so effectively, as to guarantee that this is the last prize fight to take place in the United States," Roosevelt editorialized. ROOSEVELT HOPES RENO KILLED PRIZE FIGHTING blared the *Atlanta Constitution* headline less than two weeks after the fight.

Before all of prize fighting could be challenged, however, there was the film that needed burying. Three days after the fight, newspapers began listing the localities that had banned the Jeffries–Johnson film from their theaters.* The list grew by the day. The places outlawing the film included: Kentucky, Maryland, the District of Columbia, Indianapolis, Atlanta, Minneapolis, Little Rock, Nashville, Charlotte, New Orleans, and Birmingham. Chicago was nearly there; a crusade led by the Women's Christian Temperance Union was organizing, reported one newspaper looking to broaden the movement beyond the South. There was even an international component: OPPOSITION TO [the fight] PICTURES IN ENGLAND, AUSTRALASIA, AFRICA, AND INDIA, the *New York Tribune* headlined.

In the midst of this posturing—racially biased, athletic moralizing by mayors, governors, and foreign dignitaries—Roosevelt took control. This was his turf, after all. On July 16, Roosevelt's editorial in *Outlook* was simply titled "The Recent Prize Fight." It was a short piece, just one page of magazine copy.

---

* The white fighter was almost always listed first during these discussions.

But in less than one thousand words, Roosevelt reclaimed the scepter as the leader of athletic culture in the United States, and he gave America a refresher on his résumé. Roosevelt cited his positions as assistant secretary of the Navy, police commissioner of New York City, governor of New York State, and president of the United States. In each of these roles, Roosevelt carefully explained, he had supported boxing. "I have always been fond of boxing, and have always believed in it as a vigorous manly pastime," Roosevelt declared.

But the goodness of fighting in any sort of public arena was now gone. "The betting and gambling upon the result," Roosevelt scolded—failing to mention that gambling had nearly always been part of the prizefighting world—"are thoroughly unhealthy, and the moving picture part of the proceedings has introduced a new method of money-getting and of demoralization."

Then Roosevelt gave ammunition to the segment of the American populace who despised Jack Johnson simply for his race. The Jeffries–Johnson fight had "provoked a very unfortunate display of race antagonism," Roosevelt wrote. Such a conflict undercut athletics altogether. The former president ended with two directives, (1) make the Johnson–Jeffries fight "the last prize fight to take place in the United States," and (2) find a method to "stop the exhibition of moving pictures taken thereof."

Neither proved entirely actionable. As Roosevelt would realize, being an ex-president was a bit like being a vice president. Mostly show; little direct power. Sure, people listened and, sure, the press still reported, but the power to actually enact change came in fits and starts. Still, all was not lost. Although Roosevelt's quick foray into the Jeffries–Johnson fight failed to produce any actual change, it did make one thing abundantly clear: Roosevelt's voice still reverberated loudest when it came to athletics in the United States.

TWELVE

ONE LAST RACE

It has always seemed to me that in life there are two ways of achieving
success, or, for the matter of that, of achieving what is commonly called
greatness. One is to do that which can only be done by the man of exception
and extraordinary abilities. Of course this means that only one man can
do it, and it is a very rare kind of success or of greatness...But most of us
can do the ordinary things, which, however, most of us do not do.

—THEODORE ROOSEVELT

Nineteen seventeen. "I feel like a goose being here," Roosevelt wrote to
Quentin. "Here" was Jack Cooper's Health Farm in Stamford, Connecticut, a place dedicated to restorative health practices and intense
physical training—for those who could pay for such services. Roosevelt arrived
on October 8, 1917. And with him to this bucolic farm (which specialized in
"profuse sweating"), TR brought a series of lingering losses.

He had lost the three-sided presidential election of 1912, nearly lost his life
in the Amazon to malaria, lost the chance to serve in World War I, and lost (or
at least married off; they did not come home for Christmas anymore) sons
Ted, Kermit, and Archie, and daughter Ethel. All of these defeats had occurred
since he had left the White House in 1909. But there was one thing that Roosevelt simply could not lose: the stubborn extra weight (although the malaria

had "helped" thin TR considerably for a short time after his return), especially around his midsection, that had been steadily accumulating over the decades. Roosevelt was thirty-five pounds overweight, obese by today's standards, as he turned himself over to Jack Cooper.

To a certain extent, it really only mattered where Theodore was *not* at this time. Roosevelt's four sons (the aforementioned three plus Quentin) were off to Europe's Great War. Even Ethel was headed for France as a Red Cross nurse. Their "great adventure," as Roosevelt naively and jealously called World War I, had begun.

On April 6, 1917, the United States had declared war on Germany, joining Europe's cataclysmic conflict. Four days later Roosevelt was in Washington intent on convincing President Wilson of his usefulness for the war effort. He knew it was a long shot, but he couldn't help himself. "I doubt whether the President will let me go; and surely he will try his best to cause me to fail if he does let me go," Roosevelt wrote to his sister. The pitch that Roosevelt could make, though, was an appealingly simple one: drafting and training an army would take a long time, so let a volunteer army take up the cause immediately. This volunteer force, of course, needn't follow such strict guidelines on age or physical fitness. The immediate message that America was coming could be put into action much sooner.

Wilson was no pushover; he knew what he was dealing with in Roosevelt. Having been forced into a war that he desperately tried to avoid, the president chided Roosevelt that the "Charge of the Light Brigade" days were over. There would be no San Juan Hill to take. Instead, it would be miles and miles of trenches, filled with gases and chemicals, bombarded for weeks at a time by unrelenting artillery fire. Still, Roosevelt pushed back. The values of courage and patriotism had not changed much at all, he countered.

Wilson gave Roosevelt forty-five minutes to make his pitch, then scooted him out the door. Woodrow Wilson was not about to send his political rival, an out of shape near-sixty-year-old at that, to Europe to fight for the United States. While not impervious to Roosevelt's infectious energy, Wilson did not seriously consider giving Roosevelt a position in the rapidly expanding military. Old men need not apply for these positions. Similarly, Secretary of War Newton Baker had no use for the Roosevelt-led Rough Riders. Baker wrote to Roosevelt, apologetically but firmly, that he could not possibly send the former president off to Europe. Baker tried to let Roosevelt down easily. This was to be "the bloodiest war yet fought in the world," and Baker did not intend to send any Americans into it without proper training. Furthermore, Baker did not see a place for ceremonial officers. Baker planned to send leaders "who had devoted their lives exclusively to the study and pursuit of military matters."

In Roosevelt's eyes, the Great War represented life-culminating opportunity: to command his own sons in a modernized version (although there would still be horses involved) of the Rough Riders. There was a mixture of courage, paternalism, bloodthirstiness, and delusion at work here. "If I had been given a free hand," Roosevelt seethed in a letter to Kermit, sent from Cooper's, "I would have guaranteed to have had 100,000 men in the trenches by September." Instead, Roosevelt found himself in the hands of Jack Cooper.

Even after Wilson's no, Roosevelt tried to gather support for his Rough Riders redux. Jules Jusserand offered his blessing ("Jusserand asked specifically that I be sent") and suggested that TR be sent to the lines in France immediately. LET ROOSEVELT GO, urged newspaper editorials. The ex-governor of Indiana, Samuel Ralston, sent Wilson a telegram quoting the Bible: "Isaiah said, 'Here I am; send me,' Ex-President Roosevelt is saying the same thing." Songwriters quickly scribbled down ditties supporting their former president as warrior. John L. Sullivan, a bit punchy but still a voice, offered to hold a rally to get the word out that the Rough Riders should be riding again.

None of this support mattered. *Your day has passed* was the general sentiment from Washington. The charges against Roosevelt were simple: too old and too inexperienced. Roosevelt hated Wilson for keeping him from the fight. To Fanny Parsons (a family friend), he wrote: "I shall not be allowed to go to France...neither the French nor the English can afford to antagonize the utterly selfish, treacherous, and vindictive man." Trying further to explain Wilson's decision, Roosevelt felt compelled to slander the president as a "physically timid" man.

* * *

Aging closes off opportunities for everyone. Coping with the reality of being slower, softer, weaker, and of lesser hearing and sight is an acquired skill. Roosevelt was still working on it. He mostly preferred to ignore the aging issue altogether. By 1917, though, even Roosevelt had to admit that his strength was waning. "The machine was skidding a bit," Roosevelt admitted to a reporter. "The driving gears were slipping a little." Edith, with serious health problems of her own (she had suffered through miscarriages in 1902 and 1903), gently but constantly prodded Roosevelt to do something about his weight. For most of their marriage Edith had indulged Roosevelt's overeating, but she felt she could allow it no more. The trip to Cooper's was a long overdue and last-ditch effort.

The physical decline was evident to even the most casual observer by this point. The former president arrived at Cooper's looking puffy and strained. His mustache had thinned and grayed. Fleshy cheeks and a jowly neck stretched his collar. The shortly cropped hair was making a controlled retreat. Behind the glasses, always the spectacles with TR, the creases had become thickly set, permanent markers of a lifetime of winking and smiling. Dark circles ran under the gleaming, still sparkling (although one looked a bit cloudy) eyes.

If he couldn't be in the trenches of Europe, Stamford in October wasn't entirely unpleasant. A "clean, healthy, and sanitary" hamlet of 40,000 residents, Stamford sat on the New England side of the Long Island Sound, fifty miles north of New York City. October's briskness had arrived. The woods surrounding Cooper's Health Farm shouted out bright reds and oranges.

Once on the grounds at the Health Farm, Roosevelt commanded the situation. "I came here for a general overhauling, Jack...Go to the limit—and I'll like it."

Then the men got down to the root of the problem. Roosevelt could not control, or exercise his way out of, his appetite. "Jack," Roosevelt confessed right at the start, "I have an abnormal appetite, and it is always on the job." Roosevelt was worried that he was at an impasse. Perhaps, back deep in his mind, too, was Dudley Sargent's diagnosis all those years ago. "How are you going to reduce my weight except at the expense of injury to my vital organs?" Roosevelt asked.

"Oh that will be simple enough," Cooper replied. "I'm going to allow you to eat your head off, if you want...But I will ask you to do a special turn for me."

"Ah, ha!" Roosevelt responded. "I thought there would be a twist to that. But I'm game. What is it?"

"Take a five-mile walk every morning before breakfast to burn up the excess fuel you have taken on the day before."

"Oh! That's easy! I was afraid you were going to ask me to do something strenuous," Roosevelt said, dismissing Cooper's simple plan with a reference to his own marquee line.

It was anything but easy though. Over the days that followed, Roosevelt went to boot camp. One would wish, for his sake, that he'd had modern day athletic conveniences such as Gatorade, spandex undershorts, and talcum powder. He did not; he worked himself raw. Perhaps it was the only way to assuage the gaping hole Roosevelt felt at the world leaving him behind.

* * *

Roosevelt was too young to retire to a life of chopping wood and taking Edith out for boat excursions at Sagamore Hill. But what was a former president of the United States to do? The Jimmy Carter model of ex-presidential global service had not yet been unveiled. Roosevelt joked that his only utility as a former US president in Africa was to "scare rhinos away." Roosevelt's immediate predecessor, obviously, never had the chance to consider a post-presidency. Indeed of the five presidents that came before Roosevelt, James Garfield (assassinated), Chester Arthur, Grover Cleveland, Benjamin Harrison, and William McKinley (assassinated), only Cleveland made headlines after leaving office. And he did so by winning a second, nonconsecutive term as president. Although it took a while before he admitted it, Roosevelt liked the Cleveland approach.

Just to be clear: a lot happened (Africa, New Nationalism, the Bull Moose run of 1912, the River of Doubt, World War I, etc.) between the time Theodore Roosevelt left the White House in the midst of a blizzard in March 1909 and the cool October 1917 day he showed up at Jack Cooper's in New England. Important things. Personal things. International things. Political things. Things that scholars have devoted whole books to analyzing. We know this.

Here's the flyover version.

Arriving back home in the United States (just before the Fight of the Century), Roosevelt decided to do what he had always done: write. From his public, intellectual perch at *Outlook* beginning in 1910, Roosevelt gradually set about undermining the presidency of William H. Taft. Slowly but surely. Roosevelt became convinced that Taft, loveable as he was, had little interest in carrying on the increasingly progressive agenda that Roosevelt thought he had handed off.

Serious political fissures emerged but so too did simple differences in persona. Almost immediately upon taking occupation of the White House, Taft had Roosevelt's prized tennis court bulldozed under. Strangely Roosevelt learned of this change while sitting at Taft's desk in the White House, during a spontaneous visit to the White House in 1910 when Taft happened to be traveling. Roosevelt took it well. "He inspected all the changes and expressed great admiration. He sat down at the President's desk and said how natural it seemed to be there. He looked at the new tennis court and said he thought the change was a good one," Archibald Butt (who worked as a military aide to both Roosevelt and Taft) reported. And as if anticipating the critique that might be coming, Butt added: "There was no jealousy, no carping, no envy." One has to wonder. The tennis court space did not go to waste; the Oval Office was erected on the space previously occupied by Roosevelt's tennis court.

Taft did not box or wrestle. He did not scramble through Rock Creek Park. There were no visits from fighting masters. As Alice pointed out with her typical candor and bite, "President Taft weighed too much to indulge in the vigorous activity of his predecessor. His only form of exercise was golf." You didn't want to mess with Alice. Taft became "the President who golfed too much." And he did his golfing as one might expect a three-hundred pound, morbidly obese man to do. He strolled leisurely through the green fairways of Chevy

Chase Country Club. He sweated profusely in Washington's blanketing humidity. He rarely broke one hundred and even scored a twenty-seven on one hole.

When not relaxing on the golf course, Taft went to baseball games. The contrast here is too simple to take very seriously but too tempting to ignore. While TR charged onto Franklin Field at the Army–Navy football game in 1901, Taft sat comfortably in the stands of Washington's Senators for the opening game of the 1910 season. Deciding that he need not even leave his presidential box at Nationals' Stadium to establish a new tradition, Taft declared the Major League Baseball season open with a gentle toss from the stands to Walter Johnson. Later Taft autographed the ball for Johnson, and here too the tone was less than aggressive: "For Walter Johnson, with the hope that he may continue to be as formidable as yesterday...William H. Taft."

Roosevelt, despite his promise to Henry Cabot Lodge ("When I am through with anything I am thru with it, and am under no temptation to snatch at the fringes of departing glory. When I stop being President I will stop completely."), never really stopped seeing himself as a political candidate. Roosevelt assumed that "because it was I who made him President," he could supplant Taft if need be.

TR began laying the groundwork almost immediately. In 1910, shortly after returning from Europe, TR embarked upon a 5,500-mile nationwide speaking circuit. In 1911, there was another ambitious speaking tour, this time taking the ex-president through the US South and then out west. Tellingly Roosevelt refused to endorse Taft when cornered by press covering the trip. By January 1912, the scale had tipped. Roosevelt stopped trying to talk himself out of running. On February 24, Roosevelt declared, due to the increasing calls for his candidacy, "I will accept the nomination for President if it is tendered to me." He almost had no choice.

Large swathes of the electorate had soured on Taft, but the machine politics of the era so protected incumbency that as popular as Roosevelt was, he had almost no chance to secure the Republican Party nomination. While the details are worth considering, the system was, basically, rigged. Roosevelt challenged Taft just as the American electoral system was beginning to emphasize state primaries. In states that held primary contests, Roosevelt cleaned up. He won 270 delegates to Taft's 48 (Robert La Follette of Wisconsin secured 36). The popular vote favored Roosevelt during the contest for the Republican nomination, although by a closer margin: Roosevelt: 1,157,397; Taft: 761,716; and La Follette: 351,043.

But none of this mattered. The contest came down to the Republican convention, held in Chicago in 1912. Even with the system working against him, Roosevelt gave little thought to letting his party's convention decide the matter. "He was very nearly obsessed with power, more so in the period after he left the White House than during the years in office," wrote one biographer. When Taft secured the GOP nomination, Roosevelt became the nominee of the Progressive Party. This development insured two things: a rollicking 1912 general election and, almost certainly, the victory of Democrat Woodrow Wilson.

Unlike 1904, Roosevelt campaigned exhaustively in 1912. Even Taft begrudgingly admired the effort. "I look upon him," Taft wrote to Elihu Root, "as I look upon a freak almost in the zoological Garden, a kind of animal not often found." This was a compliment, one thinks.

The tale of the 1912, three-sided campaign veers nearly into unbelievable territory when one gets to the part about Roosevelt being shot and then insisting upon finishing his speech. The attack occurred in mid-October, just outside Milwaukee, Wisconsin. Roosevelt was caught doing what he always did: waving to an adoring crowd. As he waved, a shot rang out. A would-be assassin, less than thirty feet away, aimed for TR's chest. John F. Schrank, a bartender from New York, shot Roosevelt in defense of the United States' tradition of presidents serving only two terms—of all the inane reasons. The bullet tore through Roosevelt's jacket, then a thick speech manuscript, then through an iron glasses case Roosevelt carried in his breast pocket. Only then did it get to Roosevelt. Slowed significantly, the bullet lodged several inches deep in Roosevelt's chest. It broke his fourth rib.

Staggered by this "mule kick," as Roosevelt described the pain, Roosevelt sensed a political opportunity. The potential for drama and public courage was too much to resist. Only TR. "You get me to that speech," Roosevelt demanded of his entourage, rejecting the entirely sensible demands for a trip to a nearby hospital. "It may be the last I shall deliver, but I am going to deliver this one." It was a quintessential Roosevelt moment, an opportunity for over-the-top physical courage—with an audience on hand to appreciate it. Drama, with real conviction behind it, had long been a Roosevelt specialty. At the Milwaukee Auditorium once more several doctors tried to convince TR to head to the hospital. "I will make this speech, or die; one way or the other," came Roosevelt's reply.

Interestingly, by this point Roosevelt's vision for the moment seemed to extend to his handlers. "I have something to tell you," began the event's chairman solemnly, introducing Roosevelt. "Colonel Roosevelt has been shot. He is wounded." With this, the room exploded. How does one respond to news of an assassination...but wait, isn't that the former president right there? Roosevelt stepped to the dais. He held up a hand to quell the pandemonium. "Friends, I shall ask you to be as quiet as possible. I don't know whether you fully understand that I have just been shot," Roosevelt began, making sure the audience understood that he had been, you know, shot. He unbuttoned his jacket to reveal a bloody wound. "But it takes more than that to kill a Bull Moose." Calmly, Roosevelt withdrew his prepared, now punctured, remarks. "The bullet is in me now, so that I cannot make a very long speech." Roosevelt then spoke for more than an hour.

ATTEMPT MADE TO KILL ROOSEVELT, read the next day's headline. Roosevelt had been lucky. The bullet stayed shallow, deflected by the contents of Roosevelt's jacket. The specialists in Chicago quickly ascertained that the situation was serious but not life threatening. At this point, with another assassination seemingly avoided, the narrative surrounding the event began to swing in a different direction, one that Roosevelt undoubtedly appreciated: *Who could believe the physical condition of this fifty-three-year-old? What a man!* This became the substory. An emergency room attendant declared that Roosevelt was "one of the most powerful men I have ever seen laid on an operating table." The rhetoric only escalated from there. Roosevelt, claimed another MD, survived primarily due to his "magnificent physical condition" and "regular physical exercise." He was "a physical marvel."

Roosevelt ran hard in 1912, and he inspired "a deep and genuine religious fervor" from a sizable portion of the American electorate. It was an "election that changed the country." Roosevelt even took a bullet. It wasn't nearly enough. Splitting the Republican block of voters fatally, Roosevelt won a million more votes than Taft but a million less than Woodrow Wilson. The day after the election, Taft woke up early to go golfing.

*　　*　　*

Of course the workouts at Jack Cooper's started early during Roosevelt's 1917 stay. Don't workouts always start early? Didn't Rocky run up the steps of the Philadelphia Art Museum at dawn? The wake-up call for Roosevelt at Jack's Farm came at 5:45 each morning. With barely time for a cup of coffee, and no time for grooming, Roosevelt ("The Colonel" or "Colonel Roosevelt" as Cooper insisted on calling his most high-profile visitor) got moving. The surroundings were as pleasant as the tasks were continuous. "The first exercise of the day was the walk over the half mile 'track' around the Health Farm lake, which, aside from the benefit of the open air and the varying action given the muscles by the rugged, uneven nature of the path, the charm and beauty of the scenic environment made for a spiritual exhilaration which the bare walls of a stuffy gymnasium could never produce," *Physical Culture* reported. True, but this was just the warm-up. The warm up for the warm-up really. After "working up" to the necessary pace, the day began.

The question of how much could be accomplished, how many indulgences could be undone, in two weeks went unasked. As much as possible was the mantra. As much as possible. With the sun breaking through now, Roosevelt set out on his five-mile, pre-breakfast walk/jog. The pace started slow. Roosevelt's bound-up muscles were encouraged and coaxed at first. Outright confrontation came later. TR got rolling. The stroll led to a respectable walk. The moderate pace gave way to "a snappy gait" only when the former president felt ready. By mile three, the pace was brisk. Push. For the last section, Cooper wanted a bit more. "A quick-time jog" brought Roosevelt back around to the farmhouse.

At this point, when Roosevelt and most other Americans would pat them-selves on the back as having done more than enough exercise for one day, Coo-per considered his charge having caught up from the previous day. "Aside from 'burning up' the excess fuel taken into the body the day before," Cooper ex-plained to one of the nosy journalists anxious to hear about the former presi-dent's workouts that the "tramp over the hill and through the dale put the Colonel in an agreeable mood for an early introduction to the breakfast table."

Roosevelt got his well-earned breakfast. Then, after stripping off his heavy workout clothes, he rested for an hour or so. Next came the gymnasium. Coo-per had designed an exercise program just for Roosevelt. The selected exercises "considered his weight, his age, and his blood pressure, which upon his arrival was 'high.'" In a manner that would ring true to today's P90Xers and core en-thusiasts (it's always about "the core"), Cooper ordered six "abdominal exer-cises" to get things started. These were intended to "toughen up certain groups of muscles supporting the vital organs." Of particular concern were Roosevelt's heart, liver, and kidneys. The goal was direct. Get rid of the belly fat. Whether moving in this direction or lunging thusly, all the movements "were for the purpose of reducing the fatty tissues overlying the exterior muscles of the ab-dominal wall." *Lose the gut.*

Cooper was an inventor as much as a trainer. Particularly sadistic was an early version of his: "the Reducycle." It was as if an exercise bicycle and a sauna had a bastard child. The US Patent Office described it as "a sweat-cabinet and an exercising apparatus." From the outside, the Reducycle looked like an oak paneled Jack-in-the-Box, standing about four feet high. Inside the box, a make-shift exercise bike (with brake for resistance), a canister for hot water, and an electric heater operated in dangerously close proximity. The unlucky subject, in this case Roosevelt, would climb into the box and pedal away on the ma-chine with only his head protruding from the top of the contraption. The subject's shoulders and neck were draped with a leather canvas to hold in the heat. Using the propulsion of the pedals, the Reducycle created heat and steam in order to eliminate "wastes and poisons" and "body odors." Advertisements in the *Western Osteopath* claimed Cooper's Reducycle did wonders: "reduces high blood pressure, builds up and strengthens the vital forces of the body by bringing the hill climbing muscles into play, WITHOUT OVERTAXING THE WEAK HEART." Roosevelt could lose two pounds in a half hour on this cruel machine.

To break the monotony, the morning gym session also featured "playful" interludes. Roosevelt played handball. He engaged in "ball tossing" and "ball bouncing." He also worked the punching bag. "Profuse sweating" was the goal here, too, "in order to reduce the size of the 'bulk.'" After seventy-five minutes or so, Roosevelt was released into the hands of the "rubber." The rubber was what Roosevelt insisted on calling the Farm's masseuse.

After the gym work, Roosevelt discarded his drenched clothes and dried himself thoroughly. He did this drying in preparation for the "the electric light bath." This was, basically, vitamin D shock therapy. *Physical Culture* could not wait to give its readers all the details.

The 'light' bath is a marble lined box, studded with thirty-two candle-power incandescent electric lamps. The marble seat is just of a height to permit a man's head to project through the opening in the hinged top, the space about the neck being sealed with towels to retain the heat.

Once sealed around the patient's torso, the cooking began. The temperature started near body temperature, about 102 degrees Fahrenheit, a number reached by considering the heat Roosevelt brought to the box from his exercising session. Using the surrounding incandescent lights, the temperature inched steadily higher. Attendants placed "Cold packs" on Roosevelt's head. The thirty-minute session was a battle between hot and cold, sweating and hydrating. With the temperature approaching 120 degrees, Roosevelt downed glass after glass of cold water. The staff forced Roosevelt to consume a glass every two minutes, recognizing the peril they were putting his body under. Losing God-knows-how-much sweat, Roosevelt consumed about a gallon of water during the sweatbox session.

Cooper, who had no formal medical training, saw the light bath and Redu-cycle as especially important for Roosevelt. He described these practices as the "ideal internal bath" for the former president. It was a "cleanse" in the modern-day health and diet industry vernacular. The point was to flood the circulatory system and push out impurities through the pores of the skin. In terms of measurable progress, the practice also helped to lower blood pressure. But there were risks too. Cooper and his staff paid close attention to "not shocking the Colonel's nervous system." Not too much at least. So after leaving the box, Roosevelt was moved directly to a warm shower.

Cooper had won Roosevelt's respect, as most boxers typically had over the course of Roosevelt's adult life. During his time at the camp, the Colonel told nearly everyone that he wrote to that Cooper was "a retired welter weight skin glove fighter." But as impressive as this title was, was his ability to navigate the criminal element. Cooper had "an intimate knowledge of [boxing's] under-world" *and* "an impartially friendly attitude towards both [that underworld] and the upper world from which his sporting patrons came."

Cooper's long history as a boxer and trainer had taken a rather amazing turn. The prospect of a former fighting champ training the president of the United States would have seemed inconceivable thirty years prior. The fight game had changed. A faux-fighting business emerged out of the concerns of a softening society. The concept of a gentleman boxer was no longer an oxymo-ron. In fact, it was sort of the goal. Although certainly a criminal element ex-isted still in fight circles, respectability could be had. For Jack Cooper's part, this meant trading in his fight gym in New York City for the bucolic Health Farm in Connecticut. Where he had previously trained Jim Jeffries for his fight against Jack Johnson, Cooper now took on overweight socialites. Those who could pay had access to a champion, a champion who promised to challenge but not break them.

Awkwardness pervaded almost every part of this process. Standing in the shower, Roosevelt "was given a thorough scrubbing down with pure soap." The water temperature was reduced gradually until it reached between forty and forty-five degrees. Finally the water treatment ended. A rubdown followed.

But then, wait, more water. "A stream of water from a hose at an eight-pound pressure at the nozzle was placed on the base of his spine for fifteen seconds." With Roosevelt stunned, the jet stream next went "up and down the spine." Then up and down each leg, front and back. "This left the body in a healthy pink glow, which gradually changed to a deeper red, followed by another profuse sweat." This treatment was followed by another dry-off and rubdown. Hopefully Cooper's Health Farm had fluffy towels.

The world that Roosevelt was sweating through with Jack Cooper, on the outskirts of Stamford, harnessed the power of isolation. But it was also very much a part of a bigger movement. The idea of getting away in order to "cure" oneself of modernity, basically, had become big business. The target was the nonacute pain of American life: fatigue, weight gain, loss of libido, hair thinning, bloatedness, dizziness. The list went on and on. So too did the list of facilities that sprung up across the United States. Strangely a case could be made for each of the American climate zones having special restorative powers. The Florida Nature Home and Recreation Resort, in Tangerine (really), Florida, boasted that it was a "climatic institute of the first order" and that it utilized "all drugless methods." It offered "sun and air baths," the latter of which was basically selling air for those desperate enough to purchase it. On the very same classifieds page in a 1917 issue of *Physical Culture* (the *Men's Health* of its day), the Theodore Caldwell Health Home of Pasadena, California, promised a "magnificent situation near the mountains" and "above the sea fog." The facility offered its most popular health camp during grape season, providing something that Tangerine could not match.

The resorts revealed a desperation for health among the American populace, but in a genteel and orderly way. The side effects of city life and less physical work were creating physical and mental deterioration. The "recreation resorts" and "health farms" and "physical culture health homes" and "natural life resorts"—there were countless derivations of the Come-Here-And-Get-Healthy brand—also demonstrated the morphing of sports in the United States. Experts and facilities were becoming increasingly important. Jack Cooper went by a purposeful title: Professor Jack Cooper. This "professor," a former prizefighter and brawler, operated in a middle ground between violence and respectability. He had to be both.

Jack Cooper's Health Farm owed some debt of gratitude to one of the strangest health advocates in American history: Bernarr Macfadden. The name is as good a place as any to start. Born Bernard McFadden, Bernarr changed his name because he wanted his given name to sound more like the roar of a lion and his surname to be more masculine. Seriously. Macfadden—like Roosevelt (and Sargent, Gulick, and Coubertin)—had grown up weak and sickly. And then, as he recounted hundreds of times during his lifetime as a promoter of physical culture, he found health through a dedicated fitness program. Macfadden started the magazine *Physical Culture* in 1899. It was a reporter from this magazine who showed up to interview Jack Cooper and Theodore Roosevelt shortly after their time together in the fall of 1917. *Physical Culture* wanted all the details on the techniques used by Cooper on Roosevelt. No other news outlet really cared.

Bernarr became the first fitness celebrity in America. He amassed a fortune of nearly $30 million by selling literature, inventions, and experiences related to fitness. He was fabulously quirky and outspoken. It was as if, in a modern sense, Kim Kardashian, Lance Armstrong, and Jimmy Swaggart were combined in one very toned, very tanned body—one with an exceptionally coiffed head of hair. *Time Magazine* nicknamed him "Body Love Macfadden." Macfadden seems to have been equal parts innovative and far ahead of his time, and just plain crazy. He espoused drinking as much milk as possible, completely avoiding bread ("the staff of death" he called it—and we think the paleo diets of today are tough!), abstaining from medicines and drugs, and sleeping on hard floors. He detested prudishness, and his magazines faced obscenity charges. Oh, and he refused to wear hats because he believed it would damage his hair.

When he wasn't putting himself on the cover of *Physical Culture,* or any of the other dozens of publications that his company produced, Macfadden tried to start a "Physical Culture City" (in New Jersey of all places) and even a religion emphasizing health. "Cosmotarianism," which was based on Macfadden's teachings, did not take, despite its promise that converts might well live to 150 years of age. Macfadden was not a man of half measures. He married four times and had eight children: Byrne, Byrnece, Beulah, Beverly, Brewster, Berwyn, and Braunda. And Helen.

While there is fascinating craziness to Macfadden, he led the wave of establishing health retreats like the one Roosevelt found himself a part of in 1917. Throughout Roosevelt's lifetime, and well beyond, Bernarr was roaring about physical fitness and health in his own clanging manner. He urged Americans to fight back against their weakness and fatigue. Every revolution needs its wild man; Bernarr was one for the athletic upheaval that occurred during these first decades of the twentieth century.

*   *   *

Finally lunch. After a morning of straining, Roosevelt ate as much as he wanted; he'd earned his calories. Always sociable, the ex-president of the United States lingered at the table chatting with the staff and Cooper for nearly an hour. Then he was given a "period of undisturbed relaxation." Time for a nap.

The sheer all-dayness of the endeavor was part of its effectiveness. After resting for a time, the "gymnasium clothes" went back on. A three-mile walk through the grounds and around the lake reengaged muscles that must have assumed the day's work had ended. From the trails, Roosevelt reentered the gym, that torture chamber. The trainers again focused on "the toughening up of the abdominal muscles." Roosevelt lunged, contorted, and contracted. There were muscles buried in there somewhere. Next, Roosevelt shadowboxed, returning to his favorite sport in a safe, noncontact fashion. Cooper favored some strange exercises too. He made sure that Roosevelt had a daily dose of "kicking the medicine ball" back and forth across the building. Here was the former president of the United States, undoubtedly fatigued and probably still pink from his morning pounding, kicking a heavy ball here and there. Cooper also required that Roosevelt have "a go at the double bouncing ball."

Demonstrating remarkable foresight, Jack Cooper crafted a physical training plan for Roosevelt focused on strengthening heart and lungs. The diagnosis was adept, even if the method of treatment left something to be desired. "Special breathing exercises" were meant to stimulate the lazy parts of the lungs and diaphragm. "The breath must be drawn down into the lowest part of the lungs," read one breathing directive. "This requires the expansion of the stomach region." Cooper pushed Roosevelt deep into oxygen debt. Deep breathing was clean breathing: "The act of breathing diaphragmatically, which is the only proper way of breathing is therefore, apart from its functions in insuring for the lungs the fullest intake of oxygen and the most complete elimination of carbonic acid gas, an important and vital process." A deep breath workout, far from only a byproduct of aerobic exercise, was a focus. "A part of your health-building regime must be deep breathing," explained *Physical Culture*.

Then back to the showers. Again the uncomfortableness was ratcheted up gradually. Lukewarm gave way to cold, then freezing. From the shower, Roosevelt made his way to "the slab," a cold, hard massage table. The rubber got back to his task. Using oil this time, the masseuse thoroughly treated Roosevelt's tired muscles. He dug deep, rubbing and probing. The battle against lactic acid buildup was desperate at this point. Muscle stiffening could inhibit the next steps in the process.

Amazingly at this point, at 4:45 p.m. as the sun began its retreat at the end of a shortening October day, Roosevelt was sent back to his room for a few hours of work—to catch up on his correspondence. Somehow Roosevelt still had the energy to pick up his pen. Long day, lots of exercise, late afternoon... Yawwnn. But here Roosevelt demonstrated his legendary correspondence powers. While the vast majority of Roosevelt's 150,000 lifetime letters had already been written and delivered, Roosevelt always had more to write. Roosevelt responded to urgent requests and alerted his family to his survival. The letters, compared to Roosevelt's usually effusive epistles, are a bit tired.

Having walked, run, chased balls, punched, sat through a sweatbox session, and taken two showers, TR wrote his sons. "Dearest Archie," he began, as usual, on October 14, 1917. "I have come down here for a fortnight to see if I could get into somewhat better condition." Roosevelt evidenced none of his usual enthusiasm. "I lead a life of welcome monotony, and exercises bore until I feel as if I should scream," Roosevelt wrote, talking about the Cooper's experience, one hopes. "I am losing weight a little."

Roosevelt blamed Edith for his trip to Cooper's Health Farm. At least to his boys. To Quentin: "I have come up here for two weeks at mother's urging to see if I can't get off a little weight, which I will do, and also get a rest, which I won't, and which I don't need anyhow." So there. To Kermit, he peddled the same story: "I am here for a fortnight to endeavor to lose ten or fifteen pounds, which I shall do." Then the blame. "Darling Mother thinks it will 'rest' me, which it won't." Then Roosevelt launched into his direct and at least a bit reckless criticism of Woodrow Wilson. "The trouble with the Administration, or rather Wilson, is that winning the war is entirely subordinated to questions of personnel and men of private malice."

Roosevelt reported for a "family style" dinner with Cooper and the Farm staff at 7:00 p.m. Not surprisingly, Cooper reported that Roosevelt's "magnetic personality and irrepressible spirits" charmed the entire group. By the end of the day, Roosevelt had to have been exhausted. The post-White House years had been fatiguing.

Following dinner Roosevelt donned his "workout" clothes one last time. These clothes, incidentally, lacked the qualities usually held to be important when selecting exercise gear. There was no elasticity, no breathability, and certainly no wicking away of sweat. Roosevelt preferred to dress as some sort of cross between a military man and a spur-of-the-moment hiker. His usual attire: "Khaki Knickerbockers, an olive-drab army shirt, reddish-brown woolen stockings, and tan army shoes."

The last workout of the day commenced at 9:00 p.m. With the sun having set, Roosevelt was taken to the nearby highway for a three-mile jaunt. Again a gradual workup to speed occurred. Food had to be digested; tired muscles and tendons had to be reengaged diplomatically. So, the ex-president of the United States, usually accompanied by Cooper himself for this workout, walked down a road in rural Connecticut in the darkness. Once a good lather had been worked up, the pace quickened. Although speed was not the goal here, just movement forward—survival really. A "snappy half walk, half run" wrapped up the workout.

Basically, Jack Cooper believed in sweating the weight off his clients. Make a client sweat, then cooldown, then take a massage. Repeat this process as many times as possible in a given day. The final push back to the Farm ensured Roosevelt of more "profuse perspiration." The staff again rushed in to help the Colonel with the cooldown. "He was stripped, carefully rubbed dry and again given a thorough massage." The last step was meant to "prevent soreness and stiffening of the muscles," although it is difficult to imagine that this could be avoided.

*   *   *

Roosevelt's two weeks at Jack Cooper's ended with a race. The entrants in this race included Roosevelt (who actually knew that it was a race), the mayor of New York City, a former boxing champion, a trainer, several curious newspapermen, and one little girl and one little boy.

Kept at bay to this point ("He's very spry and responds quickly to treatment... Next week he'll be ready to see you," Cooper had announced), the press finally gained access to Jack Cooper's facility on October 21, 1917. "Reporters flocked to Stamford (even from Philadelphia and Boston)," the *St. Louis Post-Dispatch* reported, "and camera men by the dozen and a couple of movie operators and probably a hundred miscellaneous persons from the town motored out to the health farm." Rural Connecticut had never seen so much action.

Roosevelt greeted the assemblage wearing his workout gear for the day—faded "gray-green" knickers, "gray-gold" stockings, simple shoes, and a brown flannel shirt.

The press fell right back into their old TR-as-Super-Active writing habits. The *New York Times* covered the story on the front page. REDUCED IN WEIGHT AND GIRTH, came the special from Stamford. Roosevelt was at it again. Reporters got the stats first: Roosevelt weighed in at 202 pounds. His waist measured 42¾ inches. The "before" measurements (although there was room to debate these) had been 216 pounds and 46 inches, so some real progress had been made.

But why had the press come at all?

Yes, on a simple level ex-presidents stay in the public eye for the rest of their lives, but one still has to wonder what the press had to gain by showing up to watch Theodore Roosevelt run a lap around a pond. Such frivolousness stood in stark contrast to the times. The nation stood at the precipice of what seemed to be a generation-defining war. If there was a time that the nation's newspapers should have ignored an old ex-president, it was 1917. The nation's future lay in the hands of its fittest and strongest. Its draft-eligible. This was the time for new leaders. Roosevelt had been out of the White House for nearly a decade. And yet the press assembled at Cooper's Farm.

The reverential, almost fantastical tone of the reports that came from the reporters who watched Roosevelt at Cooper's evidenced that Roosevelt had taken up residence in America's psyche by this point.

Roosevelt had become synonymous with action and vigor. He meant doing something rather than complaining about, well, everything. Jack Cooper's was "quite the centre of the countryside yesterday," reported a New York paper. "In front of it were drawn up automobiles and taxicabs, and around the tree shrouded entrance was a group of people seeking to get a glimpse of the man who typifies so much that is vigorous and healthy in American life." Roosevelt had traveled to Cooper's to continue his assault against physical weakness—a struggle that he had been fighting since his father issued that challenge in his wood-paneled library four decades prior. It was Roosevelt's sheer ability to keep moving forward that Americans found so appealing. "Ain't he a wonder," whispered a Stamford police officer overseeing the scene.

Roosevelt radiated enthusiasm. About Jack Cooper (and Cooper's food and drink), he could not say enough: "Jack Cooper can put a man in the best condition for a boxing contest of any man I know...He can also build up clergymen and priests and ex-Presidents and less important folk. There's a bully table here and the best spring water I ever drank." Perhaps it was just that Roosevelt was always so ridiculously engaged in his own life. He was always present and trying.

Always engaging and interacting. "The Colonel's eyes gleamed as he fanned about the strenuous stuff," said one reporter. The sheer effort Roosevelt expended in connecting with those around him and with ideas from all directions created awe among his contemporaries. The onslaught of Strenuous-Roosevelt-reporting from early in his presidency captured the fascination of a nation. It seemed like a good idea to be present at all times, to be so engaged and positive, but man it looked tiring. Who could live that way? Just Roosevelt.

The attraction also had something to do with Roosevelt's vulnerability. Roosevelt had an open relationship with weakness. He did not retreat from physical ailments, but instead he talked about them. He loved a plan that might lead to some progress. He went to places like Cooper's to address his frailties. This doggedness appealed to even the most jaded of reporters. It was Roosevelt's struggle that appealed to a broad cross section of Americans. Especially when placed against the backdrop of all of Roosevelt's successes. Roosevelt had written all of his thirty-eight books by this point. He had served, obviously, as president. He had won the Nobel Peace Prize. He had enjoyed every conceivable plaudit. But here he was. "Fourteen pounds," the *St. Louis Post-Dispatch* reported, "each one an enemy bitterly battled against—succumbed to the Colonel's two weeks of tramping, shadow boxing and weight pulling...He's going home today or tomorrow in 'fine shape, by Jove, fine!'"

To a certain extent, America also enjoyed Roosevelt as a caricature of strenuousity. Who could really believe some of the stories about this president? Was someone actually living that life? "The Colonel is up here to reduce the mileage around his waistline," wrote Arthur "Bugs" Baer, one of New York's best-known humor columnists. "He is built like a safe. And the old boy is so brown that you couldn't tell him from an autumn leaf if it were not for his accent." Roosevelt was, basically, a superhero on a weight loss crusade. "Ted merely ran about a million miles, pulled weights for a few hours, juggled a few pianos, published some calisthenics, wrestled with his trainer, swam around Cooper Lake and tossed off a couple of speeches." It was lucky for Germany that Wilson refused to send Roosevelt. "Right now the Colonel is too healthy for one little war. They will have to build an annex war to accommodate him."

As much as anything, however, Roosevelt still mattered because he had the extraordinary ability to put into words the ordinary struggles inherent in human existence. As the *Boston Globe* explained it, Roosevelt was "the coiner of telling phrases which have become so much a part of the nation's vocabulary that few people remember their author." "The Strenuous Life," obviously. But also the "Square Deal" and the "Big Stick." Roosevelt could somehow articulate just how real and difficult life's challenges were. Then, from that place of acknowledgment, he could produce in one the desire to fight, not retreat. He would say, basically, *this is hard, and it should be hard, and we might not make it...but we will make it!* Roosevelt mixed his truth-telling with a splash of defiant optimism. To the New York *Sun,* Roosevelt's time at Cooper's was simply following his long-held pattern: exercise, feel better, and then talk about it. After time with "a real trainer of men" (Cooper in this case), "he comes back refreshed and tells people about it with a smile."

The Strenuous Life had gained a rhetorical partner in 1910 when Roosevelt delivered his "Citizen in a Republic" speech. Roosevelt had delivered this speech, often referred to as the "Man in the Arena," in Jusserand's France. While the speech offered lofty ideas about democracy and citizenship, it also offered an explanation for something like Roosevelt's visit to Jack Cooper's Health Farm. The Man in the Arena was an explanation of the value of doing something, anything, even if it looked strange and uncomfortable.

The speech, which today (more than a century later) is plastered on all manner of merchandise, used in Cadillac commercials, and tattooed on Miley Cyrus's forearm (yes this feels like a crime of some sort), gave the credit to those who struggled. To those who took risks. To those were not afraid to look ridiculous. Like a fifty-eight-year-old former president at a health farm in Connecticut. "It is not the critic who counts," Roosevelt said. "Not the man who points out how the strong man stumbles, or where the doer of deeds could have done them better."

Take heart, Roosevelt (again, working "as America's greatest 'phrase-maker'") told a world of beleaguered strivers. Take heart, he reminded himself, even as he slowed with old age, even as he "felt like a goose" sometimes.

The credit belongs to the man who is actually in the arena, whose face is marred by dust and sweat and blood, who strives valiantly; who errs, who comes short again and again, because there is no effort without error and shortcoming; but who does actually strive to do the deeds; who knows great enthusiasms, the great devotions, who spends himself in a worthy cause; who at the best knows in the end the triumph of high achievement, and who at worst, if he fails, at least he fails while daring greatly, so that his place shall never be with those cold and timid souls who neither know victory nor defeat.

* * *

The hangers-on turned out just to stand near the former president on that late-October media day in 1917. William Warren Barbour, a former boxer who Roosevelt had tried to convince to take on Jack Johnson, traveled from New York City to visit Roosevelt at Cooper's. Barbour's bio read similar to TR's: he had suffered from tuberculosis as a child; he cured himself through sports and exercise. The *New York Times* noted that a Mr. A. McAfee, "a copper dealer," and William Ziegler Jr., "the baking powder man," also arrived for the press scrum because, well, why shouldn't there be a copper dealer and baking powder man present? Mostly they came because they were friends of Roosevelt. "If I had been allowed to raise a division, Mr. McAfee would have held a commission under me, and Mr. Ziegler would have been with me," Roosevelt told the assembled reporters, still not letting go the prospect of traveling to Europe to fight.

The guest with the most at stake on media day at Cooper's Farm was New York City Mayor John Mitchel. Mitchel journeyed to Jack Cooper's while in the midst of a stiff reelection challenge. Twenty years Roosevelt's junior, the rail-thin, narrow-shouldered Mitchel was a reformer. He advocated tirelessly, and aggressively, for a more scientific management of New York City. Among his ambitious reforms, Mitchel tried to combine vocational and more traditional academic educational programs. This effort managed to infuriate nearly all groups involved in the process. Mitchel came to Stamford behind in the polls with less than two weeks until Election Day. Standing with Roosevelt seemed like a sure-win press event. Instead, he got a beatdown.

After posing for pictures, Roosevelt, Barbour, and Mitchel headed for the trail that circled the facility. Roosevelt wanted to show everyone where he had been doing some of his best work. Several young boys, three police officers, and a gaggle of officials—the type who never miss a ribbon cutting—crowded in behind the principal actors. Without any warning, Roosevelt broke into a jog. The group scrambled to keep up. It was a Is-This-a-Race?...This-is-a-Race! situation. The lake loop required "a dash up and down hills." It led the walk-runners "through cabbage patches along the borders of a lake." It was a half mile around.

Roosevelt seized control of the pace. He gradually pushed the tempo. After two minutes, the group had already separated. "That army trailed out into a long and lagging tail to the Colonel's kite," the New York *Sun* reported.

What was happening? Mitchel, for one, began doubting his plan for an easy campaign boost simply by making the trip out to see Roosevelt training. His endorsement was literally running away from him. *Hey!* A small incline brought the runners to the halfway point. Some struggled to keep moving, then there was Mitchel.

Mitchel struggled to the top.

There, he "gave up," the *Brooklyn Daily Eagle* reported. Mitchel "did not even straggle," the *New York Tribune* pointed out. He just quit at the quarter mile mark. What a quitter. Mitchel trudged back to the start, defeated. The *Washington Post* caught it all. Of the race, the paper ran a simple TR headline: OUTSPRINTS MAYOR MITCHEL.*

The second half of the trail brought about "a winding sprint around the pond and up another little hill." Roosevelt kept pushing until the end—all the way through the unmarked (because it was not technically a race) finish.

---

* It was the start of a bad run for Mitchel. He went on to lose the November mayoral election. Then, eight months later, after volunteering to serve in the US Army Signal Corps, Mitchel fell out of his airplane to his death during a training exercise. *Washington Post*, October 22, 1917.

One more time, the press reveled in the narrative of a strenuous Roosevelt. "He was slightly warm; the other were winded...Col. Roosevelt hit up so fast a pace that Mayor Mitchel turned back before half," the *Post* reported. "The little army of newspaper men and onlookers were all winded when the dash was over." Roosevelt, on the other hand, looked great. He was young again. "At the finish those who also ran were convinced that the Colonel was just as young as he used to be." If only.

But this was a man doing something to beat back old age. "'De-e-lighted!' How else [to] describe Theodore Roosevelt's joyful relief at the disappearance of his—his—well, his aldermanic front?" In reporting on the race and Roosevelt's time at Cooper's, there was a concerted effort made to allay any fears that Roosevelt might actually be slipping. Sure, he was at a health farm, but that did not mean he was actually unhealthy. Of this, America received assurance. COL-ONEL IS "PATIENT" AT HEATH FARM IN CONNECTICUT, BUT IS FAR FROM BEING A SICK MAN, read one headline. Under another headline—T.R. HOPES TO SEE LESS OF HIMSELF—was another calming passage: "The Colonel is what is technically described as a 'patient' at Jack Cooper's health farm...There is absolutely nothing the matter with him except the extent of his girth."

Roosevelt's victory over Mayor Mitchel provided proof that age wasn't such an inevitable foe after all. Yes, the two runners that finished closest behind Roosevelt were "the little girl and the boy scout," and sure the six and a half minutes it took to cover half a mile wasn't exactly a record. But Roosevelt had still won.

As the gaggle of reporters gathered around the sweating victor, Roosevelt provided one final piece of information for his athletic biography. "The last boxing I did was in Washington," Roosevelt said. "I boxed with my aides most of the time, but one day a young Captain of Artillery came along and broke some blood vessels in my left eye," Roosevelt recalled. The blow was serious. "I have never been able to see out of it since, although I don't believe many people know it." As details spilled out, reporters nailed down the injury to 1906. So, wait!...Roosevelt had been doing all of this—the tennis, the Rock Creek scrambling, the training, etc.—with only one eye? Of course he had. Because one Roosevelt eye, metaphorically speaking, equaled two ordinary eyes.

"When the Colonel is aroused the light of that eye makes up for any deficiencies there might be in the other—it glares," explained the New York *Sun*.

The press could not believe that Roosevelt had covered up such a glorious injury for so long. "Bless his wild, hot heart!" wrote one North Carolina paper. "Almost anybody else would have made some sort of capital cut of it, but the Colonel did not squeal." Or at least he hadn't until 1917.

When Jack Cooper had a chance to tell his side of the story, he reported that Roosevelt had been a joy to train. Roosevelt did not take his training passively; he had theorized even as he sweated. The mind-body paradigm still worked. "If it were within my power, I would make a new commandment," Roosevelt had declared to the trainer. It would read:

Thou and thy children and they children's children shalt frequently and regularly practice some approved form of physical culture; not for thine own good alone, but for the good of thy offspring, aye, for the good of the community, for the Nation, the State and society and for all humanity. Selah!

Roosevelt could make no such edict, but his advocacy still mattered.

In a way though, the fact that Roosevelt decided in 1917 to announce a long-ago injury is a bit sad. Did he really need more attention? But the whole undertaking at Jack Cooper's—the training, the "race," and the revelation of a bygone boxing injury—provided a bookend to Roosevelt's time as the Strenuous Life president. That Roosevelt would submit to such training evidenced his willingness to keep fighting against his physical limitations. The race made clear his athletic showmanship and competitiveness. Okay, so Mayor Mitchel didn't know there was going to be a race. But Roosevelt still won. And the injury announcement? It highlighted Roosevelt's vulnerability. The ex-president of the United States could not resist being seen as the athletic warrior one more time, even as the nation faced real military conflict abroad.

As he left Cooper's, Roosevelt thanked Jack Cooper profusely. "I've had a perfectly corking time here," he said. And then Roosevelt, with one foot out the door, made a telling statement; he wished he was Jack Cooper. "I could get as much pleasure out of this sort of thing as you do. I scarcely know what I could more enjoy than the practice of taking under my care and treatment the weak and debilitated." Roosevelt continued: "The very peak of gratification would come in that final, hearty handclasp as they left to go out again into the world, and they would say to me: 'I'm feeling fit and fine and full of pop, old man; great, bully, perfectly splendid—you couldn't have done more or better for me!'" Here was Roosevelt's wish for America—crystalized into one glorious hypothetical compliment for himself. Roosevelt had always hoped that he and his Strenuous Life philosophy would create a nation "full of pop" and ready to "go out again into the world."

Newspapers across the nation on October 22, 1917, put Roosevelt's boxing injury on the front page alongside news of the fighting in Europe. ROOSEVELT BLIND IN LEFT EYE; INJURED DURING BOXING MATCH ran right next to stories on submarine attacks and advertisements for war bonds. It was the closest Roosevelt would get to the Great War. He would be dead in fifteen months.

EPILOGUE

Do what you can, with what you have, where you are.

—THEODORE ROOSEVELT

I arrived in Dickinson, North Dakota, via the Theodore Roosevelt Regional Airport. I checked into the Rough Riders Hotel in Medora, which is adjacent to the Theodore Roosevelt National Park. In the hotel room I found an "Official Badlands Teddy Bear." For dinner: Theodore's, a fine steakhouse. The nearby Bully Pulpit Golf Course beckoned, but alas I did not bring my clubs. No time, I was here on a Roosevelt fact-finding mission.

The annual Theodore Roosevelt Conference is hosted by the Theodore Roosevelt Center at Dickinson State University. The region is the future home of the Theodore Roosevelt Presidential Library. Over a couple of days each fall, eminent Roosevelt scholars share their work with appreciative Roosevelt aficionados. A field trip to Roosevelt's cabin on the Elkhorn River typically punctuates the gathering. It is, hands down, the most delightful conference I've ever attended.

But I'll admit, there was a point when the sheer Teddyness of the experience overwhelmed me. It came during a Q&A session. People lined up to ask their questions. Many attendees seemed to enjoy their time with the microphone more than offering a specific query, but we were all having fun. Then Theodore Roosevelt stood up to ask a question. Yes Roosevelt—looking rugged in his full Rough Rider getup. Ok, so it was a Roosevelt impersonator who, at least from the looks and sounds of it, was excellent at his impersonating. He, in spot-on voice and cadence, asked the Roosevelt scholar a very specific question about Roosevelt's legacy.

And thereby Mt. Rushmore exploded. At least Roosevelt's head alongside Lincoln, Jefferson, and Washington rattled a bit on its South Dakota perch.

Not even I could miss the obvious point: Why does Roosevelt still resonate today? On the one hand, we know more than ever that he had serious flaws. The case can be made (and has been) that Roosevelt was a misogynistic, racist, war-mongering tyrant. Despite his blemishes, however, there is a Roosevelt, caricatured as ably by Robin Williams in the film *Night at the Museum* as anywhere else, which still sells. The Strenuous Life still draws attention.

Perhaps this connection stems from the fact that our concerns and worries are not so very different from those of the early twentieth century, even if the games we play seem so much bigger, louder, and more serious.

And we have gone bigger. Imagine taking Roosevelt into our athletic spaces. Just for fun. Picture Roosevelt, for example, at Louisiana State University's "Death Valley" Stadium for an LSU–Alabama football game. From the field (he'd have a field pass—*Bully!*) he would look up at the 102,321 fans and out toward the field at three-hundred-pound athletes smashing into each other.

Then perhaps a visit to a youth soccer tournament. After paying $20 to park, Roosevelt would walk to the edge of the long green pitch, goals and kids (*wow, so many girls!*) and collapsible chairs and umbrellas as far as the eye can see. He'd chat with a father wearing his daughter's team colors. "You gotta play club, man. It's the only way for your daughter to get a scholarship."

And then maybe we'd give him the Lawrence Murray treatment (remember that civil servant left for dead during a tramp with Roosevelt?). What if we signed TR up for the Rock 'n' Roll Marathon in San Diego, California? On race day Roosevelt would wait in the long line, in the dark of early morning, for a shuttle bus to the start. He would chat up the anxious runners around him. *Where are you from? Is Lycra supposed to cling like this?* Fast-forward five hours. Finish line in view, a weary Roosevelt would sprint it in. Done, Roosevelt would then adjourn to In-N-Out for dinner. Yes, he might even wear his finisher's medal to the restaurant.

You get the idea. I'll stop before I have to return my American Historical Association membership card.* Such speculation is obviously well beyond the scope of critical inquiry. But the broader point here is to compare. What's the same? Or to put it more accurately, where can we today observe connections to the origins of sports covered in this book?

Start with the institutions. The NCAA, Major League Baseball, and the Olympic Games have grown into athletic behemoths. The NCAA oversees college football most significantly, but also an additional 400,000 intercollegiate athletes. Baseball is a $10 billion a year sport. The Olympic Games occurs every four years (just like Coubertin wanted it) and still produces a rare brew of international goodwill and blood-thirsty nationalism each go-round.

The debate over safety in football is ongoing too. How much violence is too much violence (recent headline: CTE FOUND IN 99% OF STUDIED BRAINS FROM DECEASED NFL PLAYERS) when it comes to sports? In 2018, following the death from football-practice induced heatstroke of a Maryland football player, the *Washington Post*'s legendary sports columnist Sally Jenkins issued a shot across the bow of the NCAA. "Prehistoric college football coaches are killing players. It's past time to stop them," she wrote. The article tallied its own "death harvest." Twenty-seven college football players have died in training since 2000.

Youth sports seem poised to take over the world. The PSAL is still flourishing; it offers the children of New York City thirty-three competitive sports in which to participate. According to the National Federation of State High School Associations, participation in high school sports has increased every year (to nearly eight million) for the past twenty-nine years. And school-based sports are just a start. Club sports, youth sports camps, personal coaches, leagues at every time of the year—these are just part of the youth sports complex that orders the lives of most American children.

---

* The American Historical Association (AHA) is history's largest professional organization. It publishes best practices, advocates for archival access, and hosts a conference each January (usually in a lovely winter destination like Chicago) where scholars share their latest work—usually by reading their papers directly to the audience.

Buzz Bissinger wrote *Friday Night Lights* in 1989 about Odessa, Texas, an out of the way place with a football addiction. "I found those Friday night lights, and they burned with more intensity than I had ever imaged," he said. The book told a great story; Bissinger also meant it as a warning on mixed priorities. The nation did not get the message. Instead the book became a Hollywood movie and then a television ("Clear eyes, Full hearts, Can't lose") series. "We've gone from *Friday Night Lights* to Every Night Lights," the *New York Times* editorialized.

In terms of the actual games, baseball, basketball, boxing, football, golf, swimming, tennis, track and field, and wrestling all still have devoted followings. This is not to say that what's popular hasn't evolved somewhat. The rise of soccer in America, especially on the youth level, occurred towards the end of the twentieth century. And basketball, while invented at the turn of the century, has exploded into a global game.

While the US Men's soccer team has struggled to compete internationally, the US *Women's* soccer team has become a world leader. The team won three World Cups and four Olympic gold medals during the past twenty years. And therein is perhaps the biggest change in the American sports landscape. Girls and women have joined their male counterparts in almost every conceivable athletic venue. Well, with the exception of those uniquely American games: football and baseball.

The passage of Title IX legislation in 1972 marked a watershed moment in toppling the male-centric hierarchy created in American sports during the Roosevelt era. This is not to say that things are equal. Girls' teams often get stuck with inferior equipment and attract less attention. Female athletes at the college level still received less scholarship support. Women's professional sports do not draw nearly the spectatorship or revenues that men's sports do. But a gender revolution has occurred in American sports.

Certainly the racial complexion of American sports has changed. African American athletes have achieved a dominance in sports today, at least in certain areas. About 50% of Division I basketball players (men and women) and football players are African American. Eighty-one percent of the players in the

NBA and 70% of those in the NFL are African American. Since the 1940s, a series of African-American athletes have been among the most famous in the United States, achieving broad cultural resonance and popularity. Jesse Owens, Joe Louis, Bill Russell, Muhammad Ali, Jim Brown, Michael Jordan—this list goes on and on.

But to say that the racial tensions inherent in the 1910 "Fight of the Century" have disappeared completely would be inaccurate. Consider the strange case of Colin Kaepernick—a biracial NFL quarterback who knelt during the national anthem to protest police brutality against people of color. Kaepernick won *Sports Illustrated*'s 2017 Muhammad Ali Legacy Award. Nike made Kaepernick the face of its newest advertising campaign. But Kaepernick is also out of a job as of this writing. No NFL team has been willing to sign Kaepernick—not long ago a Super Bowl quarterback—to even a third-string QB roster spot.

Beyond the specific sports, it's the anxieties that sound surprising similar.

Roosevelt worried about the mollycoddling of America. It was a strawman, but his point that new technologies and new ways of working had costs was shared by many Americans. Juxtapose that concern with a more current one: "Have Smartphones Destroyed a Generation?" And if yes, which generation? Concerns are growing that technology is fundamentally changing the human experience. While Roosevelt worried about the enervating effect of automobiles, we now use our smartphones to request that these automobiles come to the exact place we're standing. Is technology robbing us of our physical vitality?

Perhaps most basically, Roosevelt struggled against the effects of aging. While at Jack Cooper's, Roosevelt made a remark on the missed opportunity of American middle-agedness. "It is really distressing to rub shoulders with a world of men of forty and forty-five," Roosevelt said, "who look, act and presumably feel like old, decrepit invalids, just at the time when they should actually be entering upon the most efficient and useful period of their lives." Today, in a nation where forty-five million people start a diet each year, thirty million have diabetes, and fifty-seven million pay for a health club membership, it's safe to say that the struggle continues.

On some level, comparing oneself to Roosevelt is a recipe for disaster. Roosevelt won elections. He graduated from Harvard and wrote dozens of books. He penned thousands of letters to his children. He charged up hills and won a Nobel Peace Prize. The rest of us? We're just trying to pick the kids up on time and make sure our emails have their attachments.

But many Americans still know what it's like to win a terribly insignificant trophy and revel in that "accomplishment" for years to come. Many Americans know what it's like to wish that they had made the team. They also know the hope that comes with a new fitness plan. Likewise they understand the pangs of discouragement that come with ever-expanding waistlines and the discovery one day that what feels like a six-minute mile is actually a ten-minute mile.

Thus the Strenuous Life.

*　　*　　*

In 1918, with his sons fighting in the trenches of Europe, Roosevelt contracted an illness that nearly killed him. He had a raging fever and, just to add to the misery, a case of hemorrhoids that he just could not shake. He was hospitalized—sent to Roosevelt Hospital in New York City. There doctors worked to cool his fever and fight off an inner ear infection that looked as if it might require surgery. Things looked dire. A few careless reporters even wrote that TR had died.

He had not. He beat off the infection and returned to Sagamore Hill in March 1918, but in a severely weakened state. He worried about his sons, especially Archie who had been injured in the war. Dizziness plagued Roosevelt. He began to use a cane to make his way around. He rested every afternoon to keep his strength—mostly so that he would have the energy to play with his grandchildren.

Then on July 16, Roosevelt got word that Quentin's plane had gone down behind enemy lines. The family waited for more information. First came a report that he died. Then another that he was captured but safe. Two days later, the press confirmed Roosevelt's worst fears: Quentin was dead. Roosevelt learned the terrible news first; his immediate concern was telling Edith. "Mrs.

Roosevelt. How am I going to break it to her?" he asked a reporter. Roosevelt's youngest boy had beaten him to the grave. Roosevelt was proud of his courageous son, yes, but grief-stricken too. "It is rather awful to know that he paid with his life, and that my other sons may pay with their lives, to try to put in practice what I preached," he said in one of his last public comments on his fallen son. Roosevelt grieved in his own way, as historian Kathleen Dalton explained: "Friends viewed TR sobbing quietly in the old barn one day as he draped his arm around his horse's neck."

Painfully, life moved on. On October 27, 1918, Roosevelt celebrated his sixtieth birthday. "To-day your threescore years have tolled, and millions fain would grasp your hand," writer and historian Owen Wister wrote, "And pray that you be never old." There was no vigorous walk this year. Instead Roosevelt sat on the porch overlooking the Long Island Sound. It had been a particularly cool autumn. "I don't know that it makes any difference," he said of the landmark birthday.

Around him he had all the family he could get. Edith of course. Alice, Ethel, and Archie, who was back stateside recovering from war injuries and with his new bride Grace, returned to Sagamore Hill too. And with them, they brought the real stars of the show: the grandchildren. Richard (four years old), Edith (one year old), and Little Archie (eight months).

As always, Roosevelt had letters to write. To his sister on his birthday he wrote: "You and I have known long years of happiness. And you are as young as I am old!" He signed this one: "Methuselah's understudy." To Kermit, he wrote something similar, painting himself as old rather than young—finally. "This is my 60th birthday," he penned in his understated script. "I am glad to be sixty, for it somehow gives me the right to be titularly as old as I feel."

Perhaps most tellingly, Roosevelt penned a letter to Belle, Kermit's wife. Belle and Kermit had been married for four years and had given Roosevelt two grandsons by this time. To his twenty-six-year-old daughter-in-law, Roosevelt's love of family, his grief, and his continual irritation with Woodrow Wilson shone through. "This day I am sixty years old," he confessed. "I hope that when Kermit is as old he will be as proud of Kermit and Willard as I am of him."

Quentin's death hung over Sagamore Hill, although Roosevelt could only express it as something affecting Ethel, who after serving with the Red Cross in France, was back in the United States and "busy with her babies." Ethel, Roosevelt told Belle, "misses Quint all the time." All the time. The grief never left Roosevelt.

Neither did his will to continue the political fight against Woodrow Wilson. After a breezy, tender letter, Roosevelt wrapped up his birthday correspondence with Belle by reminding her that he had more to offer his country. "It's pretty poor business to be writing little books in these times of terrible action [Roosevelt had just finished his manuscript for *The Great Adventure*], but it is all I can do, or at least all that I am allowed to do by the people in power at Washington." Then Roosevelt signed off. "Lovingly, Kermit's father."

John J. Leary, who had written a series of stories on Roosevelt and become a confidant, visited Sagamore Hill on Roosevelt's birthday. For the piece he wrote for the *New York Tribune,* Leary settled on a telling headline: THEODORE ROOSEVELT, AMERICAN ON HIS SIXTIETH BIRTHDAY: STILL VIGOROUS, A SPARTAN IN BEREAVEMENT, GIVING HIMSELF TO THE WAR. Leary reported that Roosevelt remained hard at work. He had continued to accept speaking invitations when he could. Exercise, too, remained a priority. "The Colonel's exercise is what one might call—to use a term the Colonel made famous—a bit strenuous for a man of sixty." He rode his horses, and he rowed on the Sound, usually with Edith, when he could. Leary concluded his piece hopefully: "Apparently being sixty years old makes no difference to some men."

But it was making a difference. By November of 1918, Roosevelt could not get a proper night's sleep. The pain from his rheumatism kept him awake. He made an appearance with W.E.B. Du Bois before the Circle for Negro War Relief, but then he shut down. On November 11, Armistice Day, Roosevelt's level of discomfort finally convinced him to check back into the hospital. For six weeks, doctors poked and prodded and Roosevelt experienced pain in his limbs especially. On Christmas morning, feeling some relief but without a clear diagnosis, Roosevelt returned home to Sagamore Hill. The holiday was a startlingly quiet one; Quentin was gone, and Roosevelt had none of his usual energy.

On January 5, 1919, something strange happened. Roosevelt pulled Edith near and told her it felt like his heart might stop beating. Something was off. "I know it's not going to happen, but it is such a strange feeling," he told her. At 11:00 p.m., Roosevelt suffered through an attack in which he had considerable trouble breathing. He asked Edith to sit with him until he fell asleep. She, of course, did. Edith checked on Roosevelt again at 2:00 a.m. and found him sleeping soundly. At 4:15 a.m., Roosevelt died.

"The Old Lion is Dead." Archie sent the cable to Ted and Kermit in Europe.

The core of Roosevelt's family—Edith, Alice, Ted, Ethel, Kermit, and Archie—had to share Roosevelt in death as they had in life. The nation mourned. In some ways, the response was typical of the loss of a president. Memories of political causes and electoral victories were recounted. Newspapers quoted Roosevelt's greatest hits—a list that seemingly had no end given Roosevelt's penchant for turning a phrase.

But the obituaries connected Roosevelt to the Strenuous Life, and to athletic pursuits, in a telling way. In the days after his death, the following headlines appeared in American newspapers:

COL. THEODORE ROOSEVELT, MOST STRENUOUS
AMERICAN IS CALLED BY DEATH ANGEL.

ROOSEVELT LOVED ATHLETICS.

ROOSEVELT'S STRENUOUS, PLUCKY CAREER RUNS
SCALE OF AMERICAN STATESMANSHIP AND MANHOOD.

ROOSEVELT LIKED THE PUNCH. HIT HARD IN
ATHLETIC GAME AS IN EVERYTHING ELSE.

THEODORE ROOSEVELT, ATHLETE AND SPORTSMAN: BOXER,
WRESTLER, RUNNER, RACQUETER, HUNTER, FISHERMAN, POLO
PLAYER AND FOOTBALL AND ROWING ENTHUSIAST WAS FAMOUS
AMERICAN, WHO DIED YESTERDAY AT OYSTER BAY, N.Y.

COLONEL ROOSEVELT ARDENT BOXING FAN.

PHYSICAL TRAINING WAS CREED WITH ROOSEVELT;
STRENUOUS SPORTS BEST.

AFTER A LIFE OF STRENUOUS ACTION,
ROOSEVELT'S BODY IS LAID AT REST AT SAGAMORE.

In the *Boston Globe*'s January 6, 1919, edition, a paper that went to press just hours after Roosevelt's passing, it took two sentences in the lead story before a mention of the Strenuous Life came up.

> Theodore Roosevelt, for seven years President of the United States, died at his home at Sagamore Hill, at 4:15 this morning. The famous American, exponent of the 'strenuous life,' who had fought in the Spanish war, and risked death in hunting big game and exploring the jungles of Africa and South America, passed away peacefully in his sleep.

The first-sentence details might have explained the situation, but the Strenuous Life reference made clear to Americans what had been lost.

Roosevelt's death caught the nation by surprise. While he had been hospitalized, two decades of Strenuous Life stories had offset any suspicion that Roosevelt's end might actually be near. That Roosevelt might indeed be as mortal as the next man. Perhaps it was for the best. Roosevelt lived hard until the end; the nation never knew an old Roosevelt.

As for Roosevelt's final moments, Thomas Marshall (Woodrow Wilson's vice president) provided a nice theory on how things may have transpired. The end had happened quickly and furtively because Roosevelt could be conquered no other way. "Death had to take him in his sleep," Marshall explained, "for if he was awake there'd have been a fight."

ACKNOWLEDGMENTS

There are many people to thank now that this book is finally a reality. Two of those people are Alec Shane, the agent who took a chance on this book and me, and Keith Wallman of Diversion Books. Keith and his team at Diversion were patient throughout the process, even as we debated for weeks about exactly what to call this book of ours. Thanks for working with me to make this possible.

I am grateful for generous research support I received from my institution, the University of New Mexico. Additionally, I benefitted greatly from the expertise and kindness of the archivists at Harvard University's Theodore Roosevelt Collection, the Library of Congress Manuscript Room, and at the Theodore Roosevelt Center at Dickinson University. These "keepers of the good stuff" aided my research process both when I visited their institutions and when I cried out for help from afar.

I was fortunate to have many people read parts or all of this book. My writing group in the Honors College at UNM—Sarita Cargas, Myrriah Gomez, Amaris Ketchum, and Marygold Walsh-Dilley—made invaluable contributions to this project when it was in its earliest, most fragile forms. I was also fortunate to present portions of this research at conferences of the North American Society for Sport History and receive helpful, specific feedback.

Additionally I am grateful to Aram Goudsouzian, Michael Kazin, Brian Ingrassia, Robert Pruter, Andrew RM Smith, Johnny Smith, and David Wiggins for reading portions of this manuscript and providing all manner of corrections and suggestions. They saved me from many mistakes and encouraged me to think deeper about what it was I wanted to say with this book.

To my mom and dad, there are just too many thanks to list. My father, who read the entire manuscript, provided an overall assessment of the book which was filled with his typical wisdom and good humor. He also regularly asked me in our phone chats, with just the right mix of prodding and understanding, "Did you get anything done this week?" My mother provided a steady dose of encouragement and love. She reminded me to keep things in perspective and always make time for a nap. And both of my parents, a long time ago, taught me to love books.

To Nate and Jess, Casey and Samantha, and Wes and Kari, thanks for the hospitality on my trips back east for research. Having a place to stay and good conversations about everything besides TR made these trips seem like something close to a vacation.

I am exceedingly grateful for my three children—Carter, Tyler, and Kate—for their willingness to go along on this TR journey. Of course, they had no choice, but I appreciated their inquisitive spirits nonetheless. Now we just need to learn something about those other forty-four US presidents! Hopefully it doesn't need to be said, but I'll say it anyways: my favorite soccer and basketball games, and cross country and track meets will always be the ones in which I can watch you three.

My partner in this project, as she is in everything else, was my wife Rachael. She read every word of this darn book, often poring over this section or that page when I couldn't bear to do so myself. Her dogged persistence, keen eye, and matchless insight made completion of this book a reality. Without her, it would be still be an amorphous (or an even more amorphous) blob of words on a hard drive somewhere. I've said it before, but I've never believed it more: Rachael is basically a mix of Wonder Woman and Leslie Knope; I'm so blessed to share life with her.

ENDNOTES

INTRODUCTION

1. "spick and span" tennis getup.: *Sun* (New York), November 25, 1906; Quotes, unless otherwise noted, come from: Lawrence O. Murray, "My Initiation to the Strenuous Life," Harvard University, Theodore Roosevelt Collection.

2. to observe a White House match.: *Washington Post*, September 28, 1907.

2. the Team Roosevelt tennis experience.: *Washington Post*, December 15, 1907.

3. the great Nobel Peace Prize.": Papers of James R. Garfield, Diary 1906, December 1.

4. You must *make* your body.": Daniel Sullivan, "How Roosevelt Made his Body," *Good Health*, October 1919.

8. and 'irritable weakness.'": Clifford Putney, *Muscular Christianity: Manhood and Sports in Protestant America, 1880–1920* (Cambridge: Harvard University Press, 2001), 27.

8. the United States at the turn of the century.: Michael Kazin, Rebecca Edwards, and Adam Rothman, *The Concise Princeton Encyclopedia of American Political History* (Princeton: Princeton University Press, 2011), 673.

8. "a strategy for regeneration and renewal.": Donald J. Mrozek, *Sport and American Mentality, 1880–1919* (Knoxville: The University of Tennessee Press, 1983), 3.

9. those arriving and those already in America.: Eric Rauchway, *Murdering McKinley: The Making of Theodore Roosevelt's America* (New York: Hill and Wang, 2003), 119.

10. and tells people about it with a smile.": *Sun* (New York), October 22, 1917.

10. and the baby at every christening.": *Los Angeles Times*, March 19, 1912.

10. *I never was a champion at anything.*": Theodore Roosevelt to Pierre de Coubertin, June 15, 1903, in *Theodore Roosevelt: Letters and Speeches* (New York: Literary Classics of the United States, 2004), 266–268.

ONE: HIT THE LINE HARD

11. had to trump everything else.: *Philadelphia Inquirer*, November 30, 1901.

12. the kickoff would be pushed back.: Kathleen Dalton, *A Strenuous Life* (New York: Alfred A. Knopf, 2002), 163.

13. **to an official event more unostentatiously.":** *Philadelphia Inquirer*, December 1, 1901; Philip H. Melanson, *The Secret Service: the Hidden History of an Enigmatic Agency* (New York: Carroll & Graf Publishers, 2002), 30–32.

13. **closeness during the three-hour trip was invigorating.:** *Washington Times*, December 1, 1901.

13. **tipping them for providing safe passage.:** *Philadelphia Inquirer*, December 1, 1901.

13. **win a "smashing triumph" over Yale.:** Theodore Roosevelt to Alice Lee Roosevelt, November 30, 1901.

14. **and be somebody: get action.":** George Douglas, *The Many-Sided Roosevelt: An Anecdotal Biography* (New York: Dodd, Mead and Company, 1907), 83.

14. **TR strode forward at a disruptive clip.:** *St. Louis Post-Dispatch*, December 1, 1901.

14. **unimpeded access to the stadium.:** *St. Louis Post-Dispatch*, December 1, 1901.

14. **to keep the blood tingling," the** *Philadelphia Times* **reported.:** *Philadelphia Times*, December 1, 1901.

14. **and King Umberto of Italy in 1900.:** *Public Opinion*, September 12, 1901.

15. **McKinley died from infection on September 14, 1901.:** Morris, *The Rise of Theodore Roosevelt*, 777.

15. **meant to secure protection for the president.:** And they could not agree on one. Concerns about treating the president of the United States too much like a king continued (still, a century after overthrowing King George) to cause problems. See Melanson, *The Secret Service*, 30.

15. **in the City of Brotherly Love as well.:** Russell F. Weigley, *Philadelphia: A 300-Year History* (New York: WW Norton Company, 1982), 480–492.

15. **deserted because of a football game.":** *Baltimore Sun*, December 1, 1901.

16. **the flash of color was dazzling.":** *Philadelphia Inquirer*, December 1, 1901; Kevin Phillips, *William McKinley: The American Presidents Series: The 25th President* (New York: Time Books, 2003), 72.

16. **"more in the nature of a bathtub.":** *Los Angeles Times*, January 3, 2014; Theodore Roosevelt Birthplace, "Frequently Asked Questions," https://www.nps.gov/thrb/faqs.htm; *Boston Globe*, September 11, 2014.

17. **ran up and down the line.":** *St. Louis Post-Dispatch*, December 1, 1901.

17. **the last strains of "Hail to the Chief.":** *Philadelphia Inquirer*, December 1, 1901.

18. **the lover of true sport," the paper said.:** *Philadelphia Times*, December 1, 1901.

19. **punt the ball back to Navy on first down.:** As a point of reference, modern football teams never punt on first down. Such a move today would be considered extremely conservative and downright foolish. Part of the evolution in strategy is due to the changed role of quarterbacks. While at the turn of the twentieth century quarterbacks were the best athletes on the field and true jacks-of-all-trades (in a football sense), the quarterback position has evolved into one of a passing specialist. Not only would modern teams not want to punt on first or second or third downs, they rarely trust a quarterback to execute a kick.

20. **who might come from any direction.:** Ron Smith, *Big-Time Football at Harvard, 1905: The Diary of Coach Bill Reid* (Urbana: University of Illinois Press, 1994), xvi.

20. **the opposite slope from the British rugby.":** John Watterson, *College Football: History, Spectacle, Controversy* (Baltimore: The Johns Hopkins University Press, 2000), 19.

21. **employ similar strategies on the field.:** Michael Oriard, *Reading Football: How the Popular Press Created an American Spectacle* (Chapel Hill: The University of North Carolina Press, 1995), 45–46.

23. **grew steadily in the military academy world.:** Julie Des Jardins, *Walter Camp: Football and the Modern Man* (University of Illinois Press, 2015).

24. the first Army–Navy football contest took place.: Gene Schoor, *The Army-Navy Game: A Treasury of the Football Classic* (New York: Dodd, Mead & Company, 1967), 3–9.

24. promises well for the future," the *Times* concluded.: *New York Times*, December 1, 1890.

25. giving the West Point men a 5–0 lead.: *Philadelphia Inquirer*, December 1, 1901.

26. ended the first half tied 5–5.: *St. Louis Post-Dispatch*, December 1, 1901.

27. It was a great day for the President.: *St. Louis Post-Dispatch*, December 1, 1901.

28. in his voluminous writings.: Half-baked efforts have been made to anoint Roosevelt as the "Father" of the game. Citing the 1897 letter, the *Los Angeles Times* answered its own "Did the letter save the game?" question with some irrefutable proximity reasoning: "The letter must have worked, because in 1899, during William McKinley's first term as President, the game resumed." *Los Angeles Times*, accessed March 16, 2015, http://latimesblogs.latimes .com/sports_blog/2010/11/sports-legend-revealed-did-the-annual-army-navy-game -draw-two-us-presidents-into-the-planning-of-the.html.

28. the explosion was from the outside.": Roosevelt, *Autobiography*, 120.

29. from America's southwest territories.: *Theodore Roosevelt Cyclopedia*, 543.

29. Men of Muscle are Men of Courage.: *Daily Review* (Decatur, Illinois), October 9, 1898.

29. somehow the bullets missed him.": Morris, *The Rise of Theodore Roosevelt*, 673.

29. "I got my regiment.": Morris, *The Rise of Theodore Roosevelt*, 680.

30. and the Rough Riders stood atop Kettle Hill.: Arthur M. Schlesinger, Jr. (ed), *History of American Presidential Elections*, Vol. III (New York: Chelsea House Publishers, 1971), 1886–1887.

31. Long Island Women Worship Roosevelt's Regiment, reported one daily.: *Inter Ocean* (Chicago), August 28, 1898.

31. the difference between football and war.": John Feinstein, *A Civil War, Army vs. Navy: A Year Inside College Football's Purest Rivalry* (New York: Little, Brown, and Company, 1996), x.

31. won the next eleven contests, often trouncing Army.: The service academies have migrated towards a largely out-of-date mode of football: the option attack. Thus unlike the pass-heavy offensives of most college football programs, Air Force and Navy (and recently Army too) prefer to run the ball if at all possible. The option offense, especially the triple-option currently in vogue, is not simple; it simply leverages different matchups on the field in order to gain yardage. The option offense is believed by many football experts to be especially helpful in offsetting talent deficiencies.

31. "smelled like rotten meat") took over from 1980–2001.: ESPN.com, "The List: Worst Ballparks," accessed September 1, 2017, http://espn.go.com/page2/s/list/worstballparks/ 010503.html.

31. at Lincoln Financial Field commenced in 2002.: See also, March Beech, *When Saturday Mattered Most: The Last Golden Season of Army Football* (New York: Thomas Dunne Books, 2012); Randy Roberts, *A Team for America: The Army-Navy Game that Rallied a Nation* (New York: Houghton Mifflin Harcourt, 2011).

32. But boy, do they have spirit.": *Washington Post*, December 10, 2016.

32. between the Army and the Navy.": *Philadelphia Inquirer*, December 1, 1901; *St. Louis Post-Dispatch*, December 1, 1901.

33. that has just ended," the *Tribune* reported.: *Chicago Tribune*, December 1, 1901.

33. they went in to do or die.": *Boston Daily*, December 1, 1901.

33. a few of the victorious players.: *Philadelphia Press*, December 1, 1901.

33. up San Juan Hill," boasted one Philadelphia writer.: *Philadelphia Inquirer*, December 1, 1901.

34. meal that "shocked a nation.": Deborah Davis, *Booker T. Washington, Theodore Roosevelt and the White House Dinner that Shocked a Nation* (New York: Atria, 2012).

34. **harshly with its latest assassin.:** Eric Rauchway, *Murdering McKinley: The Making of Theodore Roosevelt's America* (New York: Hill and Wang, 2003), 39–53.

34. **arrested shortly after Roosevelt left the city.:** *New York Times*, December 2, 1901.

TWO: THE STRENUOUS (LIKE, REALLY STRENUOUS) LIFE

35. **"strenuous" more than ten thousand times.:** This estimate (a conservative one) comes from searches of the HathiTrust, Proquest Historical Newspapers, and Newspapers.com databases using a combination of search words including President, Roosevelt, Teddy, Theodore, and TR in proximity to derivations of the word strenuous.

36. **regarding Mr. Roosevelt's strenuous bravery.":** *Wilmington Messenger*, October 3, 1902; *St. Louis Post-Dispatch*, September 28, 1902; *New York Times*, December 19, 1902; *Morning Post* (Raleigh, NC), August 24, 1902; *Winona Democrat* (Winona, Mississippi), August 1, 1902; *Washington Post*, July 21, 1902; *Arkansas Democrat*, January 17, 1902; *Houston Post*, September 10, 1902.

36. **urged her countrymen to read the work.:** *St. Louis Republic*, July 15, 1902.

36. **deciding the destinies of the world.":** *San Francisco Chronicle*, November 10, 1902.

37. **of the Hamilton Club," reported the Associated Press.:** *Los Angeles Times*, April 11, 1899.

37. **even as Roosevelt motioned for quiet.:** *New York Times*, April 11, 1899; *Los Angeles Times*, April 11, 1899.

38. **but to overcome them...":** The quotations from "The Strenuous Life" speech are taken from the previously cited, Roosevelt, *The Strenuous Life*.

40. **athletically speaking, during his childhood.:** There is some discrepancy on exactly how many books Roosevelt authored. The Theodore Roosevelt Association describes TR as the author of "35-odd books;" The Theodore Roosevelt Center lists thirty-seven. The National Park Service puts the number at forty-five. See, TRA, http://www.theodoreroosevelt.org/site/c.elKSIdOWIiJ8H/b.8344387/k.2C4D/The_Author.htm; TRC, https://www.theodorerooseveltcenter.org/Research/Digital-Library/Record.aspx?libID=o274790; NPS, https://www.nps.gov/thrb/learn/historyculture/booksbytr.htm.

40. **and a speech defect.":** "Theodore Roosevelt (1858-1919) Twenty-Sixth President of the United States," *Asthma and Allergy Proc.*, Vol. 18, No. 6 (November–December 1997), 382.

40. **explain the ravages of their condition.:** Descriptions of asthma attacks, as chronicled by *Healthtalk.org.* accessed June 20, 2016, http://www.healthtalk.org/peoples-experiences/long-term-conditions/asthma/what-asthma-feels.

40. **I can't control this asthma.":** *Los Angeles Times*, June 6, 1991.

40. **attending school and making friends.:** Center for Disease Control, "National Health Statistics Reports," No. 32, January 12, 2011. The school problem continues. The CDC estimates that children missed 10.5 million days of school in 2008 due to asthma attacks.

40. **attack in November 1861.:** Carlos A. Camargo and Tweed Roosevelt, "The Misunderstood Asthma of Theodore Roosevelt," *The Journal of Clinical Immunology: In Practice*, Vol. 3, Issue 5 (September–October 2015), 696–701.

40. **from [asthma's] strangling grip.":** Dalton, 35.

41. **withdraw the overwhelmed, scared child.:** Kathleen Dalton's superb one volume biography was invaluable as I chased Roosevelt's athletic odyssey, at the risk of missing many other vital components of TR's story. Dalton provides keen and concise analysis that almost always allows the reader to grasp the particulars of the issue or event at hand, and (if necessary) continue researching to find further information. Regarding Roosevelt's childhood see, Kathleen Dalton, *Theodore Roosevelt: A Strenuous Life* (New York: Alfred A. Knopf, 2002), 15–54.

41. **neither chloroform nor "instruments."**: David McCullough, *Mornings on Horseback* (New York: Simon and Schuster, 1981), 54.

42. **throughout the state's wards.**: *New York Times*, October 27, 1858.

42. **attack was just around the corner.**: McCullough, *Mornings on Horseback*, 90.

42. **as they were convenient."**: Henry Hyde Salter, *On Asthma: Its Pathology and Treatment* (Philadelphia: Blanchard and Lea, 1864), 33.

42. **rather than his lungs.**: Camargo and Roosevelt, "The Misunderstood Asthma of Theodore Roosevelt," 700.

42. **and so off we went."**: Theodore Roosevelt to Edith Kermit Carow Roosevelt, July 10, 1869, *Theodore Roosevelt Collection*, Harvard University. Italics are mine; underlined text is Roosevelt's.

43. **shocks through his feet and head.**: McCullough, *Mornings on Horseback*, 94–95.

43. **that the blood came out."**: Theodore Roosevelt, *Theodore Roosevelt's Diaries of Boyhood and Youth* (New York: Scribner's Sons, 1928), 3, 77.

43. **caffeine stimulation could only do so much.**: Camargo and Roosevelt, "The Misunderstood Asthma of Theodore Roosevelt," 698.

43. **infirmities," was how one reporter described TR discussing his past.**: Robert Johnstone Mooney, "Boxing and Wrestling with Roosevelt in the White House," *Outlook*, October 24, 1923.

43. **in 1901 described Roosevelt as a child.**: *The Ladies' Home Journal*, Vol. XVIII, 4 (March 1901), 9.

44. **father and mother trying to help me."**: Roosevelt, *Autobiography*, 11–12.

44. **"the best man I ever knew."**: Corinne Roosevelt Robinson, *My Brother Theodore* (New York: Charles Scribner's Sons, 1921), 7.

44. **but I know you will do it."**: McCullough, *Mornings on Horseback*, 112–113.

44. **until the day of his death."**: Daniel Sullivan, "How Roosevelt Made his Body," *Good Health*, October 1919.

45. **on the second floor of the family dwelling.**: Camargo and Roosevelt, "The Misunderstood Asthma of Theodore Roosevelt," 698.

45. **swing and bar and seesaw."**: Robinson, *My Brother Theodore Roosevelt*, 50.

45. **the exponent of the strenuous life."**: Robinson, *My Brother Theodore Roosevelt*, 50; Corinne's story of a boy and his personal gym became standard biographical fodder. See, for example, Edward Emerson, *Adventures of Theodore Roosevelt* (New York: E.P. Dutton & Co., 1928), 6.

45. **"spacious and lofty hall" at Wood's Gym.**: "Gymnastics," *Aquatic Monthly and Nautical Review: Devoted to the Interests of the Yachting and Rowing Community*, Vol. 1, 8 (January 1, 1873), 582.

45. **$24 billion annually on fitness memberships.**: International Health, Racquet, and Sportsclub Association, accessed March 1, 2016, http://www.ihrsa.org/industry-research/.

46. **without having broken a sweat at all.**: *New York Times*, December 31, 1875.

46. **damage whatever in return."**: Roosevelt, *Autobiography*, 26–27.

46. **(bevis virginiansas)," Roosevelt wrote of one trip.**: *Diary of Theodore Roosevelt from August 1-31, 1871*. Theodore Roosevelt Collection. MS Am 1454.55 (7). Houghton Library, Harvard University.

47. **100 yards 12 seconds.**: *Diary of Theodore Roosevelt's Athletic Achievements*, 1875.

47. **he had the data to prove it.**: Ibid.

48. **Tom Hyer and Yankee Sullivan, and Heenan and Sayers."**: Roosevelt, *Autobiography*, 27; "Athletic: Before and After," *Turf, Field, and Farm* (March 19, 1875), 187.

48. **triumphs which would be worth relating.**: Roosevelt, *Autobiography*, 27–28.

49.   **that one caused the other.:** *Guardian*, January 6, 2012, accessed September 6, 2017, https://www.theguardian.com/science/blog/2012/jan/06/correlation-causation.

49.   **does not exist causes problems.:** *Daily Mail*, May 27, 2014.

50.   **until I got those spectacles.":** Roosevelt, *Autobiography*, 13–14.

50.   **trailing off of Roosevelt's asthma.:** David McCullough, "How Teddy Roosevelt Charged Through Asthma," *American Lung Association Bulletin*, Vol. 68, No. 1 (January–February 1982).

50.   **though there was no such understanding.:** Camargo and Roosevelt, "The Misunderstood Asthma of Theodore Roosevelt."

THREE: HARVARD AND ITS HARVARDNESS

52.   **first intercollegiate athletic competition.:** Guy Lewis, "The Beginnings of Organized Collegiate Sport," *American Quarterly*, Vol. 22, 2, Part 1 (Summer 1970), 224.

52.   **for affluent northeasterners.:** *Outing*, June 1, 1901.

52.   **also attracted dozens of participants.:** William E. Harding, *The American Athlete. A Treatise on the Rules and Principles of Training for Athletic Contests and the Regimen of Physical Culture* (New York: Richard K. Fox, Police Gazette, 1881), 9.

52.   **consisted solely of kicking the ball.:** Mark F. Bernstein, *Football: The Ivy League Origins of an American Obsession* (Philadelphia: University of Pennsylvania Press, 2001), 9–11.

52.   **which made, counted for one point.:** Bernstein; Thomas G. Bergin, *The Game: The Harvard-Yale Football Rivalry, 1875–1983* (New Haven: Yale University Press, 1984), 4.

53.   **crowded around the field.:** Bernstein, 11.

53.   **drunkenness as they celebrated their team's victory.:** The actual charges were for singing and yelling in the streets, but alcohol was almost certainly involved. Bernstein, 11.

53.   **had been assembling for decades.:** Harvard University, *Annual Report of the President of Harvard University to the Overseers on the State of the University for the Academic Year 1876-1877* (Cambridge, MA: Press of John Wilson and Son, 1878). See also, Werner Sollors, Caldwell Titcomb, and Thomas A. Underwood, *History of African-American Experience at Harvard and Radcliffe* (New York: NYU Press, 1993).

54.   **prettier or more tasteful wall paper.":** Theodore Roosevelt to Anna Roosevelt. September 30, 1876, Theodore Roosevelt Collection. Houghton Library, Harvard University.

54.   **than the average male freshman today.:** Sareen S. Gropper et al., "The Freshman 15—A Closer Look," *Journal of American College Health*, Vol. 58, No. 3 (November 2009), 223–231.

54.   **with Roosevelt weighed 217 pounds.:** Harvard College, *Class of 1880, Secretary's Report*, 14.

54.   **remembered one of Roosevelt's Harvard classmates.:** Hagedorn, *The Life of Theodore Roosevelt*, 58.

54.   **came off to some as "lady-like.":** Dalton, *Theodore Roosevelt: A Strenuous Life*, 64; *Outing*, December 20, 1903.

54.   **My name's Roosevelt. What's yours?'":** Donald George Wilhelm, *Theodore Roosevelt as an Undergraduate* (Boston: J.W. Luce and Co., 1910), 54.

55.   **weights, and sparred regularly.:** "Athletics and Gymnastics at Harvard," *Outing*, Vol. II, 6 (September 1883), 419.

55.   **at least competent athletically.:** *Personal diary of Theodore Roosevelt, 1878*, 1878 Theodore Roosevelt Papers, Library of Congress Manuscript Division.

55.   **four competitors, "thrown by Davis.":** *Diary of Theodore Roosevelt from January 7 to December 27, 1877*. 1877 Theodore Roosevelt Collection. MS Am 1454.55 (11). Houghton Library, Harvard University.

55.   **past one o'clock when we separated.":** Letter from Theodore Roosevelt to Corinne Roosevelt Robinson, October 28, 1877. Theodore Roosevelt Collection. MS Am 1540 (17). Houghton Library, Harvard University.

55.   **a prolonged period of grief.:** Serge Ricard (ed), *A Companion to Theodore Roosevelt* (New York: Wiley-Blackwell, 2011), 12.

56.   **It seems as if it was years ago.":** Ricard, *A Companion to Theodore Roosevelt*, 12.

56.   **impunity because I was decent.":** "Letter to Edward S. Martin," November 26, 1900 in Albert B. Hart and Herbert R. Ferleger (eds) *Theodore Roosevelt Cyclopedia* (New York: Roosevelt Memorial Association, 1941), 581.

56.   **probably repeat this every day.":** *Personal diary of Theodore Roosevelt, 1878*, 1878 Theodore Roosevelt Papers, Library of Congress Manuscript Division.

57.   **victories over other collegiate teams.:** *New York Times*, October 7, 1878.

57.   **our athletic meetings a success.":** Theodore Roosevelt, Letter to the *Harvard Advocate*, Harvard University "Athletics Subject File."

57.   **I drink very little.":** *Personal diary of Theodore Roosevelt, 1878*, 1878 Theodore Roosevelt Papers, Library of Congress Manuscript Division.

59.   **nothing like a modern athletic structure.:** "Athletics and Gymnastics at Harvard," *Outing*, Vol. II, 6 (September 1883), 419.

59.   **(rather entitled sounding) contemporaries.:** Donald George Wilhelm, *Theodore Roosevelt as an Undergraduate* (Boston: JW Luce and Co., 1910), 53–54.

59.   **"densely packed" crowd for the fighting festival.:** *Boston Globe*, March 23, 1879.

59.   **she remained cool to his charms.:** Paul Grondahl, *I Rose Like a Rocket: The Political Education of Theodore Roosevelt* (New York: Free Press, 2004), 57.

60.   **spectacles lashed to his head.":** Carleton B. Case, *Good Stories about Roosevelt: The Humorous Side of a Great American* (Chicago: Shrewesbury Publishing, Co., 1920), 8.

60.   **their destination," the Boston Globe reported.:** *Boston Globe*, March 23, 1879.

60.   **Hanks won the second round.:** Henry Beach Needham, "Theodore Roosevelt–An Outdoor man," *McClure's Magazines*, Vol. XXVI, 3 (January 1906); There is some debate on whether this round by round detail is completely accurate. We know that Hanks won convincingly; the rest is up for some debate. See Harvard University file on Athletics and the George Doubleday letter.

60.   **"punishing Roosevelt severely.":** *New York Times*, March 23, 1879.

60.   **he showed himself a fighter.":** Hermann Hagedorn, *The Boy's Life of Theodore Roosevelt* (New York: Harper and Brothers, 1918), 58.

61.   **the past week...":** *Personal diary of Theodore Roosevelt, 1879*, Theodore Roosevelt Papers, Library of Congress Manuscript Division.

61.   **and hisses from the gallery.":** Owen Wister, *Roosevelt: The Story of a Friendship* (New York: The MacMillan Company, 1930), 5.

61.   **and the bout continued.:** Owen Wister, "Theodore Roosevelt: The Sportsman and the Man," *Outing*, Vol. XXXXVIII, 3 (June 1901), 243; Morris, *The Rise of Theodore Roosevelt*, 91.

62.   **present to the American people.":** Wister, "Theodore Roosevelt: The Sportsman and the Man," 244. Several different versions of the hit-after-the-bell story eventually emerged. Wister in *Roosevelt: The Story of a Friendship* recounted, incorrectly it appears, that Hanks had been the sucker puncher. Jacob Riis, the journalist who would pierce Americans' poverty malaise with his *How the Other Half Lives*, added a satisfying, victorious ending to the story. Roosevelt, as Riis described it in his 1904 account, had been unable to get his glove on and thus was struck while unprepared. Roosevelt's response, according to Riis: "I guess you made a mistake. We do not do it that way here." Then Roosevelt offered his hand and proposed the fight continue. "The next moment [Roosevelt's] right shot out and took the

man upon the point of the jaw, and the left followed suit. In two minutes he was down and out." See Jacob Riis, *Theodore Roosevelt: The Citizen* (Washington DC: Johnson, Wynne Company, 1904), 30–31.

62.   **blocked his path since childhood.**: Biographies published during Roosevelt's lifetime tell competing versions of Roosevelt's Harvard boxing career. As a result, many contemporary Roosevelt biographies do so as well. Most all contain elements of a tournament bout and a sucker punch episode. Many combine the Hanks and sucker punch fights into one contest, seemingly drawing on Owen Wister's account (in which Wister himself admits he cannot remember who Roosevelt was fighting when the sucker punch occurred). The various accounts are similar but not entirely coherent. It's my best guess that the Hanks fight and the sucker punch fight were actually different fights. That the *Boston Globe's* March 23, 1879, story, which is very detailed, mentions nothing of a sucker punch leads me to this still-tentative conclusion. For examples of the early points of diversion see, the Wister stories mentioned previously, Hermann Hagedorn, *The Life of Theodore Roosevelt* (London: G. G. Harrap & co., ltd., 1919), 62–63 and Donald George Wilhelm, *Theodore Roosevelt as an Undergraduate* (Boston: JW Luce and Co., 1910), 56.

62.   **from the moment he first saw her.**: Morris, *The Rise of Theodore Roosevelt*, 81–82; Dalton, 71. Morris's description of Alice Lee is a tribute to a beautiful, charming, young woman. It's vivid and powerful, and even a bit voyeuristic.

63.   **how bewitchingly pretty she is!"** : *Personal diary of Theodore Roosevelt, 1880*, 1880 Theodore Roosevelt Papers, Library of Congress Manuscript Division.

63.   **intense jealous man she called 'Teddy.'"**: Dalton, *A Strenuous Life*, 70–77.

64.   **with racially bigoted derision.**: Dudley Sargent, *The Autobiography of Dudley Sargent* (Philadelphia: Lea and Febiger Press, 1927), 161.

64.   **new venue to fit his plans.**: Sargent, *The Autobiography of Dudley Sargent*, 166.

64.   **the factors in human progress."**: Dudley Sargent, *Physical Education* (Boston: Ginn & Co., 1906), 19–20.

65.   **wasn't his life's work.**: Brenda Butler Boynton, "A Biographical Sketch of Dudley Allen Sargent," Master's Thesis, Boston University School of Education, 1941, 6.

65.   **matter of course," Sargent concluded.**: Sargent, *Physical Education*, 19–20.

65.   **and training to attain condition.**: Bruce L. Bennett, "Contributions of Dr. Sargent to Physical Education"; Dudley Sargent, *Battle-Ball* (Cambridge, MA, 1894).

65.   **were called." Roosevelt took his place.**: These were the observations of Pierre de Coubertin during his visit to Harvard. Norbert Muller (ed), *Pierre de Coubertin, 1863–1937, Olympism: Selected Writings* (Lausanne, Switzerland: International Olympic Committee, 2000), 82.

65.   **and legs, all are taken."**: *Boston Weekly Globe*, November 2, 1881.

66.   **average college aged man blew a thirty.**: Dudley Sargent, *An Anthropometric Chart, Showing the Relation of the Individual in Size, Strength, Symmetry and Development to the Normal Standard* (Cambridge, MA: 1886).

66.   **caused by Roosevelt's asthma.**: Muller, *Pierre de Coubertin*, 81–82; John Miller, *The Big Scrum: How Teddy Roosevelt Saved Football* (New York: Harper Perennial Press, 2011), 94–95.

66.   **helped me in afterlife."**: Roosevelt, *Autobiography*, 18.

67.   **too sacred to be written about."**: *Personal Diary*, 1880. And yes, Springfield, Massachusetts, is the home of James Naismith and basketball's invention.

67.   **walk," Alice wrote to Corinne.**: Stacy A. Cordery, *Alice: Alice Roosevelt Longworth from White House Princess to Washington Power Broker* (New York: Viking, 2007), 11.

68.   **deficient in brains and birth."**: *Diary kept by Theodore Roosevelt during the New York Assembly*, 1882. Theodore Roosevelt Birthplace National Historic Site.

68.   and happiest of all little mothers.": Cordery, *Alice*, 14.

68.   into a semiconscious state.: Cordery, *Alice*, 15.

69.   if he exerted himself too fully.: Hagedorn, *The Boys' Life of Theodore Roosevelt*, 64.

69.   Valentine's Day, both women died.: Morris, *The Rise of Theodore Roosevelt*, 229; Dalton, *A Strenuous Life*, 88–89.

70.   the light went out from my life forever.: *In memory of my darling wife Alice Hathaway Roosevelt and of my beloved mother Martha Bulloch Roosevelt*, 1884. Theodore Roosevelt Birthplace National Historic Site.

FOUR: THE TENNIS CABINET

71.   loved Roosevelt since childhood, accepted.: Dalton, *A Strenuous Life*, 104.

71.   Nor could Edith resist him.": Morris, *The Rise of Theodore Roosevelt*, 308.

72.   visit my sins upon poor little Edith.": Letter from Theodore Roosevelt to Anna Roosevelt, September 20, 1886.

72.   remained with Edith throughout her life.: Sylvia Jukes Morris, *Edith Kermit Roosevelt: Portrait of a First Lady* (New York: Vintage Books, 1980), 20.

73.   simmering romance turned cold.: Morris, *Edith Kermit Roosevelt: Portrait of a First Lady*, 58.

73.   consoling the mourning Roosevelt family.: Morris, *Edith Kermit Roosevelt: Portrait of a First Lady*, 70.

73.   it was so obviously true.: Roosevelt, *Autobiography*, 117; Arthur M. Schlesinger, Jr. (ed), *History of American Presidential Elections*, Vol. III (New York: Chelsea House Publishers, 1971), 1886–1887.

74.   bold, predictive fellow called out.: Morris, 707.

74.   during the summer of 1899.: *New York Times*, July 13, 1899.

74.   referencing an undetermined cabinet post.: *Chicago Daily Tribune*, July 20, 1899.

74.   we want Teddy.": Corinne Roosevelt Robinson, *My Brother Theodore Roosevelt*, 197.

74.   more than half of the states in the Union.: Morris, *The Rise of Theodore Roosevelt*, 769.

75.   persuasion was usually enough for TR.: Paul Grondahl, *I Rose Like a Rocket: The Political Education of Theodore Roosevelt*, 3.

76.   and necessary sanitary conditions.": Morris, *The Rise of Theodore Roosevelt*, 19.

76.   "unreasonable and abnormal extent.": Charles Moore and the United States President, *Restoration of the White House: Message of the President of the United States Transmitting the Report of the Architects* (Washington: Government Printing Office, 1903), 8.

76.   than Washington had ever anticipated.: Gilson Willets, *Inside History of the White House: the Complete History of the Domestic and Official Life In Washington of the Nation's Presidents And Their Families* (New York: The Christian herald, 1908), 48.

76.   members of the profession of architecture.": Moore and the US president, *Restoration of the White House*, 9.

77.   and a room for the press.: Moore and the US president, 11.

77.   playing background and a screen.": A. Wallis Myers, *The Complete Lawn Tennis Player* (Philadelphia: G.W. Jacobs & Co., 1908), 39–40.

77.   that the president needed to watch his weight.: "Perhaps Edith had read about his prodigious eating..." Edmund Morris, *Theodore Rex*, 236.

77.   getting fat," he wrote as the court was being built.: Theodore Roosevelt to Theodore Roosevelt Jr., October 31, 1902.

78.   found at nearby country clubs.: *Washington Post*, December 15, 1907.

78. reported matter-of-factly in his *Autobiography*.: Theodore Roosevelt, *The Autobiography of Theodore Roosevelt: Condensed from the original edition, supplemented by letters, speeches, and other writings, and edited with an introduction by Wayne Andrews* (New York: Charles Scribner's Sons, 1959), 32.

78. wrote in a typical update to Kermit.: Theodore Roosevelt to Kermit Roosevelt, May 14, 1905, Theodore Roosevelt Papers.

78. I beat Ted and Church two deuce sets.": Letter from Theodore Roosevelt to Kermit Roosevelt, December 4, 1904. Theodore Roosevelt Collection, Harvard University.

79. "leader of all sports among the young girls.": *Wilkes-Barre News*, February 2, 1902.

79. and athletics sports," the paper concluded.: *Washington Times*, February 17, 1906.

79. the dash of her father and brothers.": *Atlanta Constitution*, September 29, 1907; *Tampa Tribune*, March 18, 1906.

79. *New York Times* picked up on the story.: *New York Times*, April 27, 1903.

80. used at the Potomac Speedway.: *Washington Post*, April 25, 1903.

80. carnival of graft and extravagance.": In *Outlook*, April 9, 1904.

80. on the White House grounds.": "Is the President Extravagant?" *Outlook*, 76.15 (April 9, 1904), 868.

80. article into the congressional record.: *Congressional Record*, House of Representatives, April 25, 1904, 5575–5576.

80. strung with good quality of cat gut.": "The Court and its Mission," *Puck*, 61.1577 (May 22, 1907), 11.

81. And golf is fatal.": Stephen R. Lowe, *Sir Walter and Mr. Jones: Walter Hagan, Bobby Jones, and the Rise of American Golf* (Chelsea, MI: Sleeping Bear Press, 2000), 4.

81. the back-screen of a tennis court...": William Bayard Hale, *A Week in the White House with Theodore Roosevelt: A Study of the President at the Nation's Business* (New York: G.P. Putnam's Sons, 1908), 9.

82. stopping on account of the elements.: Letter from Archie Butt to Pamela R. B. Butt Mother, June 16, 1908, in *The Letters of Archie Butt*, 37.

82. whose tastes are similar to his own.": *Sporting Life*, July 8, 1905.

83. Leslie Shaw was a horseman.: *Sporting Life*, July 8, 1905.

83. later the Tennis Cabinet.: Harold Pinkett, "The Keep Commission, 1905-1909: A Rooseveltian Effort for Administrative Reform," *Journal of American History*, Vol. 52, No. 2 (September 1965), 297–312; *Detroit Free Press*, November 25, 1906.

83. or in the ranch country.": UPI, March 1, 1909.

84. several of the men kidded as they left the White House.: Jusserand, *What Me Befell*, 331.

85. receive a silver cup like Bacon.": Jusserand, 332.

85. shows you wherein you are wrong.": *Sun* (New York), November 25, 1906.

85. put somebody else in your place.": *Citizen* (Howard, KS), March 29, 1905.

85. Mr. Garfield's play," Roosevelt said.: *Baltimore Sun*, May 25, 1906.

85. invitation to the White House court.: *Springville Journal*, January 3, 1907.

86. in the United States (*What Me Befell: The Reminiscences of J.J. Jusserand*).: Jean Jules Jusserand, *A Literary History of the English People* (New York: G.P. Putnam's Sons, 1926); Jean Jules Jusserand, *What to Expect of Shakespeare* (London: British Academy, 1911); Jean Jules Jusserand, *With Americans of Past and Present Days* (New York: Scribner's Sons, 1916); Jean Jules Jusserand, *What Me Befell: The Reminiscences of J.J. Jusserand* (Boston: Houghton Mifflin Co., 1933).

86. he received transfer to the United States.: Jean Jules Jusserand, *Les sports et jeux d'exercise dans l'ancienne France* (Paris: Plon-Nourrit et Cie., 1901).

87. devotee of the lost art of walking.": Jusserand Memorial Committee, *Jean Jules Jusserand*, 28.

87. if I could lend it to him.": Jusserand Memorial Committee, *Jean Jules Jusserand*, 41.

87. became one of the Tennis cabinet…": National Geographic Society, *Souvenir Record of Testimonial Dinner Given in Honor of the Ambassador of France and Madame Jules Jean Jusserand: By the People of the City of Washington, January 10, 1925* (Washington: Press of Judd & Detweiler, 1925), 41.

87. for the anniversary of the "cession.": Jules Jean Jusserand, *What Me Befell: The Reminiscences of J.J. Jusserand* (Boston: Houghton Mifflin Co., 1934), 244.

87. I'd like to lie down and die.": *Evening Star* (Washington DC), April 4, 1906; Paul F. Boller, *Presidential Anecdotes* (New York: Oxford University Press, 1996), 194–195.

87. but played very hard.": *Tennis* (April 1976), 31.

87. National Tennis Tournament at Newport.": W. Draper Lewis, *The Life of Theodore Roosevelt* (Published for the United Publishers of the United States and Canada, 1919), 170.

88. his sweater and his heavy trousers.": *Washington Post*, December 15, 1907.

88. neither new nor fashionable.": Myers, *The Complete Lawn Tennis Player*, 40.

88. simple for a competent player.: Myers, 40.

89. doing anything is to do it hard.": Edmund Morris, *Theodore Rex*, 529.

89. sports-obsessed American's view of diplomatic history.: See, *Sports Illustrated*, October 15, 1990, http://www.si.com/vault/1990/10/15/122886/the-ultimate-tennis-club-in-washington-the-white-house-is-the-place-to-play.

89. provided a multitude of distractions.: Arthur F. Winnington Ingram, *The Call of the Father* (New York: Thomas Whittaker, 1907), 2.

89. a few tennis players to boast of.": *Washington Post*, September 28, 1907.

90. bishop departs for his native shores.: *Washington Post*, September 28, 1907.

91. didn't sound very Rooseveltian at all.: Benjamin Rader, *American Sports: From the Digital Age of Folk Games to the Age of Televised Sports* (Upper Saddle River, NJ: Pearson Prentice Hall, 2009), 196.

92. insult on the class front.: *Los Angeles Times*, March 28, 1999.

92. women could compete.: Alan Guttmann, *A History of Women's Sports* (New York: Columbia University Press, 1991), 124.

92. control over the sporting world.": Susan Cahn, *Coming on Strong: Gender and Sexuality in Twentieth-Century Women's Sport* (Cambridge: Harvard University Press, 1994), 30.

92. *Chicago Tribune* reported, matter of factly.: *Chicago Tribune*, February 11, 1906.

FIVE: CREATING THE ROOSEVELT ATHLETIC LEAGUE

93. girls' branch resemble the boys.": *Evening World* (New York), January 26, 1906.

94. who knew how to get things done.: *Brooklyn Life*, February 22, 1898. Many years later in a moving obituary, Wingate was described as a "great citizen" of Brooklyn. "He was so active, alert and youthful in his point of view up to almost the end of his earthly sojourn, that in spite of his years his friends were as little prepared for it as though he had been many years younger and he was so far from having outlived his usefulness as a man of affairs that the loss to the community was far more than a sentimental one." *Brooklyn Life and Activities of Long Island*, March 31, 1928.

94. Edward M. Shepard and many others.": George W. Wingate to Theodore Roosevelt, August 16, 1905.

95.   the powerful Guggenheim family.: Edmund Morris, *Theodore Rex*, 29.

95.   school-based athletics moving forward.: Robert Pruter, *The Rise of America High School Sports and the Search for Control, 1880–1930* (New York: Syracuse University Press, 2013), 32–45, 47, 67.

96.   presented the Junior Basketball Trophy.: Crampton and Emanuel, *The Official Handbook of the Public Schools Athletic League, New York City*, 152–167.

96.   *work, and full of promise."*: Jacob Riis to Theodore Roosevelt, August 15, 1905.

96.   during this Progressive period.: Nell Irvin Painter, *Standing at Armageddon, The United States, 1877–1919* (New York: W.W. Norton and Co., 1987), xii.

97.   continent, but overseas as well.": Crampton and Emanuel, *The Official Handbook of the Public Schools Athletic League, New York City*, 13; Pruter, *The Rise of American High School Sports and the Search for Control*, 68–70.

97.   up from 25 percent in 1870.: Steven A. Riess, *Sport in Industrial America, 1850–1920* (Malden, MA: Wiley-Blackwell, 2013), 14.

97.   powerful corporations than ever before.: Painter, *Standing at Armageddon*, 177.

97.   opportunities for their own development.": Luther Halsey Gulick and Wm. C.J. Kelly (eds), *Official Handbook of the Public Schools Athletic League* (New York: American Sports Publishing Company, 1904), 11.

97.   back to the 1850s in Europe.: Clifford Putney, *Muscular Christianity: Manhood and Sports in Protestant American, 1880–1920* (Cambridge, MA: Harvard University Press, 2001), 11.

98.   "establishment of institutional control.": Robert Pruter, *The Rise of America High School Sports and the Search for Control, 1880–1930* (New York: Syracuse University Press, 2013).

98.   nonacademic change in American children.: Technically, the PSAL existed outside of the New York City school system. "This work cannot be done by the existing school organization…and yet because of the very close relation of the work to the schools, it has been thought desirable that this organization should be initiated by those who are close to the school work." Athletics would complement classroom work. As plans unfolded, it became clear that the support of teachers, mostly on an unpaid basis, would be necessary to carry out the plans of the PSAL. Athletics became another opportunity—and another responsibility—for school teachers. Luther Halsey Gulick and Wm. C.J. Kelly (eds), *Official Handbook of the Public Schools Athletic League* (New York: American Sports Publishing Company, 1904), 11.

98.   into vigorous athletic sports.": Luther Halsey Gulick, MD, *Health of School Children, Statement of the Endeavors of the Board of Education to Conserve the Health of Children Under Its Care* (New York: William Wood & Co., 1906), 21.

99.   1908–1909: 7,049: Crampton and Emanuel, *The Official Handbook of the Public Schools Athletic League, New York City*, 89.

99.   compared to European children.: Patricia A. Eisenman and C. Robert Barnett, "Physical Fitness in the 1950s and 1970s: Why did One Fail and the Other Boom?" *Question*, Vol. 31, No. 1 (March 1979), 114–115.

100. but on a national scale.: Newsletter, *President's Council on Physical Fitness and Sports*, Vol. 5, No. 2 (August 1968); President's Council on Physical Fitness and Sports, *The Presidential Fitness Award Program, Instructor's Guide* (Washington, DC, 1986).

100. endurance, strength, speed, and agility.: *The Presidential Fitness Award Program, Instructor's Guide*, 3–6.

101. and a brief congratulatory message.": *The Presidential Fitness Award Program, Instructor's Guide*, 5–16.

102. my sit-n-reach to defeat ISIS.": "The Sad, Sad Stories of the Presidential Fitness Test," *SB Nation*, accessed February 22, 2018, https://www.sbnation.com/2015/7/31/9038201/the-sad-sad-stories-of-the-presidential-fitness-test.

103. **a large part of this activity.":** Luther Gulick, *Physical Education by Muscular Exercise* (Philadelphia: P. Blakiston's Son & Co., 1904), 4.

103. **direct the form of play.":** Luther Halsey Gulick, *A Philosophy of Play* (New York: C. Scribner's Sons, 1920), v.

103. **rich efficient life is an end.":** Luther Gulick, *The Efficient Life* (New York: Doubleday, Page & Co., 1907), xv.

103. **Oberlin College in Ohio in 1880.:** Ethel Josephine Dorgan, *Luther Halsey Gulick, 1865–1918* (New York City: Teachers College, Columbia University, 1934), 1.

104. **buildings" made from Ohio sandstone.:** Geoffrey Blodgett, "Oberlin College Architecture: A Short History," http://www2.oberlin.edu/external/EOG/gbslides/AShortHistory.html.

104. **a stop on the Underground Railroad.:** Nat Brandt, *The Town that Started the Civil War* (Syracuse, NY: Syracuse University Press, 1990).

104. **quality-efficiency," he concluded.:** Luther Gulick, *The Efficient Life*, 10.

105. **and physical education instructors.:** *Cambridge Tribune*, Vol. XXXVII, No. 13, May 30, 1914.

105. **enable him to inspire others.":** Dorgan, *Luther Halsey Gulick*, 6. Dudley Sargent struggled, bitterly at times, to explain how a man so scattered, so intellectually adulterous, so ready to depart one task for another accomplished so much. Gulick was an "ardent, impulsive" man, according to Sargent; a man who was "not particularly fond of study; and he hated petty details and all routine work." Additionally, Gulick had the stupefying tendency to start something—a game in a crowded gymnasium for example—then work to get others interested, explain the rules, split up teams, drum up enthusiasm for the contest at hand, and then with all that accomplished, "almost immediately drop it and take up something that furnished more excitement for his playful impulses."

105. **undesirable traits to their offspring.":** Dorgan, *Luther Halsey Gulick*, 8.

106. **uncontrollable desire to experiment.":** Dorgan, *Luther Halsey Gulick*, 18.

106. **throw on the nature of the player?":** Luther Gulick, *A Philosophy of Play* (New York: Scribner's Sons, 1920), xi.

107. **the tendons in his own hand.:** Dorgan, *Luther Halsey Gulick*, 35.

107. **the building blocks to learning.:** Dorgan, *Luther Halsey Gulick*, 65.

109. **fell under the jurisdiction of the PSNYC.:** A. Emerson Palmer, *The New York Public School; Being a History of Free Education in the City of New York* (New York: The Macmillan Company, 1905), 316.

109. **in order to undo Gulick's hire.:** Dorgan, 74.

109. **"without the power of health.":** *Fifth Annual Report of the City Superintendent of Schools to the Board of Education of the City of New York, For the Year Ending July 31, 1903* (New York), 301.

109. **especially for children.:** While this saying became common in the past few years, it's probably not actually true. At least not literally. See, Jeff K. Vallance et al., "Evaluating the Evidence on Sitting, Smoking and Health: Is Sitting Really the New Smoking?" *American Journal of Public Health*, Vol. 108, No. 11 (2018), 1478.

109. **from long sitting at a desk.":** Ibid.

110. **and home hygiene.":** Luther Gulick and Leonard P. Ayres, *Medical Inspection in Schools* (New York: Russell Sage Foundation, reprint, 1917), 70; J. Thomas Jable, "The Public Schools Athletic League of New York City: Organized Athletics for City Schoolchildren, 1903–1914," 217–238; Steven A. Riess (ed), *The American Sporting Experience: A Historical Anthology of Sport in America* (New York: Leisure Press, 1984).

111. **knapsack carried upon the back.":** Department of Education, City of New York, *Sixth Annual Report of City Superintendent of Schools for the Year Ending July 31, 1904* (New York), 261.

111. **Nazis at the 1936 Olympic Games.:** Susan D. Bachrach, *The Nazi Olympics: Berlin 1936* (New York: Little Brown and Company, 2000).

111. **novel race evoked considerable laughter.":** *New York Times*, December 9, 1903.

112. **ever taken place in the United States.":** *New York Times*, December 27, 1903.

112. **fog descended over much of the city.:** *New York Times*, December 27, 1903.

113. **"specially devoted to colored children.":** A. Emerson Palmer, *The New York Public School; Being a History of Free Education in the City of New York* (New York: MacMillan Company, 1905), 141.

113. **abolishing racially segregated schools all together.:** Palmer, *The New York Public School; Being a History of Free Education in the City of New York*, 177–178.

113. **before the start," readers learned.:** *New York Times*, December 27, 1903.

113. **fellows in the track events.":** *New York Times*, December 27, 1903.

114. **auspicious "Indoor Records" heading.:** *New York Times*, December 27, 1903; *Official Handbook of the Public Schools Athletic League*, 56.

115. **behalf will come later on.":** *New York Times*, November 29, 1903.

115. **but the boys I like better.":** *Argus Leader* (Sioux Falls, SD), April 6, 1903.

115. **program was being rolled out.:** *New York Tribune*, November 29, 1905; *Evening World* (New York), January 26, 1906.

115. **participated in twenty athletic events.:** C. Ward Crampton and Emanuel Haug (eds), *The Official Handbook of the Public Schools Athletic League, New York City* (New York: American Sports Publishing Company, 1909), 19–20; *Brooklyn Eagle*, February 6, 1911.

116. **should differ from those of boys.":** *New York Tribune*, November 29, 1905.

116. **nine hundred teachers, in PSAL activities.:** *Brooklyn Eagle*, February 6, 1911.

116. **Roosevelt to Wingate in its entirety.:** The PSAL was so anxious to reprint the letter that George Wingate wrote to Roosevelt's secretary, William Loeb, requesting a new copy of Roosevelt's letter with darker print and "a good black signature." That way the printers could create a strong facsimile. George Wingate to William Loeb, September 6, 1905.

116. **to be a better citizen.":** PSAL, 1905, 17.

117. **and several basketball courts.:** *New York Times*, September 16, 1905.

117. **into comparative insignificance.":** *New York Times*, December 23, 1905.

117. **just as much as the boys.":** Theodore Roosevelt to Ruth Granger, April 26, 1911.

SIX: 1904

119. **under no matter what provocation.":** Theodore Roosevelt to Kermit Roosevelt, April 9, 1904.

119. **not actually been elected to the office.:** Lewis L. Gould, *The Presidency of Theodore Roosevelt* (Lawrence: University of Kansas Press, 1991), x; For more on Roosevelt's innovations with the press, see: Doris Kearns Goodwin, *The Bully Pulpit: Theodore Roosevelt William Howard Taft, and the Golden Age of Journalism* (New York: Simon & Schuster, 2013).

119. **the Roosevelt Corollary to the Monroe Doctrine.:** Roosevelt, *Autobiography*, 210; Typical of this: "His Accidency, President Roosevelt, is fond of parade and gold lace. He has matured a plan to increase the number of handsome young officers in brilliant filigree at his receptions next winter..." *Wilmington Messenger*, April 6, 1904; Four men before Roosevelt had assumed the presidency due to the death (whether by assassination or natural causes) of the president: John Tyler, Millard Fillmore, Andrew Johnson, and Chester Arthur. None were subsequently elected in the own right.

120. **that madman and the Presidency?":** William Horner, *Ohio's Kingmaker: Mark Hanna, Man and Myth* (Ohio University Press, 2010); Theodore Roosevelt to Henry Cabot

Lodge, May 27, 1903, Theodore Roosevelt Papers, Library of Congress Manuscript Division.

120. **if they can prevent my nomination.":** Theodore Roosevelt to Ted Roosevelt, January 29, 1904.

121. **trying to hold Roosevelt back.:** Roosevelt, *Autobiography*, 202.

121. **there were the Democrats.:** Arthur Schlesinger, Jr. (ed), *History of American Presidential Elections, 1789–1968*, Vol. III (New York: Chelsea House Publishers, 1971), 1965–1992.

121. **fire and fury of the Great Commoner.:** Arthur Schlesinger, Jr. (ed), *History of American Presidential Elections, 1789–1968*, 1965.

122. **packed a powerful political punch as well.:** I know that's a lot of alliteration. It happened unintentionally at first; then I couldn't force myself to undo it.

122. **galloping alongside the railroads.:** Dalton, *Theodore Roosevelt*, 241.

122. **was jammed with 2500 spectators.:** Donovan, *The Roosevelt that I Know*, 213.

123. **earlier in Albany," Donovan said.:** Donovan, *The Roosevelt that I Know*, 13.

123. **I had besought him to do so.":** Letter from Theodore Roosevelt to Kermit Roosevelt, January 19, 1905, Theodore Roosevelt Collection. MS Am 1541 (101). Houghton Library, Harvard University.

124. **"he seemed oblivious to all things else.":** William McKinley Mooney, "Boxing Lessons from Theodore Roosevelt," *Leslie's Illustrated Weekly*, Vol. 133, No. 3442 (October 22, 1921), 348.

124. **But don't betray that to a soul.":** Robert Johnstone Mooney, "Boxing and Wrestling with Roosevelt in the White House," *Outing*, October 24, 1923.

124. **to be good at everything.:** *St. Louis Magazine*, accessed November 4, 2018, https://www.stlmag.com/dining/st-louis-style-pizza/.

125. **makes upon progress of man.:** David R. Francis, *The Universal Exposition of 1904* (St. Louis: Louisiana Purchase Exposition Company, 1913), 19–20.

125. **St. Louis planned to outdo them all.:** James B. Gilbert, *Whose Fair? Experience, Memory, and the History of the Great St. Louis Exposition* (Chicago: University of Chicago Press, 2009), 20.

126. **enterprise," and he got to work.:** Francis, *Universal Exposition*, v.

126. **would include more than one thousand buildings.:** Francis, *Universal Exposition*, 46–47.

126. **around $200 million in 2019 dollars.:** *The Piker and World's Fair Guide* (St. Louis: National Publishing Co., 1904), 21.

127. **and an estate in the countryside.:** Allen Guttmann, *The Olympics: A History of the Modern Olympics* (Urbana: University of Illinois Press, 1992), 7.

127. **lost himself in the heroism of *Tom Brown's Schooldays*.:** While separated by an ocean, Roosevelt and Coubertin actually cherished the same book as boys: *Tom Brown's Schooldays*. This bestseller, written by Thomas Hughes and published in 1857, presented a clear, heavy-handed narrative on the usefulness of physical development and aggressiveness. The book sparked an entire genre of schoolboy literature. J.K. Rowling cited the work as an inspiration for her *Harry Potter* series. It touched the malleable souls of both Coubertin and Roosevelt as they stood on the cusp of manhood. In the book, a pivotal cricket match offered a powerful—more powerful than any moment in class or even at church—moment for growing up. "This is worth living for," the team captain preached to his teammates. "The whole sum of school boy existence gathered into one straining, struggling half-hour; a half-hour worth a year of common life."; *The Guardian*, July 9, 1999; Thomas Hughes, *Tom Brown's Schooldays* (London: Walter Scott Publishing, 1857), 99; Guttmann, *The Olympics: A History of the Modern Olympics*, 9.

127. **learned to box, fence, and row.:** Nobert Muller, *Pierre de Coubertin, 1863–1937* (Lausanne: International Olympic Committee, 2000), 24.

128. **opened up new learning opportunities.**: Muller, *Pierre de Coubertin*, 129.

128. **for poorer areas of the city.**: John J. MacAloon, *This Great Symbol: Pierre de Coubertin and the Origins of the Modern Olympic Games* (Chicago: University of Chicago Press, 1981), 127.

128. **doubt its sympathy on this occasion.":** Pierre de Coubertin to Theodore Roosevelt, November 15, 1901.

128. **Honorary President at the Chicago Olympian Games.":** Theodore Roosevelt to Pierre de Coubertin, December 7, 1901.

129. **leadership of the Paris games of 1900.":** Pierre de Coubertin to Theodore Roosevelt, December 23, 1901; Theodore Roosevelt to Pierre de Coubertin, January 9, 1902; October 4, 1902.

129. **his desire for Roosevelt's support.**: Pierre Coubertin to Theodore Roosevelt, June 2, 1903.

133. **as well as ride and swim.":** Theodore Roosevelt to Pierre de Coubertin, June 15, 1903.

133. **stealing the Olympics from Chicago.**: There is a long and sordid tale here. For more see, George Matthews, *America's First Olympics*, 14; Theodore Roosevelt to William R. Harper, Charles R. Crane, John Barton Payne, LaVerne W. Noyes, and Henry J. Furber, May 28, 1902; John E. Findling, "Chicago Loses the 1904 Olympics," *Journal of Olympic History*, Vol. 12 (October 2004), 27.

133. **were delayed until 1905?:** Matthews, 30.

133. **shared the hosting duties of a 1904 Olympiad? :** The Chicago Cubs and St. Louis Cardinals maintain one of the best, most widely appreciated, rivalries in United States sports culture. The clubs compete regularly as members of the National League Central Division in Major League Baseball. The two Midwest teams have played more than 2,300 games against each other. The regular season records reflect an amazing parity; the Cubs have won 51% of the contests. But, in the all-important category of World Series titles, St. Louis has hammered its Chicago rivals. The Cardinals have eleven World Series titles, the Cubs have just three. Whatever true animosity exists between the cities (it's always difficult to assess the true impact of a sports rivalry beyond the newspapers and stands) can be connected back to 1904 to a certain extent. In that election year, Chicago hosted the Republican National Convention. St. Louis welcomed the Democrats. Then the two cities tussled over control of the Olympic Games. Business leaders from both cities made expensive bids to get and hold onto the Games.

134. **on physical health and training.**: Louisiana Purchase Exposition Company Collection, Executive Committee Meeting Minutes, 1269. Missouri History/Archives.

134. **very few things were left out.**: *Universal Exposition Saint Louis, 1904, Programme of Olympic Games and World Championship Contests* (Saint Louis: Department of Physical Culture, 1904), 3; Louisiana Purchase Exposition Company Collection, Executive Committee Meeting Minutes, 1269. Missouri History/Archives, 1520.

134. ***working* presidency," he made clear.**: Theodore Roosevelt to James E. Sullivan, March 15, 1904.

134. **conquered by the United States.**: Charles J.P. Lucas, *The Olympic Games, 1904* (St. Louis, MO: Woodward & Tieran Printing Co., 1905), 17.

135. **was the twenty-four-plus mile marathon.**: The current distance, 26.2 miles, was not codified until the 1908 Games in London.

135. **wrote a firsthand account of the Olympic Games.**: Charles J.P. Lucas, *The Olympic Games, 1904* (St. Louis, MO: Woodward & Tieran Printing Co., 1905), 17–20.

137. **for perpetrating an athletic fraud.**: Despite a story in recent years in the *Los Angeles Times* (August 10, 2010), *Smithsonian Magazine*, *Time Magazine* (July 24, 2012), and other publications, Alice Roosevelt was not on hand to nearly crown Lorz champion. This myth

begun it seems by Bill Henry's *An Approved History of the Olympics* (Southern California Committee, 1984).

138. **and all in the archery competition.**: *St. Louis Republican*, September 25, 1904; International Olympic Committee, "Factsheet Women in the Olympic Movement," https://stillmed.olympic.org/Documents/Reference_documents_Factsheets/Women_in_Olympic_Movement.pdf.

138. **teams would never have it so good.**: Mark Dyreson, *Making the American Team: Sport, Culture, and the Olympic Experience* (Urbana: University of Illinois Press, 1997).

138. **victory," the *Los Angeles Times* concluded.**: *Los Angeles Times*, November 9, 1904.

138. **stress for Roosevelt's Republicans.**: "Republicans Lasso the Nation," the disappointed *Atlanta Constitution* reported; *Atlanta Constitution*, November 9, 1904.

138. **SAYS HE WILL NOT RUN AGAIN.**: *New York Times*, November 9, 1904.

139. **the machinery building, the electricity building.**: *St. Louis Post-Dispatch*, November 26, 1904.

139. **I cannot possibly do both."**: *New York Times*, February 21, 1980.

140. **emblematic of the AAU of the US."**: James E. Sullivan to Theodore Roosevelt, July 15, 1904, Theodore Roosevelt Collection, Harvard University, Olympics Subject File.

140. **any idea that I was at all lame."**: Letter, Theodore Roosevelt to Kermit Roosevelt, November 29, 1904, *Letters to Kermit from Theodore Roosevelt* (New York: Charles Scribner's Sons, 1946).

140. **Officials worried about the weather.**: *Washington Post*, March 3, 1905.

140. **unelected president of the United States.**: Donovan, *The Roosevelt that I Know*, 17–19.

SEVEN: TED'S DANGEROUS FOOTBALL ADVENTURE

142. **"would not sign such a petition."**: Theodore Roosevelt to Charles W. Eliot, April 4, 1904, *The Letters of Theodore Roosevelt*, 767.

142. **one Eliot biographer noted, diplomatically.**: Henry James, *Charles W. Eliot, President of Harvard University 1869–1909* (New York: Houghton Mifflin Company, 1930), 767.

142. **substitute or something of that kind."**: Roosevelt scribbled in "or even the second" as an addendum to the typed letter.

143. **in the Roosevelt family library.**: Robert W. Walker, *The Namesake: A Biography of Theodore Roosevelt, Jr.* (New York: Brick Tower Press), 17.

143. **"small, nervous, grim, pug-ugly" boy.**: Edmund Morris, *Theodore Rex*, 252.

143. **time we were very, very small."**: In *The Namesake*, NEED TO GET ORIGINAL.

144. **but he wouldn't disgrace me."**: John J. Leary, *Talks with TR, from the Diaries of John J. Leary* (Boston: Houghton Mifflin Co., 1920), 233–234.

145. **live up to his father's expectations."**: Walker, *The Namesake*, 29.

145. **great temptation to push him."**: Walker, 29.

145. **into a curriculum at Groton.**: Eric Burns, *The Golden Lad: The Haunting Story of Quentin and Theodore Roosevelt* (New York: Pegasus Books, 2016), 92; Dalton, *A Strenuous Life*, 89.

145. **reported in November 1900.**: Theodore Roosevelt to ES Martin, November 22, 1900, *Theodore Roosevelt's Letters to His Children*, Joseph Bucklin Bishop, ed. (New York: Charles Scribner's Sons, 1919), 18.

146. **non-football player, just as the boys did."**: Frank Ashburn, *Peabody of Groton, A Portrait* (New York: Coward McCann, Inc, 1944), 100; For a more general study of sport and boarding schools, see: Axel Bundgaard, *Muscle and Manliness: The Rise of Sport in American Boarding Schools* (New York: Syracuse University Press, 2005).

146. **yesterday," he wrote TR in 1903.**: Kermit Roosevelt to Theodore Roosevelt, October 11, 1903.

146. **Lowell Textile, and Rindge Manual.**: *The Grotonian*, Vol. XXII, (November 1905).

146. **from losing its original beauty."**: Letter from Endicott Peabody to Theodore Roosevelt, January 11, 1902, Theodore Roosevelt Papers, Library of Congress Manuscript Division. http://www.theodorerooseveltcenter.org/Research/Digital-Library/Record.aspx?lib ID=o36670. Theodore Roosevelt Digital Library. Dickinson State University.

147. **—Your loving Ted."**: Letter from Theodore Roosevelt, Jr to Theodore Roosevelt, undated, Theodore Roosevelt, Jr. Papers, Library of Congress.

147. **to make the game a bit safer.**: John Watterson, *College Football: History, Spectacle, Controversy* (Baltimore: The Johns Hopkins University Press, 2000), 60–62.

148. **good by [sic] your loving Ted."**: Ted Roosevelt to Theodore Roosevelt, October 1903, Theodore Roosevelt Jr. Papers, Library of Congress.

149. **dangerous to the Romans?" TR asked.**: Theodore Roosevelt to Ted Roosevelt, October 4, 1903, *A Bully Father: Theodore Roosevelt's Letters to His Children* (New York: Random House, 1995), 126–128.

149. **second squad instead of the third."**: Theodore Roosevelt to Ted Roosevelt, October 4, 1903, *A Bully Father: Theodore Roosevelt's Letters to His Children* (New York: Random House, 1995), 129.

150. **mine by Sire George Trevelyan."**: It was hard to be this man's namesake. It was Ted's lifetime and posthumous burden. After all, Edmund Morris, Roosevelt's biographer extraordinaire, summed up teenage Ted as having "all of his father's purposeful force, but imagination and intellect were denied him;" Edmund Morris, *Theodore Rex*, 251–252; Theodore Roosevelt to Ted Roosevelt, November 28, 1903, *Theodore Roosevelt's Letters to His Children* (New York: Charles Scribner's Sons, 1919), 80.

150. **finished the game" with grit.**: Morris, 252.

150. **none of them actually does."**: Theodore Roosevelt to Henry Beach Needham, July 19, 1905, *The Letters of Theodore Roosevelt*, Vol. 4 (Cambridge: Harvard University Press, 1951), 1281.

151. **and settled career in life."**: Theodore Roosevelt to Theodore Roosevelt, Jr., in Robert Walker, *The Namesake*, 45.

152. **more than thirty thousand fans for big games.**: Ingrassia, *The Rise of Gridiron University*, 139–143; Ronald A. Smith, "Commercialized Intercollegiate Athletics and the 1903 Stadium," *The New England Quarterly*, Vol. 78, No. 1 (March 2005), 42–44.

152. **best and is most fit for."**: James, *Charles Eliot*, 230.

152. **than being rendered obsolete by it.**: James, *Charles Eliot*, 184–196.

152. **institution profited from greatly.**: To put this in modern context, if the president of the University of Alabama came out as an advocate for football abolition today, it would create a firestorm of interest because of the very gains UA experiences each fall when the Nick Saban-led Tide roll to victory after victory.

153. **and outlawing coaching salaries.**: Smith, *Pay for Play*, 24.

153. **was roughly as dangerous as crew.**: Walter Camp, *Football Facts and Figures: A Symposium of Expert Opinions on the Game's Place in American Athletics* (New York: Harper & Brothers, 1894), vii–vix.

154. **to younger players as well.**: Henry Beach Needham, "The College Athlete: How Commercialism is Making Him a Professional," *McClure's Magazine* 25 (June 1905), 115–128; and "The College Athlete: His Amateur Code: Its Evasion and Administration," *McClure's Magazine* 25 (July 1905), 260–272.

154. **calls for immediate treatment."**: Endicott Peabody to Theodore Roosevelt, September 16, 1905, Library of Congress.

155. **reforms could be agreed upon.**: For one of the earliest scholarly treatments of Roosevelt's role in football reform (and one that has stood the test of time), see Guy Lewis, "Theodore Roosevelt's Role in the 1905 Football Controversy," *Research Quarterly*, Vol, 40, No, 4 (1969), 717–724.

155. **rain in the forecast.**: *Washington Post*, October 9, 1905.

155. **have mucker [dirty] play."**: Theodore Roosevelt to Kermit Roosevelt.

155. **view," before heading for the White House).**: Smith, *Big-Time Football at Harvard, The Diary of Bill Reid*, 193.

155. **rules, for that will help."**: Miller, *The Big Scrum*, 187–188.

156. **heavy close formation plays."**: *Philadelphia Inquirer*, October 10, 1905.

156. **had happened in previous years."**: Smith, *Big-Time Football at Harvard, The Diary of Bill Reid*, 194.

157. **the action would open up.**: Julie Des Jardins, *Walter Camp: Football and the Modern Man* (New York: Oxford University Press, 2015), 176–181.

157. **because he had an injured ankle.**: Smith, *Big-Time Football at Harvard, 1905*, 194.

157. **"football confab" to continue.**: *Hartford Courant*, October 10, 1905.

157. **an agreement on the matter."**: Smith, *Big-Time Football at Harvard, 1905*, 194.

158. **characterized as a "little meeting?"**: Miller, *The Big Scrum*, 189.

158. **to this matter than anything else."**: Smith, *Big-Time Football at Harvard, 1905*, 195.

159. **Yale met Harvard as an equal?"**: *The Harvard Graduates' Magazine*, Vol. 14 (1905–1906), 218.

159. **or regulate, or purify athletics."**: *The Harvard Graduates' Magazine*, Vol. 14 (1905–1906), 218.

159. **change in the rules next year."**: *Hartford Courant*, October 12, 1905.

159. **to abide by whatever you do."**: Theodore Roosevelt to Walter Camp, October 11, 1905, Theodore Roosevelt Papers, Library of Congress.

160. **of a nervous temperament."**: This was a syndicated article and image that appeared in newspapers across the country but not in the major dailies. The October 10 report seems to have been a reconfigured version of an October 4, 1905, *Pittsburgh Press* article with a newly acquired image added. The story and image persisted for several months. See: *Pittsburgh Press*, October 4, 1905; *Wilkes-Barre Times Leader*, October 10, 1905; *Spokane Press*, October 10, 1905; *Union Leader* (Wilkes-Barre, PA), October 10, 1905; *Alexandria Times-Tribune* (Alexandria, IN), November 8, 1905; *Star and Enterprise* (Newville, PA), November 8, 1905; *Fairmount News* (Fairmount, IN), December 13, 1905; *Covina Argus* (Covina, CA), December 16, 1905.

160. **1894's *System of Phrenology*.**: Mattieu Williams, *A Vindication of Phrenology* (Chatto & Windus, 1894), 49–50.

160. **eagerly waiting for you."**: Theodore Roosevelt to Ted Roosevelt, October 2, 1905.

161. **his work in a determined fashion."**: *Boston Globe*, October 5, 1905.

161. **wrote to Kermit on October 17, 1905.**: Theodore Roosevelt to Kermit Roosevelt, October 17, 1905, Theodore Roosevelt Papers, Library of Congress.

161. **read the widely distributed story.**: *Boston Globe*, October 29, 1905.

161. **honor of the family all right!"**: Theodore Roosevelt to Ted Roosevelt, November 1, 1905.

161. **as well as offensive play."**: *Harvard Crimson*, November 13, 1905.

162. **yet," he informed his father.**: Ted Roosevelt to Theodore Roosevelt, undated, Theodore Roosevelt Jr. Papers, Library of Congress.

163. **a member of a "second eleven."**: *Harvard Crimson*, November 18, 1905.

163. **Young Roosevelt will be at Left End for Harvard Freshman.**: *Pittsburgh Press*, November 18, 1905.

163. **Harvard had failed to score.**: *Harvard Crimson*, November 18, 1905.

164. On the defense the Harvard team was weak.": *Harvard Crimson*, November 20, 1905.
164. earned his opponent's respect.: *Washington Post*, November 19, 1905.
164. dragged him along with them.": *Washington Post*, November 19, 1905; *Boston Daily Globe*, November 19, 1905.
165. he arose and played on.: *Washington Post*, November 19, 1905.
165. done for the day.: *Washington Post*, November 19, 1905.
166. improve upon it a little now.": Theodore Roosevelt to Ted Roosevelt, November 19, 1905.
166. family credit in great shape.": Theodore Roosevelt to Ted Roosevelt, November 27, 1905.
166. So there was that.: *New York Times*, November 25, 1905.
166. kept by the *Chicago Daily Tribune*.: *Chicago Daily Tribune*, November 26, 1905.
167. pain at all," he told his mother.: Ted Roosevelt to Edith Roosevelt, November 21, 1905.
167. the position of class president.: *Washington Times*, November 20, 1905.
167. is strenuous," the press reported.: *Washington Times*, November 20, 1905; *Washington Post*, November 21, 1905; *Pittsburgh Press*, November 20, 1905.
167. mercifully, gave up football.: Walker, *The Namesake*, 38, 47, 49, 52.
168. look to the rest of the world.: Ingrassia, *The Rise of Gridiron University*, 57.
168. Intercollegiate Athletic Association of the United States (IAAUS).: "1905 Harvard Football File," *Harvard University Archives*; Ingrassia, *The Rise of Gridiron University*, 58.
169. Quill–Burr matter be kept confidential.: Watterson, *College Football*, 70–72.
170. beyond the first decade of the twentieth century.: John S. Watterson, "Political Football: Theodore Roosevelt, Woodrow Wilson and the Gridiron Reform Movement," *Presidential Studies Quarterly*, Vol. 25, No. 3 (Summer 1995), 555–564.

EIGHT: "WALKING"

171. Ethel and Edith at the Episcopal Eye and Ear Hospital.: Excellent, I know.
171. it to his bedridden daughter.: Theodore Roosevelt to Kermit Roosevelt, October 27, 1907, Theodore Roosevelt Papers.
172. front, on the left side.: Christian F. Reisner, *Roosevelt's Religion* (New York: The Abingdon Press, 1922), 248, 334. Most of the nation's press, including the *Washington Post*, reported that Roosevelt attended church on his birthday. Roosevelt's own letter to Kermit insinuates the same. Several Washington newspapers, however, reported that Roosevelt actually skipped church on his birthday, choosing instead to work for a few hours.
172. and yells about me.": Theodore Roosevelt to Kermit Roosevelt, October 27, 1907, Theodore Roosevelt Papers.
173. the fight against extra pounds.: *Washington Post*, October 28, 1907; *New York Times*, October 28, 1907.
173. good physically by the trip.": *Washington Herald*, October 28, 1907.
174. tramp through the rain.": *Washington Times*, October 28, 1907.
174. diplomatic work could wait.: Edward Van Every, *Muldoon, The Solid Man of Sport; His Amazing Story as Related for the First Time by him to his Friend, Edward Van Every* (New York: Frederick A. Stokes, 1929), 285; *New York Times*, September 9, 1907.
174. better in my life.": *Washington Post*, May 23, 1907.
174. you had to swim it.": Speech to Recreation Congress, October 19, 1926, as quoted in Robert W. Walker, *The Namesake*, 20.
175. one contemporary described it.: James Morgan, *Theodore Roosevelt: The Boy and the Man* (New York: Grosset & Dunlap, 1919), 227.
175. if it came in our way.": Roosevelt, *Autobiography*, 32.

175. **that I could hardly stand.":** Percy Sykes, *The Right Honourable Sir Mortimer Durand: A Biography* (Lahore: Al-Biruni, 1977), 275.

175. **of walking, riding, etc.":** Theodore Roosevelt to Henry John Elwes, August 10, 1903, Theodore Roosevelt Papers, Library of Congress.

175. **stopped asking altogether.:** Theodore Roosevelt to Hermann Speck von Sternburg, May 13, 1904.

176. **the assistant secretary of the Navy.:** John S.D. Eisenhower, *Teddy Roosevelt and Leonard Wood: Partners in Command* (Columbia: University of Missouri Press, 2014), 21.

176. **along the cliffs," Roosevelt said.:** Roosevelt, *Autobiography*, 33.

176. **wrote one White House reporter.:** Gilson Willets, *Inside History of the White House: The Complete History of the Domestic and Official Life in Washington of the Nation's Presidents and their Families* (New York: The Christian Herald, 1908), 395–396.

177. **rocks in the bed of the creek.":** Murray, *Introduction to the Strenuous Life*, 6.

177. **thorns, and the rest.":** Jusserand, *What Me Befell*, 332.

178. **made with human legs.:** Murray, *Introduction to the Strenuous Life*, 7–8.

178. **asked me to a 'walk.'":** Murray, 329.

179. **"the gospel of walking.":** Jim Reisler, *Walk of Ages: Edward Payson Weston's Extraordinary 1909 Trek Across America* (Lincoln: University of Nebraska Press, 2015), 8; *Weston and his Walks; Souvenir Programme of the Great Transcontinental Walk, Ocean to Ocean in Ninety Days* (Walter H. Moles, 1910).

180. **whole world heard about it.:** Matthew Algeo, *Pedestrianism: When Watching People Walk Was America's Favorite Spectator Sport* (Chicago: Chicago Review Press, 2014).

180. **chance of breaking the record.:** *New York Times*, December 26, 1896; *New York Times*, December 27, 1896; *Sun* (New York), December 27, 1896.

180. **apologized to his onlookers.:** Reiser, *Walk of Ages*, 101.

181. **can beat my former record.":** *Boston Globe*, October 30, 1907.

181. **Walking will cure all.":** Quoted in Reisler, *Walk of Ages*, 100.

181. **an athlete if he tries.":** *Buffalo Commercial*, November 14, 1907.

182. **the *Chicago Tribune* reported.:** *Chicago Tribune*, November 27, 1907.

182. **walker went back inside.:** *Chicago Tribune*, November 28, 1907.

183. **the serious pedestrian class.:** *Buffalo Commercial*, November 14, 1907.

183. **desist, which they all did.":** Jusserand, *What Me Befell*, 333.

184. **shoreline of the Potomac River.:** Roosevelt, *Autobiography*, 47.

184. **craggy, sharp shoreline.:** John C. Reed, Robert S. Sigafoos, and George W. Fisher, *The River and the Rocks: The Geologic Story of Great Falls and the Potomac River Gorge* (Washington, DC: US Geological Survey Bulletin 1471, 1980), 13.

184. **the terrain "with horror.":** Jusserand, *What Me Befell*, 335.

185. **like again," Camp concluded.:** James Scott Brown, *Robert Bacon, Life and Letters* (New York: Doubleday, Page & Co., 1923), 29.

185. **men clamoring up first.:** Jusserand, *What Me Befell*, 335.

185. **thoroughly enjoy it.":** Roosevelt, *Autobiography*, 45–50.

186. **forgotten your gloves?":** Jusserand, *What Me Befell*, 335.

186. **greasy mud.":** Jusserand, *What Me Befell*, 335.

NINE: BASEBALL'S GREAT ROOSEVELT CHASE

188. **delight of Nationals fans.:** In 2013, the Nationals added William H. Taft to the mascot race.

188. **Teddy doesn't win.":** https://dcist.com/story/18/09/05/racing-presidents-oral-history/.

189. nor has he ever been.": *Evening Star* (Washington, DC), September 30, 1907; *Baltimore Sun*, May 7, 1906.

189. large measure of brains.": *Spalding's Official Base Ball Guide for 1903*, 283.

189. with the National Pastime.: *Spalding's Official Base Ball Guide for 1903*, 367.

190. "Czar of Baseball.": Eugene Murdock, *Ban Johnson: Czar of baseball* (New York: Praeger, 1982).

190. weaned on an icicle.: Joe Santry and Cindy Thomson, "Ban Johnson," *Society for American Baseball Research*, https://sabr.org/bioproj/person/dabf79f8.

190. whole bunch to the game.": *Sporting Life*, April 21, 1906.

190. a pass laced with gold.: *Washington Post*, April 6, 1906.

190. at the grounds in the capital.": *Sporting Life*, April 28, 1906.

191. party" at American League Park.: *Washington Post*, April 8, 1906.

191. the team," Sullivan crowed.: James E. Sullivan, *The Olympic Games at Athens, 1906* (New York: American Sports Publishing Company, 1906), 45.

191. Rough Rider-baseball connection.: Henry Chadwick (ed), *Spalding's Official Base Ball Guide for 1905* (New York: American Sports Publishing Co., 1905), 26–27.

191. foot ball fields of America.'": *Spalding's Official Base Ball Guide for 1905*, 27.

192. social position may be.": Letter From Theodore Roosevelt to Paul H. Lacey, January 16, 1904, Library of Congress.

192. guided baseball's development.: *Spalding's Official Base Ball Guide for 1906* (New York: American Sports Publishing Co., 1906), 24.

192. opportunities is a mystery.": *Sporting Life*, May 25, 1907.

192. piece of artistic workmanship.": *Sporting Life*, May 25, 1907.

193. perfect physical development.: William B. Mead and Paul Dickson, *Baseball: The President's Game* (New York Farragut Publishing Co., 1993), 17–19.

194. no 'molly coddles.'": *Sporting Life*, May 25, 1907.

194. organized in base ball history.": *Sporting Life*, May 25, 1907.

194. typical game for Americans.": T.H. Murnane, *Official Guide of the National Association of Professional Base Ball Leagues, 1908* (New York: American Sports Publishing Co., 1908), 5.

194. as compliments, sort of.: *Official Guide of the National Association of Professional Base Ball Leagues, 1908*, 5.

194. game during his time as president.: He did, though, greet several baseball clubs at the White House when they came to Washington for their games. And this fit Roosevelt's persona to a certain extent. He enjoyed meeting with most anyone who appeared at his door. His curiosity led him to listen closely to his visitors. Roosevelt appreciated new ideas and information. But with baseball, Roosevelt never came close to investing the same type of attention that he would for most all other sports that had some level of popularity during the period.

195. at all—wearing glasses.: There's a website for this. The top ten glasses wearing ballplayers: William White, Specs Toporcer, Chick Hafey, Clint Courtney, Chris Sabo, Tom Henke, Pete Mikkelsen, Eric Sogard, and Joseph Kelly. Oh and some guy named Reggie Jackson. "Top 10 Professional Baseball Players with Glasses, http://baseballreflections.com/2017/06/23/top-10-professional-baseball-players-glasses/.

195. call "super vision.": Visual Acuity definition according to the American Optometric Association; "Visual Training Gave These Baseball Players Better Vision," *Huffington Post*, https://www.huffingtonpost.com/2015/05/18/visual-training-perfect-vision_n_7306758.html.

195. the game's greatest hitters.: Lou Pavlovich, Jr., "The Baseball Vision of Barry Bonds," *Collegiate Baseball News*, 2014, http://baseballnews.com/the-baseball-vision-of-barry-bonds/.

195. **unlikely mix from the start.**: Roosevelt's exact prescription remains unknown because, despite having dozens of pairs over the course of his lifetime, no pair of his glasses made it into an archival collection. For more on the controversy surrounding TR's vision problems, see: Milton Bruce Shields and Louis Victor Priebe, "Theodore Roosevelt's Vision," *Theodore Roosevelt Association Journal*, Vol. XXXII, No. 4 (Fall 2011), 7–13.

195. **liner of his Rough Rider hat.**: Morris, *The Rise of Theodore Roosevelt*, 667.

195. **haziness during his presidency.**: "Theodore Roosevelt's Vision," 10; Robert van de Berg et al., *Investigative Ophthalmology and Visual Science*, Vol. 49, No. 3 (March 2008), 882–886.

195. **literally rather than metaphorically.**: Edmund Lindop and Joseph Jares, *White House Sportsmen* (Cambridge: Houghton Mifflin Co., 1964).

196. **not even at Harvard."**: William B. Mean, Paul Dickson, *Baseball: The President's Game* (New York: Walker Books, 1997), 20.

196. **"an effeminate man."**: *Atlanta Constitution*, February 28, 1907.

196. **out the window," he said.**: *Los Angeles Times*, October 22, 1934; *The Baseball Almanac*, accessed February 15, 2009, http://www.baseball-almanac.com/prz_qtr.shtml.

197. **"national decadence" of professional sports.**: Theodore Roosevelt, "Professionalism in Sports," *The North American Review*, 1890.

197. **over other people's lives."**: Curt Flood, "Why I am Challenging Baseball," in *The Complete Armchair Book of Baseball*, edited by John Thorn (New York: Galahad Books, 1985).

197. **to play the national game."**: Edmund Lindop and Joseph Jares, *White House Sportsmen* (Cambridge: Houghton Mifflin Co., 1964), 105–106.

197. **otherwise-fine Executive Mansion lawn.**: Eric Burns, *The Golden Lad: The Haunting Story of Quentin and Theodore Roosevelt* (New York: Pegasus Books, 2016).

198. **this deity occasionally.**: Marc Bloch, *The Historian's Craft: Reflections of the Nature and Uses of History and the Techniques and Methods of those Who Write It* (New York: Vintage, 1964).

198. **Pirates of the National League.**: *Boston Globe*, October 1, 1903.

198. **"Baseball Extra" after each game.**: *Boston Globe*, October 3, 1903.

198. **clubs from Pittsburgh and Boston.**: *Louisville Courier-Journal*, October 14, 1903; *San Francisco Call*, October 14, 1903; *Steven's Point Journal*, October 2, 1903.

199. **simply a master pitcher.**: Reed Browning, *Cy Young: A Baseball Life* (Boston: University of Massachusetts Press, 2003).

199. **Leach, an infielder for the Pirates.**: Lawrence S. Ritter, *The Glory of their Times: The Story of the Early Days of Baseball Told by the Men Who Played It* (New York: Perennial, New Enlarged Edition, 2002), 26–27.

200. **and 530 feet to center.**: Roger Abrams, *The First World Series and the Baseball Fanatics of 1903* (Boston: Northeastern University Press, 2003), 16.

200. **on the Boston grounds."**: *New York Times*, October 3, 1903.

201. **without influencing the result."**: *New York Times*, October 4, 1903.

201. **at Pittsburgh's Union Station.**: Abrams, *The First World Series*, 106.

202. **on the day of Game Eight.**: Theodore Roosevelt to William Howard Taft, October 13, 1903, *The Letters of Theodore Roosevelt*, Vol. III, "The Square Deal, 1901–1903," (Cambridge, Harvard University Press, 1951), 619.

203. **all the offense Dineen needed.**: Abrams, *The First World Series*, 166.

203. **in some newspapers.**: *Central New Jersey Home News* (New Brunswick, NJ), May 18, 1903.

203. **waiting mitt, told the story.**: Louis P. Masur, *Autumn Glory: Baseball's First World Series* (New York: Farrer, Straus, and Giroux, 2004), 215.

204. **want to foster at Harvard."**: *Harvard Gazette*, April 19, 2012.

204. **doubling every few years.**: *Wall Street Journal*, October 25, 2018; No one was suggesting, as the *Wall Street Journal* did in October 2018, that the game was in need of "insane ideas to save baseball."

204. **ballooned to 7,236,290.**: Thorn and Palmer, *Total Baseball*, 144–145. The merger of the AL-NL occurred in1901 and does not skew this pattern.

204. **sport of choice for farmers.":** David Vaught, "Abner Doubleday, Marc Bloch, and the Cultural Significance of Baseball in Rural America," *Agricultural History*, Vol. 85, No. 1 (Winter 2001), 15.

204. **dishonesty of players," formed in 1876.**: *Chicago Daily Tribune*, February 7, 1876.

206. **authoritative way and for all time.":** Henry Chadwick (ed), *Spalding's Official Base Ball Guide, 1908: Thirty-First Year* (New York: American Sports Publishing Company, 1908), 35.

206. **famous Delmonico's Restaurant.**: *Pittsburgh Daily Post*, August 9, 1889; *St. Louis Post-Dispatch*, April 9, 1889.

206. **American in its origin.":** Quotes from Thorn, *Baseball in the Garden of Eden*, 11–15.

207. **secretary of the Special Commission.**: *Spalding's Official Base Ball Guide, 1908*, 35.

207. **alongside eventual appointees.":** Thorn, *Baseball in the Garden of Eden*, 174.

207. **the commission had produced.**: *Spalding's Official Base Ball Guide, 1908*, 35. Unfortunately, a fire destroyed the commission's records in 1911.

208. **something like cricket.**: Thorn, *Baseball in the Garden of Eden*, 8.

208. **the game of Base ball?":** Thorn, *Baseball in the Garden of Eden*, 9.

208. **preserved for 65 years.":** Thorn, *Baseball in the Garden of Eden*, 9.

209. ***Otsego Farmer* picked up on the theory.**: Thorn, *Baseball in the Garden of Eden*, 9.

209. **product," the New York *Sun* said.**: *New York Tribune*, March 20, 1908; *Press and Sun-Bulletin* (Binghamton, NY), April 17, 1908; *Baltimore Sun*, April 19, 1908.

210. **Yours truly. Abner Graves.":** Thorn, *Baseball in the Garden of Eden*, 280.

210. **any other foreign game.":** *Spalding's Official Base Ball Guide, 1908*, 36.

210. **the Origin of Base Ball.":** *Spalding's Official Base Ball Guide, 1908*, 36.

210. **Doubleday invented the game.**: Will Irwin, "Baseball Before the Professionals Came," *Collier's Magazine*, May 8, 1909, 12–13; David Vaught, "Abner Doubleday, March Bloch, and the Cultural Significance of Baseball in Rural America," *Agricultural History*, Vol. 85, No. 1 (Winter 2011), 1–20.

210. **is the 'Father of Baseball.'":** *New York Times*, November 13, 2010.

TEN: LEGACY

211. **only a modicum of solace.**: Butt, *Letters of Archie Butt*, December 10, 1908.

212. **arduous and exacting task.":** Butt, *Letters of Archie Butt*, May 15, 1908.

212. **gouty..." Roosevelt said in 1908.**: Theodore Roosevelt to Alfred E. Pearch, July 28, 1908, Theodore Roosevelt Papers.

212. **cut a less than athletic figure.**: "Sure! He's Great Big," Library of Congress Prints and Photographs Division.

212. Archie Butt, *The Letters of Archie Butt* (New York: Doubleday, Page and Company, 1924), 71.

212. **the New York *Sun* explained.**: *Sun*, June 22, 1908.

213. **The courts bought it.**: "On the "Student-Athlete Experience," see: NCAA Research "The Best Part of My Student-Athlete Experience is..." and "If I Could Change One Thing About My Student-Athlete Experience..." http://www.ncaa.org/about/resources/research/best-part-my-student-athlete-experience; Taylor Branch, "The Shame of College

Sports," *The Atlantic*, October, 2011; Chuck Slothower, "Fort Lewis' First 'Student-Athlete,'" *Durango Herald*, September 25, 2014; Johnny Smith, "The Job is Football: The Myth of the Student-Athlete," *The American Historian*, August 2016.

213.   **for a single athletic contest.":** Craig Lambert, "The Mystique of Red Top," *Harvard Magazine*, May–June 2010.

214.   **intervene in their futures.:** *Boston Globe*, June 16, 1908.

214.   **the remainder of the year.:** *Boston Globe*, June 16, 1908.

214.   ***Topeka State Journal* reported it.:** *Topeka State Journal*, June 22, 1908.

215.   **a blow at Harvard athletics.":** Theodore Roosevelt to Charles Eliot, July 10, 1908, Theodore Roosevelt Papers.

216.   **Morgan and Fish remained suspended.:** *New York Times*, June 23, 1908.

216.   **the New York *Sun* reported.:** *Sun*, June 24, 1908.

216.   **Charles Morgan Jr. and Harvard university.":** *San Francisco Examiner*, Jun 23, 1908; *Baltimore Sun*, June 23, 1908; *Salt Lake Herald*, June 24, 1908; *Sun* (New York), June 24, 1908; *Boston Globe*, June 23, 1908.

217.   **with all my heart," Roosevelt wrote.:** Theodore Roosevelt to Charles Eliot, November 23, 1908, Theodore Roosevelt Papers, Library of Congress.

218.   **the American–British rivalry.:** *Forth Olympiad; Being the Official Report of the Olympic Games of 1908 Celebrated in London Under the Patronage of His Most Gracious Majesty Kind Edward VII and by the Sanction of the International Olympic Committee* (London: British Olympic Council, 1909), 19–20.

218.   **resounded through the stadium.":** Pierre de Coubertin, *Olympism*, 425.

218.   **and promoting nationalism.":** George R. Matthews, "The Controversial Olympic games of 1908 As Viewed by the *New York Times* and the *Times* of London," *Journal of Sport History*, Vol. 7, No. 2 (Summer 1980), 40.

219.   ***of His Most Gracious Majesty King Edward VII.:*** British Olympic Council, *The Fourth Olympiad Being the Official Report, The Olympic Games of 1908* (London: The British Olympic Association, 1909), 99.

219.   **athletic idol of the British.":** Matthews, 48.

219.   **1906 Scottish Championships.:** British Olympic Council, *The Fourth Olympiad*, 57.

219.   **which he could never regain.":** *New York Tribune*, July 24, 1908.

220.   **bunched," the *New York Tribune* reported.:** *New York Tribune*, July 24, 1908.

220.   **the race had been declared void.":** *New York Tribune*, July 24, 1908.

221.   **"willfully obstructed" Halswelle.:** British Olympic Council, *The Fourth Olympiad*, 55.

222.   **a doctor (British) had confirmed.:** *New York Tribune*, July 24, 1908.

223.   **victory as ours on this occasion.":** Theodore Roosevelt to James E. Sullivan, August 24, 1908, Theodore Roosevelt Papers.

224.   **failed to come up to Carpenter's time.":** Not one of Roosevelt's better points. Few runners can match a race time when running alone.

225.   **could play out so simply.:** See Theodore A. Cooke to Theodore Roosevelt, September 8, 1908, November 2, 1908, Theodore Roosevelt Papers; Theodore Roosevelt to George C. Buell, August 18, 1908; Theodore Roosevelt to Lord Desborough, July 3, 1908, August 28, 1908, Theodore Roosevelt Papers; Theodore Roosevelt to Theodore A. Cook, November 17, 1908, Theodore Roosevelt Papers.

225.   **his half-century birthday.:** Theodore Roosevelt to Kermit Roosevelt, October 27, 1908, Theodore Roosevelt Papers.

226.   **with nothing to say.:** Patricia O'Toole, *When Trumpets Call: Theodore Roosevelt After the White House* (New York: Simon & Schuster, 2005), 9.

226. **Ethel's signaled its close.:** Dalton, *Theodore Roosevelt*, 330–344; *New York Times*, November 15, 1908; *New York Times*, December 29, 1908.

226. **finishing of the Panama Canal.":** Theodore Roosevelt to William Howard Taft, February 26, 1909, Theodore Roosevelt Papers.

227. **on the base of the sculpture.:** Art of Sagamore Hill, accessed November 1, 2018, https://artsandculture.google.com/exhibit/nQLiVHOCgDXMJA.

227. **Roosevelt understood.:** Kermit Roosevelt, *The Happy Hunting-Grounds* (London: Hodder & Stoughton, 1920), 175–176; *Scribner's Magazine*, Vol. 68, No. 3 (September, 1920), 272; David A. Wolff, *Seth Bullock: Black Hills Lawman* (Pierre, SD: South Dakota State Historical Society, 2009).

228. **hair thinner as the years progressed.:** It can still be purchased, for $6.90, on Amazon.com: https://www.amazon.com/President-Roosevelt-Photograph-Theodore-crouching/dp/B018DXEDJO.

228. **do right *because* it is right.":** Theodore Roosevelt to Jules Jusserand, August 3, 1908.

228. **to work because we have played.":** Theodore Roosevelt to Gifford Pinchot, February 24, 1909; March 2, 1909; Theodore Roosevelt to Gifford Pinchot and James R. Garfield, March 3, 1909.

ELEVEN: WAIT...JACK JOHNSON?

229. *wallopitiveness than Theodore Roosevelt.*: *Boston Globe*, June 28, 1908.

230. **"breed well or fight well.":** Theodore Roosevelt, *North American Review*, July 1895.

230. **Kathleen Dalton described it.:** Dalton, *The Strenuous Life*, 126.

230. **and a backward one (blacks).:** *New York Times*, February 14, 1905.

231. **at the center of the issue.:** Edmund Morris, *Theodore Rex*, 453.

231. **By Negro Soldiers, read the headline.:** *Brownsville Herald*, August 14, 1906.

231. **black troops gone from their midst.:** John D. Weaver, *The Brownsville Raid* (College Station: Texas A&M Press, 1992, Originally published in 1970), 281–283.

231. **salaries, honors, and pensions.:** Frank N. Schubert, "The 25th Infantry at Brownsville, Texas: Buffalo Soldiers, the 'Brownsville Six,' and the Medal of Honor," *Journal of Military History* (October 2011), 1217–1224.

232. **our scorn as our Judas.":** *New York Herald*, November 20, 1906.

232. **fair chance in the Brownsville affair.":** In Ward, *Unforgiveable Blackness*, 247; *Washington Post*, November 7, 1910; *Pittston Gazette*, November 7, 1910. The Brownsville decision would haunt Roosevelt for the rest of his political life and beyond. The decision begot a congressional investigation, headed by Senator Joseph Foraker—a longtime nemesis of Roosevelt's—that lasted until 1910. In 1972, the US Congress would reverse Roosevelt's decision and restore the men's records to show honorable discharges. No financial restitution, however, was made with the soldiers' estates. See, while somewhat dated, James A. Tinsely, "Roosevelt, Foraker, and the Brownsville Affray," *The Journal of Negro History*, Vol. 41, No. 1 (January 1956), 43–65, is a useful synopsis of the struggle between Congress and the president over Brownsville.

233. **and the world in general!":** Jack Johnson, *Jack Johnson: In the Ring and Out*, Edition with afterword and appendices (New York: Proteus Publishing, 1977), 26.

233. **described this monumental change.:** Randy Roberts, *Papa Jack: Jack Johnson and the Era of White Hopes* (New York: The Free Press, 1983), 5.

233. **lynched by a marauding mob.:** *Chicago Tribune*, August 18, 1908.

233. **law enforcement than the latter.**: Theresa Runstedtler, *Jack Johnson, Rebel Sojourner: Boxing in the Face of the Global Color Line* (New York: University of California Press, 2012).

233. **cast only with white women.":** Johnson, *Jack Johnson*, 65.

233. **to me to hold me own.":** Johnson, *Jack Johnson*, 32–33.

234. **"Colored Heavyweight Champion of the World.":** Geoffrey C. Ward, *Unforgivable Blackness: The Rise and Fall of Jack Johnson* (New York: Vintage Books, 2006), 52–55.

234. **to defeat his black opponents.**: Roberts, *Papa Jack*, 43.

235. **America until he defeats Jack Johnson.":** *Chicago Tribune*, December 8, 1907.

235. **proud to be his," Roosevelt said.**: Leary, *Talks with TR*, 119.

235. **a bare-knuckle one.":** Elliott J. Gorn, *The Manly Art: Bare-Knuckle Prize-Fighting in America* (Ithaca: Cornell University Press, 1986), 229.

235. **even a hint of an offer.":** Leary, *Talks with TR*, 119.

236. **to an African American.":** Christopher Klein, *Strong Boy: The Life and Times of John L. Sullivan, America's First Sports Hero* (Guilford, CT: Lyons Press, 2013), 189. Klein argues that this obligation stemmed from Sullivan's Boston roots, and that Sullivan "embodied the bigotry that flowed through Irish America."

236. **but I am all right.":** Theodore Roosevelt to John L. Sullivan, October 30, 1908, Theodore Roosevelt Papers; John L. Sullivan's weight had ballooned to 335 pounds by 1907, see *New York Times*, May 9, 1907.

236. **uphold American supremacy.":** Emphasis added; see, John J. Leary, *Talks with TR, from the Diaries of John J. Leary Jr.* (Boston: Houghton Mifflin Company, 1920), 118–119.

236. **showed up at their doorstep.**: Roosevelt, *Autobiography*, 338. At first glance, connecting the GWF with Jack Johnson's pursuit of the heavyweight title might seem to be the work of an over-tenured academic. What could the one possibly have to do with the other? But Theresa Runstedtler, a historian at American University, makes a compelling case for the rejoinder. "The gleaming white metal bodies of the Great White Fleet became traveling symbols of the U.S. nation's strength," Runstedtler explains. The press attention surrounding the GWF repeated, over and over, ideas of American supremacy and dominance, almost always in a manner which presumed that the America in question was white. That *Physical Culture* (a magazine interested in fitness and boxing) covered the GWF crew only made the connection more clear. "The proposed interracial match," Runstedtler concludes, "must have seemed like it would provide the perfect climax to the U.S. fleet's Pacific tour, for boxing had long followed the transoceanic flows of U.S. imperialism." See, Theresa Runstedtler, *Jack Johnson, Rebel Sojourner: Boxing in the Shadow of the Global Color Line* (Berkeley: University of California Press, 2012), 52–54.

236. **summarized one newspaper.**: *Los Angeles Times*, April 28, 1908; *Washington Post*, April 28, 1908; Johnson, 51.

237. **or any other nationality.":** Adam Pollack, *In the Ring with Tommy Burns* (WIN by KO Publications, 2011).

237. **sometimes transcended racial bias.**: Ward, *Unforgivable Blackness*, 95. Burns's success as a boxing promoter and businessman secured his fortune much more than did his earnings from fighting. By 1914, Burns had an estimated net worth of half a million dollars. See, Don Morrow and Terry Jackson, "Boxing's Interregnum: How Good was Tommy Burns, World Heavyweight Boxing Champion, 1906–1908," *Canadian Journal of Sport History*, Vol. 24, Issue 2 (December 1993), 30–46.

237. **Dollars, Dollars, Dollars, in it.":** Ward, *Unforgivable Blackness*, 115.

237. **week leading up to the bout.**: *Washington Post*, December 21, 1908; *New York Times*, December 21, 1908.

237. **to take a return shot.:** Ward, *Unforgivable Blackness*, 125.

237. **fights of my career," Johnson said.:** Johnson, *Jack Johnson*, 52.

238. **read the next day's newspapers.:** *Atlanta Constitution*, December 27, 1908.

238. **financial wagers had been booked.:** *Chicago Daily Tribune*, December 27, 1908.

239. **sent the fighter on his way.:** *Washington Post*, January 14, 1909; *Evening Star* (Washington, DC), January 14, 1909. A few scholars have tried to make the Nelson–Roosevelt meeting into a presidential repudiation of Jack Johnson. It was not. Roosevelt received visitors daily. Nelson called on the White House, waited, and then enjoyed his few minutes with the president. As an example of this mischaracterization, see Jeanne Campbell Reesman, *Jack London's Racial Lives* (Athens: University of Georgia Press, 2009), 185: "President Theodore Roosevelt, the nation's foremost proponent of the 'strenuous life,' repudiated Johnson in 1909 by inviting Battling Nelson to the White House as the 'white champion of the world,'" Roosevelt did not invite Nelson, nor was Nelson known in 1909 as the "white champion of the world."

239. **But the weather left no choice.:** *New York Times*, March 5, 1909.

239. **American soil again for fifteen months.:** *Chicago Daily Tribune*, March 5, 1909; *New York Times*, November 5, 1908; *Christian Science Monitor*, March 4, 1908.

239. **and thirteen rhinos.:** Joseph Gardner, *Departing Glory: Theodore Roosevelt as ex-President* (New York: Charles Scribner's Sons, 1973), 136.

240. **audacity to perform wonders.":** J. Lee Thompson, *Never Call Retreat: Theodore Roosevelt and the Great War* (New York: Palgrave MacMillan, 2013), 6.

240. **"Jeff, it's up to you.":** Ward, *Unforgiveable Blackness*, 132–133.

241. **from 270 to 230 pounds.":** *Atlanta Constitution*, February 13, 1910.

241. **the lead-up to the fight.:** Ward, *Unforgiveable Blackness*, 155.

241. **for Gavin's wife, Alberta.:** *Washington Post*, January 16, 1910.

241. **newspapers across the country.:** *Buffalo Evening News*, January 15, 1910; *Washington Post*, January 16, 1910.

242. **"Your Champion, Jack Johnson.":** Roosevelt's letter to Davis and Johnson's call for Roosevelt to serve as referee were printed in thousands of newspapers—many with biting commentary accompanying them. See, for example, *Washington Post*, January 20, 1910 and *El Paso Herald*, January 21, 1910.

242. **afraid he may be 'jobbed.'":** *Buffalo Commercial*, January 18, 1910.

243. **made of solid gold.":** *New York Times*, April 26, 1910.

243. **vigor and frankness...":** *Washington Post*, June 10, 1910.

243. **the Republican Party.:** *Atlanta Constitution*, June 12, 1910.

243. **had not changed that much.:** *New York Times*, June 19, 1910.

244. **TR announced matter-of-factly.:** *Outlook*, July 2, 1910.

245. **was one of that sort.":** *Atlanta Constitution*, July 2, 1910.

245. **Reno, Nevada, on July 4, 1910.:** *New York Times*, April 26, 1910.

245. **fighters would take a fall.:** For an excellent description of the Johnson–Jeffries fight, see Geoffrey C. Ward, *Unforgivable Blackness: The Rise and Fall of Jack Johnson* (New York: Vintage Books, 2004), 157–212.

245. **busy post-presidency schedule.:** *Washington Post*, June 17, 1910.

245. **night before the contest.:** Roberts, *Papa Jack*, 100.

245. **rabid for a brawling spectacle.:** The site of this fight today is a salvage yard on the outskirts of Reno. While this might seem depressing, the city of Reno constructed a thorough and engaging exhibit on the fight at a nearby bus stop. Somehow this combination of historical memory and practical infrastructural improvement works brilliantly. And yes, I made my wife and children take a selfie at the spot when we visited.

246. **all possible dispute.":** Johnson, 145.

246. **best man in the world.":** Quoted in Roberts, *Papa Jack*, 114.

247. **the first black movie star.":** Dan Streible and Charles Musser, *Fight Pictures: A History of Boxing and Early Cinema* (Berkeley: University of California Press, 2008), 195.

248. **United States," Roosevelt editorialized.:** Theodore Roosevelt, "The Recent Prize Fight," *Outlook*, July 16, 1910.

248. **two weeks after the fight.:** *Atlanta Constitution*, July 14, 1910.

248. *New York Tribune* **headlined.:** *New York Tribune*, July 8, 1910; *Louisville Courier-Journal*, July 10, 1910.

248. **pictures taken thereof.":** Theodore Roosevelt, "The Recent Prize Fight," *Outlook*, July 16, 1910.

TWELVE: ONE LAST RACE

249. **a series of lingering losses.:** Theodore Roosevelt to Quentin Roosevelt, October 15, 1917, Theodore Roosevelt Papers.

250. **Roosevelt wrote to his sister.:** Theodore Roosevelt to Anna Roosevelt Cowles, May 17, 1917.

250. **Light Brigade" days were over.:** J. Lee Thompson, *Never Call Retreat: Theodore Roosevelt and the Great War* (New York: Palgrave MacMillan, 2013).

251. **pursuit of military matters.":** Thompson, *Never Call Retreat*, 179.

251. **in the hands of Jack Cooper.:** Theodore Roosevelt to Kermit Roosevelt, October 17, 1917.

251. **Rough Riders should be riding again.:** Theodore Roosevelt to Frances T. Parson, May 24, 1917; *Indianapolis Star*, May 2, 1917.

251. **a "physically timid" man.:** Theodore Roosevelt to Frances T. Parson, May 24, 1917.

252. **overdue and last-ditch effort.:** Richard M. Winans, "Roosevelt's Fighting Energy: How He Got It," *Physical Culture* (February 1918), 19–20; Sylvia Morris, *Edith Kermit Roosevelt*, 417.

252. **one looked a bit cloudy) eyes.:** In case you're wondering, yes. Yes it feels like a cheap shot to criticize the flagging physique of a fifty-eight-year-old Roosevelt. The process of growing old is only impassive when it concerns someone we don't know. As I worked on this book my grandmother and grandfather struggled through their nineties before passing away. It was heart wrenching. Somewhat relatedly, I turned forty. I wouldn't call what happened in the months leading up to this birthday a crisis. Well, maybe a small one. I tried to run a marathon, in the Nevada desert in June no less, to make myself feel better and more virile during the experience. It did not go all that well. I stumbled into the finish exhausted, still turning forty, and reminded that this might be harder than it looked.

252. **fifty miles north of New York City.:** *Annual Report of the City of Stamford, Connecticut, 1917* (Stamford, CT, 1918), 1.

252. **Go to the limit—and I'll like it.":** Unless otherwise specified, the quotes from TR's time at Jack Cooper's Health Farm are taken from the previously cited *Physical Culture*, February 1918 story. While there are varying accounts of Roosevelt's time, *Physical Culture* offered far more detail and information—not surprising given the audience of the magazine.

253. **was to "scare rhinos away.":** Gardener, 133.

254. **analyzing. We know this.:** Sometimes when you write about sports you get accused of having a myopic perspective: it's just about sports and/or sports explains everything. I get it; I'm purposely choosing to focus elsewhere in light of the overarching ideas explored by this book.

254. **no carping, no envy.":** Archibald Butt, *Taft and Roosevelt, the Intimate Letters of Archie Butt*, Vol. 2 (Garden City, NY: Doubleday, Doran & Company, Inc., 1930), 562.

254. **exercise was golf.":** Wayne Whipple and Alice Roosevelt Longworth, *The Story of the White House and its Home Life* (Boston, MA: Dwinell-Wright Co., 1937), 53.

254. **golfed too much.":** *Washington Post*, April 21, 2017.

255. **yesterday...William H. Taft.":** *Sioux City Journal*, April 16, 1910.

255. **as a political candidate.:** Theodore Roosevelt to Henry Cabot Lodge, July 19, 1908.

255. **Taft if need be.:** Gardner, 179.

255. **if it is tendered to me.":** Gardner, 214.

256. **office," wrote one biographer.:** Gardner, 220.

256. **animal not often found.":** Gardner, 268.

257. **going to deliver this one.":** Gardner, 273.

257. **spoke for more than an hour.:** *Baltimore Sun*, October 15, 1912.

257. **Roosevelt, read the next day's headline.:** *Boston Globe*, October 15, 1912.

257. **He was "a physical marvel.":** *Chicago Tribune*, October 22, 1912.

258. **"election that changed the country.":** Corinne Roosevelt Robinson, *My Brother Theodore Roosevelt* (New York: Charles Scribners' Sons, 1921), 275; James Chace, *Wilson, Roosevelt, Taft & Debs—The Election that Changed the Country* (New York: Simon and Schuster, 2004).

258. **woke up early to go golfing.:** *Chicago Tribune*, April 24, 2017.

258. **necessary pace, the day began.:** Richard M. Winans, "Roosevelt's Fighting Energy: How He Got It," *Physical Culture* (February 1918), 54.

259. **introduction to the breakfast table.":** Richard M. Winans, "Roosevelt's Fighting Energy: How He Got It," *Physical Culture* (February 1918), 54.

259. **and an exercising apparatus.":** *Official Gazette of the United States Patent Office*, March 2, 1920, Vol. 272, No. 1, 160.

260. **THE WEAK HEART.":** *The Western Osteopath*, Vol. 16, No. 12 (May 1922), 48.

260. **on this cruel machine.:** Edmond Morris, *Colonel Roosevelt* (New York: 2010), 508.

260. **the sweatbox session.:** Richard M. Winans, "Roosevelt's Fighting Energy: How He Got It," *Physical Culture* (February 1918), 54.

261. **his sporting patrons came.":** Theodore Roosevelt to Archie Roosevelt, October 14, 1917, Theodore Roosevelt Papers.

261. **overweight socialites.:** *Chicago Daily Tribune*, February 27, 1907.

262. **had fluffy towels.:** Richard M. Winans, "Roosevelt's Fighting Energy: How He Got It," *Physical Culture* (February 1918), 54.

262. **Tangerine could not match.:** *Physical Culture*, Vol. 38, No. 04, 1917.

264. **decades of the twentieth century.:** Mark Adams, *Mr. America: How Muscular Millionaire Bernarr Macfadden Transformed the Nation through Sex, Salad, and the Ultimate Starvation Diet* (New York: HarperCollins, 2009); Robert Ernst, *Weakness is a Crime: The Life of Bernarr Macfadden* (Syracuse: Syracuse University Press, 1991).

264. **the double bouncing ball.":** Richard M. Winans, "Roosevelt's Fighting Energy: How He Got It," *Physical Culture* (February 1918), 54.

265. **breathing," explained** *Physical Culture*.: *Physical Culture*, Vol. 46, No. 05, 1921.

266. **losing weight a little.":** Theodore Roosevelt to Archie Roosevelt, October 14, 1917, Theodore Roosevelt Papers.

266. **men of private malice.":** Theodore Roosevelt to Quentin Roosevelt, October 15, 1917, Theodore Roosevelt Papers; Theodore Roosevelt to Kermit Roosevelt, October 17, 1917, Theodore Roosevelt Papers.

267. **wrapped up the workout.**: Richard M. Winans, "Roosevelt's Fighting Energy: How He Got It," *Physical Culture* (February 1918), 56.

267. **this could be avoided.**: Richard M. Winans, "Roosevelt's Fighting Energy: How He Got It," *Physical Culture* (February 1918), 56.

267. **a brown flannel shirt.**: *Philadelphia Inquirer*, October 13, 1917; *St. Louis Post-Dispatch*, October 22, 1917.

268. **real progress had been made.**: *New York Times*, October 22, 1917.

268. **overseeing the scene.**: *Sun* (New York), October 22, 1917.

269. **Just Roosevelt.**: *New York Tribune*, October 22, 1917.

269. **'fine shape, by Jove, fine!'"**: *St. Louis Post-Dispatch*, October 22, 1917.

269. **to accommodate him."**: *Evening World* (New York), October 22, 1917.

270. **and the "Big Stick."**: *Boston Globe*, January 7, 1919.

270. **about it with a smile."**: *Sun* (New York), October 22, 1917.

271. **to Europe to fight.**: *New York Times*, October 22, 1917.

272. **the New York Sun reported.**: *Sun*, October 22, 1917.

273. **used to be." If only.**: *Brooklyn Eagle*, October 22, 1917; *Washington Post*, October 22, 1917; *Sun* (New York), October 22, 1917.

273. **extent of his girth."**: *Salt Lake Telegram*, October 28, 1917; *Los Angeles Times*, October 12, 1917; *Vermont Union-Journal*, October 17, 1917.

273. **Roosevelt had still won.**: *Sun* (New York), October 22, 1917; *Washington Post*, October 22, 1917.

273. **many people know it."**: *Sun* (New York), October 22, 1917.

274. **explained the New York Sun.**: *Sun*, October 22, 1917.

274. **hadn't until 1917.**: *Robesonian* (Lumberton, NC), October 29, 1917.

274. **all humanity. Selah!**: Richard M. Winans, "Roosevelt's Fighting Energy: How He Got It," *Physical Culture* (February 1918), 17.

274. **Roosevelt still won.**: *Dispatch* (Moline, IL), January 13, 1919.

275. **"go out again into the world."**: Richard M. Winans, "Roosevelt's Fighting Energy: How He Got It," *Physical Culture* (February 1918), 18.

275. **advertisements for war bonds.**: *Pittsburgh Post-Gazette*, October 22, 1917.

EPILOGUE

276. **when it comes to sports?**: https://www.cnn.com/2017/07/25/health/cte-nfl-players -brains-study/index.html.

279. **died in training since 2000.**: *Washington Post*, August 21, 2018.

279. **for the past twenty-nine years.**: National Federation of State high School Association, 2017–2018 High School Athletics Participation Survey, https://www.nfhs.org/articles/ high-school-sports-participation-increases-for-29th-consecutive-year/.

280. **I had ever imaged," he said.**: H.G. Bissinger, *Friday Night Lights: A Town, A Team, and A Dream* (New York DaCapo Press, 1990), xiii.

280. **the New York Times editorialized.**: *New York Times*, August 17, 2014.

280. **football players are African American.**: The exact percentages of African American participation are as follows. Division I Men's Basketball: 56%; Division I Football: 48%; Division I Women's Basketball: 47%.

281. **"Have Smartphones Destroyed a Generation?"**: Jean M. Twenge, "Have Smart Phones Destroyed a Generation," *The Atlantic*, September 2017.

281. **and useful period of their lives.":** *Washington Post*, January 1, 2018; National Institute of Diabetes and Digestive and Kidney Disease, "Overweigh and Obesity Statistics," https://www.niddk.nih.gov/health-information/health-statistics/diabetes-statistics; Club Industry, https://www.clubindustry.com/studies/ihrsa-reports-57-million-health-club-members-276-billion-industry-revenue-2016.

283. **her?" he asked a reporter.:** O'Toole, *When Trumpets Call*, 390.

283. **around his horse's neck.":** Dalton, *Theodore Roosevelt*, 507.

283. **of the landmark birthday.:** *New York Tribune*, October 27, 1918.

283. **and Little Archie (eight months).:** *New York Tribune*, October 27, 1918; *Brooklyn Daily Eagle*, October 27, 1918.

283. **to be titularly as old as I feel.":** Theodore Roosevelt to Corinne Roosevelt Robinson, October 27, 1918; Theodore Roosevelt to Kermit Roosevelt, October 27, 1918.

284. **"Lovingly, Kermit's father.":** Emphasis added. Theodore Roosevelt to Belle Roosevelt, October 27, 1918; Theodore Roosevelt, *The Great Adventure: Present-Day Studies in American Nationalism* (New York: Charles Scribner's Sons, 1918). Roosevelt finished writing this book after learning of Quentin's death. He dedicated the book to, "All who in this war have paid with their bodies for their souls' desire."

285. **found him sleeping soundly.:** *New York Times*, January 7, 1919.

286. **at Rest at Sagamore.:** *Rapid City Journal*, January 7, 1919; *El Dorado Republican* (El Dorado, KS), January 17, 1919; *Indianapolis Star*, January 7, 1919; *Nebraska State Journal* (Lincoln, NE), January 25, 1919; *St. Louis Star and Times*, January 7, 1919; *Anaconda Standard* (Anaconda, MT), January 26, 1919; *Santa Ana Register*, January 18, 1919; *Wahpeton Time* (Wahpeton, ND), January 9, 1919.

286. **peacefully in his sleep.:** *Boston Globe*, January 6, 1919.

INDEX

ABOUT THE AUTHOR

Ryan Swanson is an associate professor of history, in the Honors College, at the University of New Mexico. He earned his PhD in history from Georgetown in 2008 and has been studying and researching Theodore Roosevelt and his role in athletics in the United States for the past ten years. He is the author of *When Baseball Went White: Reconstruction, Reconciliation, and Dreams of a National Pastime*, which won the 2015 Society for American Baseball Research (SABR) research award, and *Separate Games: African American Sport Behind the Walls of Segregation*, which received the North American Society for Sport History (NASSH) anthology prize in 2017. Swanson has also published a wide variety of articles, both in popular and academic venues, and book chapters on the history of athletics during the nineteenth and early twentieth centuries in the United States.